MCQs in Integrated Sciences for M

Commissioning Editor: Mike Parkinson
Project Editor: Sarah Keer-Keer
Project Controller: Nancy Arnott
Designer: Erik Bigland

MCQs in Integrated Sciences for Medical Students

Dr Wai-Ching Leung
Senior Registrar in Public Health Medicine
Northern Region Public Health Medicine Training Scheme
MA MRCP(UK) MRCPCH MRCGP MRCPsych DCH DO DRCOG PGCE AdvDipEd

CHURCHILL LIVINGSTONE

EDINBURGH LONDON NEW YORK PHILADELPHIA SYDNEY ST LOUIS TORONTO 1999

CHURCHILL LIVINGSTONE
An imprint of Harcourt Publishers Limited

First published 1999

ISBN 0 443 06239 0

British Library Cataloguing in Publication Data
A catalogue record for this book is available from the British Library.

Library of Congress Cataloging in Publication Data
A catalog record for this book is available from the Library of Congress.

Medical knowledge is constantly changing. As new information becomes available, changes in treatment, procedures, equipment and the use of drugs become necessary. The author and the publishers have, as far as it is possible, taken care to ensure that the information given in this text is accurate and up to date. However, readers are strongly advised to confirm that the information, especially with regard to drug usage, complies with current legislation and standards of practice.

The publisher's policy is to use **paper manufactured from sustainable forests**

Printed in China
EPC/01

Contents

Preface

By 1998, most medical schools in the UK would have implemented the fundamental changes in the undergraduate medical curriculum recommended by the General Medical Council in 1993, albeit in different ways and to different extents. These recommendations include substantial reduction of factual information; identifying a 'core curriculum' encompassing the essential knowledge and skills; that this 'core curriculum' should be system-based and its component should be integrated across different areas of basic sciences (e.g. anatomy, physiology, biochemistry) as well as integrated with clinical areas.

In the first two years of most medical curricula, medical students will be presented with a combination of modules on general principles which are not system-based (e.g. cells, nutrition and energy, public health), as well as system-based integrated basic science modules (e.g. cardiovascular system, respiratory system). Clinical skills taught tend to be basic (e.g. taking the pulse and blood pressure, auscultation of the heart and chest), and related to the basic science modules. More detailed clinical examination skills are usually introduced in the third year.

Hence, changes in student assessments are inevitable. Firstly, objective methods such as MCQs, data interpretation and OSCE are considered more appropriate than essay questions or long cases. Secondly, new assessments should focus on a few key scientific principles which can be related to clinical practice rather than obscure facts. As a result, anatomy is likely to be examined in much less detail than previously. Thirdly, the units of assessment will be based on systems (e.g. cardiovascular system) or broad areas of general principles (e.g. nutrition and energy, public health and statistics) rather than traditional areas of basic sciences (e.g. anatomy, physiology). Lastly, students would be expected to show some understanding of the relevance of the scientific principles to clinical practice.

With these fundamental changes, there are no currently available revision books which are suitable for the new curriculum and assessment methods. Furthermore, students would have to buy numerous revision books (e.g. in anatomy, physiology and pathology). This self-assessment book aims to fill this gap. It allows students in their first two or three years to test their knowledge and understanding of the core curriculum, as well as to practise their examination techniques.

The book is in two parts. The first part (chapters 1–9), which constitutes a third of the book, deals with general principles that do not apply to a single body system. The second part (chapters 10–19) is system-based. The book has the following features:

- It is in an MCQ format.
- It covers all the basic science disciplines taught in the first two to three years of the medical curriculum using an integrated approach.
- It includes only key essential knowledge which students are expected to know.
- It includes the scientific basis for clinical examination techniques.
- It includes application of basic sciences to clinical practice.

I hope students will find this book useful in their revision and preparation for their examinations.

Finally, I would like to thank Dr Susan Laidlaw, currently a specialist registrar in public health medicine and a former psychiatrist, for her contribution to Chapter 8 on psychology and sociology.

W–C. L

Part I
General basic medical sciences

1. The cell
Questions

1.1 The following organelles may contain (DNA):

- **A** The nucleus
- **B** Lysosomes
- **C** Rough endoplasmic reticulum
- **D** Mitochondria
- **E** Golgi apparatus

1.2 The cytoskeleton:

- **A** Is only present in muscle cells
- **B** Allows the cell to change shape
- **C** Allows the cell to move
- **D** Facilitates movement of organelles from one part of the cell to another
- **E** Plays an important role in mitosis

1.3 The following have an important role in the process of translation in protein synthesis:

- **A** Double-stranded DNA
- **B** Transfer RNA
- **C** Ribosomes
- **D** Lysosomes
- **E** Cilia

1.4 The following statements about the human cell membrane are true:

- **A** It consists of a phospholipid molecule bilayer
- **B** The non-polar hydrophobic tails of the molecules are exposed to the outside
- **C** Cholesterol molecules regulate the fluidity of the cell membrane
- **D** The outside of the cell is electronegative compared to the inside
- **E** It is freely permeable to organic ions

1.5 Given that there are more negatively charged non-diffusible proteins inside cells than in interstitial fluids, the following statements are true:

- **A** Cells would swell and rupture if active transport of ions out of cells ceases
- **B** The concentrations of diffusible ions on the inside and the outside of the cell membrane are equal
- **C** The product of the concentrations of sodium and chloride inside the cell is equal to the product outside the cell
- **D** An electrical gradient exists across the cell membrane at equilibrium
- **E** The Na^+,K^+-ATPase generates a negative electrical potential inside the cell

1.6 The following statements about membrane potentials across cell membranes are true:

- **A** The equilibrium potential for chloride ion is the membrane potential at which the rates of influx and efflux of chloride ion are equal
- **B** The equilibrium potential for chloride ion increases if the chloride ion concentration is doubled both inside and outside the cell
- **C** The resting membrane potential in a motor neurone normally closely approximates the equilibrium potential for sodium ions
- **D** The resting membrane potential for sodium ions is about –90 mV
- **E** The resting membrane potential for potassium ions is about +60 mV

1.7 The following statements about protein synthesis in human are true:

- **A** Translation is the process for the synthesis of mRNA
- **B** The mRNA manufactured in the nucleus is shorter than the final mRNA which enters the cytoplasm
- **C** Amino acids are coded by a group of three bases (codon)
- **D** All codons specify particular amino acids
- **E** All amino acids are coded for by unique codons

1.8 The types of protein embedded in the cell membrane include:

- **A** Carriers
- **B** Ion channels
- **C** Hormone receptors
- **D** ATP
- **E** Enzymes

1.9 Energy is needed for the following mode of transport across the cell membrane:

- **A** Diffusion
- **B** Facilitated diffusion
- **C** By a carrier against a chemical gradient
- **D** By a carrier against an electrical gradient
- **E** Osmosis

1.10 The following statements about Na^+,K^+-ATPase are true:

A Energy is absorbed when the enzyme catalyses the hydrolysis of an ATP molecule
B It is absent in the brain
C It transports one sodium ion out of the cell for each potassium ion transported in
D Inhibition results in an increase in intracellular calcium concentration
E Inhibition may result in improved contraction of the cardiac muscle

1.11 Common examples of the mechanisms for chemical messengers outside the cell to exert intracellular effects include:

A Acting via cytoplasmic nuclear receptors to start transcription of specific mRNA
B Opening ion channels in the cell membrane
C Direct entry into the nucleus to start transcription of specific mRNA
D Inducing altered electrical potential inside the cell
E Binding to membrane receptors to initiate release of intracellular messengers

1.12 Recognised second messengers include:

A Calmodulin
B G protein
C Cyclic AMP
D Inositol triphosphate
E Noradrenaline

1.13 Gap (communicating) junctions:

A Allow small molecules to pass from the inside to the outside of a cell
B Allow small molecules to pass from the inside of one cell to another
C Are impermeable to ions
D Are important in synchronising the contraction of heart muscle
E Are essential in tissues lacking in blood supply

1.14 Proteins:

A Are only found outside cells
B May be synthesised outside cells
C May be able to bind hormones
D Are often linear in shape
E May catalyse chemical reactions

1.15 The following statements about enzymes are true:

A They catalyse chemical reactions
B They cannot act on more than one substrate
C They act by increasing the activation energy
D Only one enzyme can catalyse a given chemical reaction
E A given enzyme can only catalyse one chemical reaction

1.16 The following statements about the concentration of enzymes are true:

A Measurement may be useful in detecting liver diseases
B It may be measured by the initial rate of disappearance of substrates
C It may be measured by the initial rate of appearance of products
D It may be measured by the average rate of disappearance of substrates over a day
E It may be measured by the average rate of appearance of products over a day

1.17 The following statements about the genetic code are true:

A The code in humans differs significantly from that in other mammals
B One codon may code for more than one amino acid
C Chain termination occurs in translation when a codon codes for 'glycine'
D Frameshift mutation by one nucleotide is often silent
E Mutation of the third nucleotide in the codon is often silent

1.18 Mitosis:

A Results in two daughter haploid cells
B Occurs in cancer cells
C Occurs in neurones
D Occurs in fully formed red blood cells
E Occurs in skin cells

1.19 Isoenzymes:

A Are enzymes which catalyse different biochemical reactions
B Are physically identical
C Are chemically identical
D Are often present in different cell types
E Are usually produced by genes on different chromosomes

1.20 The following statements about the rate of enzyme-catalysed reactions in vivo are true:

A It approximately doubles for every 10°C rise in temperature between 0°C and 100°C
B It approximately doubles for every 10-fold increase in hydrogen concentration between pH 2 and pH 10

C An increase in enzyme concentration usually results in a significant increase in reaction rate
D An increase in substrate concentration always results in a significant increase in reaction rate
E It can be predicted from the value of ΔG^0 (change in free energy) of the reaction

1.21 The following statements are consistent with the Michaelis–Menten equation on enzyme reactions:

A The Michaelis constant K_m is the enzyme concentration which produces half-maximal velocity
B When the substrate concentration is very much less than K_m, the initial rate of reaction is directly proportional to the substrate concentration
C When the substrate concentration is very much more than K_m, the initial rate of reaction is inversely proportional to the substrate concentration
D When the substrate concentration is equal to K_m, the initial rate of reaction is half maximal
E The value of K_m can be easily determined by the intercepts of a plot of substrate concentration against initial velocity

1.22 The following statements about the effects of enzyme inhibitors are true:

A A non-competitive inhibitor combines with an enzyme at the same site as the substrate
B A competitive inhibitor increases the apparent Michaelis constant K_m of the enzyme
C A competitive inhibitor reduces the maximal velocity V_{max} of the reaction
D A non-competitive inhibitor increases the maximal velocity V_{max} of the reaction
E A non-competitive inhibitor increases the apparent Michaelis constant K_m of the enzyme

1.23 Mechanisms for regulating enzyme activities in vivo include:

A Secretion of inactive precursors of enzymes
B Feedback inhibition by end products
C Compartmentalisation of enzymes in different cellular organelles
D Hormonal entry from outside the cell
E Feedback regulation at allosteric sites by metabolites

1.24 Allosteric enzymes:

A Often contain a single binding site for both the substrate and the allosteric effector
B Characteristically obey the Michaelis–Menton equation
C Often result in a sigmoid substrate saturation curve
D May affect the apparent K_m of the reaction
E May affect the V_m of the reaction

1. The cell
Answers

1.1 A D

The nucleus consists mostly of chromosomes which carry the genetic message of the cell. The chromosomes are made up of DNA. Without the nucleus, the cell cannot divide and eventually dies (e.g. red blood cells). However, the mitochondria contains a small amount of DNA which codes for a small number (13) of the proteins in the ATP generating system in the mitochondria. This may be clinically important, as mutation in the mitochondrial DNA may result in rare muscular disorders with a special pattern of inheritance. Mitochondria may have been independent microorganisms which became incorporated into the cell in the course of evolution.

1.2 B C D E

The cytoskeleton is a system of fibres which maintains the shape of the cell, allows the cell to change shape and move, and facilitates movement of organelles from one part of the cell to another. The fibres vary in diameter, and include microtubules (the largest), intermediate filaments and microfilaments. The microtubules are constantly assembled and disassembled, and help to form tracks for the transport of organelles such as mitochondria and secretory granules to move to the part of the cell where they are needed. Microfilaments consist of actins, and are responsible for the movement of organelles, as well as the contraction of muscles.

1.3 B C

Translation is the process by which a polypeptide chain of a protein is formed from the processed messenger RNA, and occurs in the ribosomes. The amino acids in the cytoplasm are activated by adenosine monophosphate and an enzyme, and each activated amino acid is attached to a transfer RNA. The tRNA–amino acid complex is then attached to the processed mRNA in the ribosomes. Double-stranded DNA is only found in the nucleus. Lysosomes contain enzymes which would destroy most cellular components, and act as a digestive system for the cell. Cilia are projections from the cells.

1.4 A C

Human cell membrane basically consists of a phospholipid bilayer. Each phospholipid molecule consists of a polar hydrophilic phosphate head and two non-polar hydrophobic tails. The polar heads are exposed to the outside and the cytoplasm of the cell, whilst the non-polar tails are buried within the cell membrane. Cholesterol molecules are present to stabilise the cell membrane and regulate its fluidity by filling the gaps between the tails of phospholipid fatty acid tails whilst simultaneously preventing too close placing. The inside of the cell is almost invariably electronegative relative to the outside, although the magnitude of this resting potential varies amongst tissues. The membrane is impermeable to intracellular organic anions, and this results in an asymmetry of the distribution of permeant anions at equilibrium. This is the Donnan effect, and is the cause of the membrane potential.

1.5 A C D E

Since there are more negatively charged non-diffusible proteins inside cells, there are more osmotically active particles inside than outside cells. Hence, cells would swell and rupture if there were no active transport of ions out of cells. This active transport is carried out by Na^+,K^+-ATPase. The concentration of the diffusible ions is governed by the Gibbs–Donnan equation. For any pair of cation and anion with the same valency, the outside to inside concentration ratio of the cation is the same as the inside to outside concentration ratio of the anion. In other words, the product of the concentrations of the cation and anion inside the cell is equal to the corresponding product outside the cell. Since the distribution of positive and negative charged ions across the membrane is asymmetrical, there is an electrical gradient across the membrane at equilibrium. Furthermore, the Na^+,K^+-ATPase pumps three Na^+ out of the cells in exchange for every two K^+ into the cells. This also contributes to the electrical gradient across cell membranes.

1.6 A

The equilibrium potential for any diffusible ion is the membrane potential at which the rates of influx and efflux of the ions are equal. The magnitude of the membrane potential can be determined by the Nernst equation:

$$E_x = \frac{RT}{F} \ln \frac{[X_o]}{[X_i]}$$

Hence, doubling the concentrations of the relevant ions both inside and outside the cells would not alter its equilibrium potential. The resting membrane potential differs slightly amongst tissues. In the motor neurone, the resting membrane potential is about –70 mV, which is entirely accounted for by the chloride equilibrium potential. The equilibrium potential for sodium ions is about +60 mV, and accounts for the membrane potential of neurones at depolarisation during an action potential. The electrical potential for potassium ions is about –90 mV, and is important when tissues are hyperpolarised.

1.7 C

The process of synthesis of mRNA in the nucleus is known as transcription, whilst the synthesis of protein from mRNA in the ribosomes is known as translation. In eukaryotic cells, segments of DNA which code for protein synthesis (exons) are separated from segments which do not (introns). The mRNA molecules synthesised in the nucleus are spliced to eliminate the introns before entering the cytoplasm. Hence the final mRNA is shorter than the mRNA synthesised in the nucleus. In translation, each amino acid is coded for by a group of three bases (codon). Out of the 64 codons, only 61 code for particular amino acids, whilst the other three code for chain termination. As there are only 20 amino acids, most are coded for by more than one codon.

1.8 A B C E

There are different proteins embedded in the cell membranes, with a variety of functions. They include (a) structural proteins, (b) ion channels (which allow ions to pass in and out of the cell when activated), (c) carriers (which facilitate diffusion of substances across the membrane down an electrochemical gradient), (d) pumps (which actively transport substances across the membrane), (e) receptors (which cause physiological changes inside the cells when bound to a hormone or a neurotransmitter), (f) enzymes (which catalyse biochemical reactions at the surface of the membrane). ATP is a high-energy phosphate compound and not a protein.

1.9 C D

Diffusion is the movement of a substance from an area of higher to lower concentration (chemical gradient). Ions may also move down an electrical gradient. Osmosis is the diffusion of solvent (e.g. water) molecules from areas with a lower to a higher solute concentration. All these processes do not require energy. Diffusion down a chemical or electrical gradient may be facilitated by a protein (carrier), and no energy is required. However, transport of substances against a chemical or electrical gradient require energy, which is usually provided by the hydrolysis of ATP by Na^+,K^+-ATPase.

1.10 D E

The enzyme Na^+,K^+-ATPase is present throughout all the cells in the body, and is responsible for a large part of the basal metabolism. It catalyses the hydrolysis of ATP to ADP, and energy is released in the process. This energy is used to transport three

Na^+ out of the cell for every two K^+ transported in, and results in a net positive charge outside the cell. It may be linked to a second active transport system (e.g. for transport of glucose across the intestinal mucosa). Digoxin inhibits the enzyme. This results in a decrease in intracellular sodium concentration and hence a decrease in the sodium gradient across the cell membrane. The normal exchange of an inflow of sodium ion for an outflow of calcium ion is reduced, and the intracellular calcium level increases. This facilitates the contraction of cardiac muscle (positively inotropic effect).

1.11 A B E

The commonest mechanism for chemical messengers to exert intracellular effects is binding to a membrane receptor to initiate the release of intracellular mediators (second messengers). Other mechanisms include acting via cytoplasmic or nuclear receptors to initiate transcription of certain mRNAs (e.g. thyroid hormone), and opening of specific ion channels in the membrane (e.g. acetylcholine acting on the nicotinic receptors to open the sodium channels).

1.12 A B C D

Second messengers are intracellular mediators the release of which is triggered by extracellular chemicals (first messenger) binding to membrane receptors. An example is noradrenaline (first messenger) binding to β_1-adrenergic membrane receptors, which triggers the increase of intracellular cyclic AMP (second messenger). Many second messengers have been identified in recent years, and include cyclic AMP, cyclic GMP, calcium-binding proteins (e.g. calmodulin), G proteins, inositol triphosphate and diacyclglycerol.

1.13 B D E

Gap (communicating) junctions are channels which connect one cell to another, and are composed of polypeptides called connexin. They allow passage of small polar molecules such as metabolites and amino acids, and ions. They are essential to allow nutrients to travel from one cell to another in tissues lacking in blood supply (e.g. cornea, bone). They are also important in synchronising the contraction of cardiac or uterine muscle by allowing rapid transfer of calcium ions.

1.14 C E

Proteins may be found outside cells (e.g. immunoglobulins), in the plasma membrane (e.g. hormone receptors) and inside cells (e.g. haemoglobin). However, they are all synthesised inside cells in ribosomes. Whilst polypeptides are linear, the shape of proteins is determined by the exact nature of their folding (i.e. the tertiary structure). Most non-structural proteins are globular in shape (e.g. haemoglobin). They are capable of binding to other molecules (ligands) at specific regions (binding sites). Enzymes are proteins, or rarely RNA molecules, capable of binding to ligands and initiate the catalysis of a chemical reaction involving the ligands.

1.15 A

Although most chemical reactions are catalysed by enzymes (which are proteins), it was discovered in the mid-1980s that some RNA molecules (ribozymes) may also catalyse reactions. Most enzymes can act on more than one substrate. Different enzymes may catalyse the same chemical reaction, and different enzymes may catalyse the same reaction. Enzymes speed up reaction by lowering the activation energy barrier, but do not change the final equilibrium.

1.16 A B C

Measurement of the concentration of enzymes is often useful in the diagnosis of diseases. For example, in liver or heart diseases, specific enzymes are often released from the damaged liver or cardiac cells. Enzyme concentration is most commonly measured by the initial rate of disappearance of substrates or the appearance of products. The initial rate must be measured, as the rate of reaction decreases with time as the concentration of substrates falls. Enzyme concentration may sometimes be measured by immunological methods using antibodies to the enzyme.

1.17 E

There are three nucleotides in a codon. Hence, a trinucleotide codon codes for 64 amino acids. As there are only 20 amino acids, an amino acid may be coded for by more than one codon. Of the different codons which code for a particular amino acid, the first two nucleotides are often the same, but the third nucleotide may differ. Hence, mutation of the third nucleotide is often silent and has no effect on the functioning of the resulting protein. On the other hand, one codon only codes for one amino acid. There is one codon (AUG) which codes for 'start', and three codons which code for 'stop'. Chain termination occurs with the 'stop' codon. Frameshift mutation by one nucleotide usually results in a wholly incorrect amino acid sequence, and hence a non-functional protein.

1.18 B E

Mitosis is a type of cell division in somatic cells, and is essential for growth, tissue formation and repair. It starts with a parent diploid cell (consisting of two sets of chromosomes) and ends with two diploid daughter cells. In contrast, meiosis is the other type of cell division, which is responsible for the production of gametes. It starts with a diploid cell and ends with two haploid daughter cells. Mitosis occurs in all embryonic tissues. It also occurs in all tissues throughout life apart from fully specialised end cells such as neurones. Fully formed red blood cells do not have a nucleus and are therefore unable to undergo mitosis. Cancer cells undergo mitosis at a faster rate than normal cells. This is important in the treatment of cancer, as several cytotoxic drugs and radiotherapy act by inhibiting mitosis via different mechanisms.

1.19 D

Isoenzymes are enzymes which catalyse the same biochemical reactions, but are of physically and chemically distinct forms. They are often present in different cell types (e.g. isoenzymes of lactate dehydrogenase are present in the heart, skeletal muscle and the liver). Isoenzymes are products of genes which are closely related. Often, they are made up of the same subunits combined in different ways. Clinically, identification of the specific form of isoenzymes may pinpoint where an abnormal enzyme is produced, and hence the likely diagnosis in the patient.

1.20 C

Increase in temperature results in increase in the kinetic energy and the frequency of collision between molecules of the reactants. Hence, the rate of reaction increases with temperature below a certain threshold. However, when the temperature reaches a certain level, the energy in the enzyme molecule may exceed that needed to break the chemical bonds that maintain the secondary and tertiary structure of the molecule. As a result, denaturation occurs. Hence, the relationship between the rate of reaction and temperature is bell-shaped, and there is an optimum temperature which gives rise to a maximum rate of reaction. Similarly, there is an optimum pH for a given enzymatic reaction, and this optimum pH depends on the particular biochemical reaction and the enzyme. For most biochemical reactions in vivo, there is an excess of substrates over enzymes. Hence, the rate of reaction increases with the concentration of enzymes. However, an increase in the concentration of substrates will not increase the rate of reaction unless there are sufficient free enzymes around to react. Whilst the value of ΔG^0 (change in the free energy of the reaction) will dictate the direction of the reaction for which it will be spontaneous, it does not predict the rate of reaction. The rate of reaction depends on the magnitude of the energy barrier.

1.21 B D

The Michaelis–Menten equation describes how the initial rate of reaction varies with substrate concentration whilst keeping other factors constant. The Michaelis constant K_m is defined as the substrate concentration that produces half-maximal velocity. The Michaelis–Menten equation is as follows:

$$V_i = \frac{v_{max}\,[S]}{k_m + [S]}$$

where v_i is the initial rate of reaction, v_{max} is the maximal velocity, K_m is the Michaelis constant, and $[S]$ is the substrate concentration.

It can be easily shown that when $[S] << K_m$, v is approximately directly proportional to $[S]$. When $[S] = K_m$, v_i is approximately equal to v_{max}. When $[S] > K_m$, v_i is approximately equal to 1/2 v_{max}.

From the equation, it can be seen that a direct plot of v_i and $[S]$ would be difficult to interpret. However, rearranging the equation to

$$\frac{1}{v_i} = \frac{K_m}{V_{max}} \frac{1}{[S]} + \frac{1}{V_{max}}$$

It can be seen if we perform a double reciprocal plot of $1/V_i$ and $1/[S]$, K_m and V_{max} can be calculated.

1.22 B

A competitive enzyme inhibitor usually binds to the substrate binding site of the enzyme, whereas a non-competitive inhibitor usually binds to another site of the enzyme. In the presence of a competitive enzyme inhibitor, increase of substrate concentration will eventually overcome the inhibition. Hence, the maximal velocity is unchanged, but the Michaelis constant K_m (the substrate concentration that produces half-maximal velocity) is increased. On the other hand, for non-competitive inhibitors, the maximal velocity is reduced as increase in substrate cannot overcome the inhibition, but the K_m is unchanged as the substrate binding site of the enzyme is unaffected.

1.23 A B C E

There are many ways of regulating enzyme activities in vivo. The enzymes may be kept separate in different cellular organelles (e.g. enzymes involved in the citric acid cycle are kept in the mitochondria); enzymes may be secreted in an inactive form so that they may be activated rapidly if necessary (e.g. chemotrypsin is secreted in an inactive form), there may be direct feedback inhibition from the end products, or there may be allosteric inhibition at an allosteric site different from the substrate site.

1.24 C D E

Allosteric enzymes are enzymes whose activity is affected by effectors at allosteric sites separate from the catalytic sites. It is an important mechanism for regulating enzyme activities. It does not obey the Michalelis–Menten equation, which predicts a hyperbolic substrate saturation curve. The substrate saturation curve is often sigmoid in shape, similar to the oxygen dissociation curve of haemoglobin. It indicates the phenomenon of cooperativity between different substrate binding sites, and that the presence of a substrate molecule at a catalytic site increases the chance of a second substrate binding at a second catalytic site. Allosteric enzymes may affect either K_m or V_{max}.

2. General principles of pharmacology
Questions

2.1 The relationship between pharmacological effect and log dose for drugs A and B is shown in Figure 1. The following conclusions can be drawn from the figure:

- **A** The dose–response curve for drug A is linear
- **B** Drug B produces a higher maximal response than drug A
- **C** Drug B is more potent than drug A
- **D** The EC_{50} is lower for drug B than drug A. (The EC_{50} value is the concentration of drug which gives rise to 50% of the maximal response)
- **E** Both drugs produce the pharmacological effect by the same mechanism

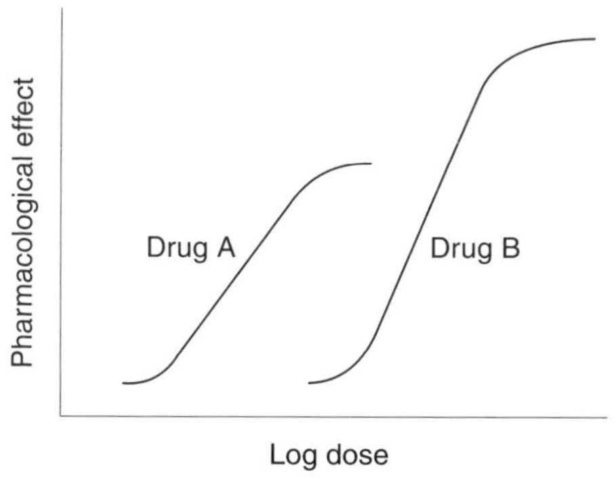

Fig. 1 Relationship between pharmacological effect and log dose for drugs A and B.

2.2 The following are the results of loss of sensitivity of target tissues to a drug:

- **A** A reduction in the concentration of the drug
- **B** A reduction in the maximal response of the drug
- **C** A reduction in the EC_{50} value
- **D** A shift of the log dose–response curve to the right
- **E** A shift of the log dose–response curve downwards

2.3 An antidepressant highly selective for its antidepressant effect:

A Achieves a higher antidepressant effect than other drugs
B Has a lower EC_{50} value than for other effects such as sedation
C Has a higher potency for depression than other drugs
D Has a higher potency than for other effects such as sedation
E Has a higher therapeutic index

2.4 The following statements about enzyme inhibitors are true:

A The therapeutic effect may be due to an increase in substrate concentration
B The therapeutic effect may be due to a decrease in the product concentration
C Non-competitive enzyme inhibitors bind to the active site of the enzyme
D Competitive enzyme inhibitors are always reversible
E The time of onset of action is always shorter for non-competitive than competitive enzyme inhibitors

2.5 The following statements about receptor agonists and antagonists are true:

A An agonist almost always results in an increase of cellular activity
B An antagonist almost always results in a reduction of cellular activity
C It is necessary for an antagonist to bind to an agonist to exert its pharmacological effects
D It is not possible for a substance to act as an agonist without binding to the receptor
E A partial agonist can produce a maximal response if present in a sufficiently high concentration

2.6 Factors associated with increased permeability of a drug to the plasma membrane include:

A A high lipid solubility
B A high water solubility
C A high molecular weight
D A high proportion of the non-ionised form of the drug
E The presence of specific carrier systems

2.7 Antagonism between two drugs:

A Is defined as the effect of two drugs together being less than either of the two drugs alone
B May be due to one drug being antagonist to another at the same receptor site
C Does not occur if the drugs act on different receptors
D May involve the release of a mediator by one of the drugs
E Is synonymous with potentiation between two drugs

2.8 **Modified-release capsules:**

A Increase the rate of absorption of the drug through the stomach
B Increase the rate at which the drug dissolves
C Are indicated if the drug may be inactivated by acids
D Consist of numerous identical small granules
E May result in a smooth sustained release of the drug

2.9 **Drug given via the following routes avoid first-pass metabolism by the liver:**

A Buccal mucosa
B The skin
C Respiratory mucosa
D Subcutaneously
E Intramuscularly

2.10 **Systemic bioavailability of a drug administered orally may be:**

A Higher than that given intravenously
B Reduced by poor gut absorption
C Reduced by liver metabolism
D Reduced by gut metabolism
E Increased by binding with other substances in the gut lumen

2.11 **The following statements about the effects of drug binding to plasma proteins are true:**

A Most drugs bind to plasma proteins irreversibly by covalent bonds
B Most drugs do not bind to plasma proteins to any significant extent
C The proportion of bound drug to total plasma concentration increases when the concentration of the drug is increased
D Protein binding may smooth the free plasma concentration of a drug
E The free concentration of a drug may be increased by the presence of another protein-binding drug

2.12 **The apparent volume of distribution of a drug:**

A Is a measure of the extent of the drug distribution in the body
B Is usually measured immediately after the drug is administered
C Cannot be greater than the total body volume
D Is usually increased by the drug binding to plasma protein
E Is usually reduced by the drug binding to tissues

2.13 **Renal clearance of a drug:**

A Is usually higher than hepatic clearance for lipid-soluble drugs
B Decreases linearly with the concentration of the drug
C Is defined as the rate of elimination of the drug by the kidney
D Can be thought of as the volume of blood cleared of the drug by the kidney per unit time
E Of creatinine is used to estimate the glomerular filtration rate (GFR)

2.14 Renal clearance is higher:

A For water-soluble than lipid-soluble drugs
B For drugs with than those without active tubular secretion
C In those with diseased kidneys than those with normal kidneys for a given drug
D For acidic drugs the lower the urinary pH
E For basic drugs the lower the urinary pH

2.15 The following statements about cytochrome P_{450} are true:

A It is largely located at the nucleus of the cell
B It is involved in the metabolism of endogenous substances
C It is involved in the oxidation of many drugs
D Activity may be increased or decreased by drugs
E A reduction of activity may lead to a lack of drug effects

2.16 Significant factors determining the steady-state concentration of a drug when regularly repeated intravenous doses of a drug are given include:

A The average rate of the drug given
B The renal clearance of the drug
C The hepatic clearance of the drug
D The volume of distribution of the drug
E Whether an initial large intravenous bolus of the drug (a loading dose) is given

2.17 The following statements about the elimination of a drug by zero-order kinetics are true:

A The rate of elimination is faster the higher the plasma concentration of the drug
B The elimination half-life of the drug is constant
C The rate of elimination of the drug is constant over time
D A steady-state concentration will be reached if an intravenous infusion is given at a rate above the current elimination rate
E It occurs more frequently for therapeutic ranges than for toxic ranges of drugs

2.18 The following are relative indications for monitoring of the plasma concentrations of a drug:

A The therapeutic effects are difficult to monitor clinically over a short time period
B The toxic effects are difficult to monitor clinically
C The therapeutic window is wide
D The therapeutic index is low
E The drug is eliminated by a first-order process

2.19 The following statements about the elderly compared with younger adults are true:

A The metabolism of drugs is higher, which results in reduced bioavailability

B The volume of distribution for water-soluble drugs is increased
C The renal excretion of drugs is lower
D The response to a given concentration of a drug is less
E The doses required for a given drug are generally smaller

2.20 True drug allergy:

A Is the commonest cause of adverse drug effects
B Exhibits a graded dose–response relationship
C Decreases in severity over time
D Can be predicted from the mechanism of the therapeutic actions of the drug
E Should be managed by a reduction in the dose of the drug given

2.21 The following statements about inverse agonists are true:

A They are full agonists of different potencies
B Their effects are inversely proportional to the concentration
C The effects are inversely proportional to their potencies
D They produce effects which are opposite to those of the agonists
E They are synonymous with antagonists

2.22 The following statements about partial agonists are true:

A They do not activate the receptors
B They produce effects which are opposite to those of the full agonists
C The maximal response is less than that of full agonists
D The effect of a combination of a full and a partial agonist together is always greater than that of the full agonist alone
E The effect of a full and partial agonist together is usually smaller than that of the partial agonist alone

2.23 The following reduce the systemic availability of an orally administered drug:

A Low lipid solubility of the drug
B Intestinal hurry
C Binding of active drugs to food
D Reduced liver metabolism of the drug
E Instability of the drug under low pH

2.24 Drugs with a half-life of:

A 10 min may be administered with a loading dose identical to the maintenance dose
B 2 h may be administered orally three times a day
C 12 h may be administered orally twice a day
D 72 h may be administered intravenously
E 120 h may be administered with a loading dose greater than the maintenance dose

2.25 Prolonged exposure to an agonist may result in:

A Upregulation of receptors
B An increase in the density of receptors on cells
C A decrease in the capacity of the receptors to respond
D An increase in the receptor occupancy
E Patients tolerant and refractory to treatment by agonists of the receptors

2.26 The likelihood of the rebound phenomenon on withdrawal of drug is higher:

A The longer the drug has been previously administered
B The shorter the half-life of the drug
C For a partial agonist than a pure antagonist
D The more abrupt the withdrawal
E For a drug with inhibitory than a drug with excitatory effects

2.27 Drug Y may increase the effect of drug X if drug Y:

A Is a purgative and drug X is given orally
B Binds to drug X in the gut lumen
C Is an enzyme inducer and drug X is metabolised in the liver
D Is an enzyme inhibitor and drug X is metabolised in the liver
E Inhibits the active reabsorption of drug X across the renal tubular epithelium

2. General principles of pharmacology
Answers

2.1 **B**

The relationship between pharmacological effects and the drug concentration is usually hyperbolic (see Fig. 2). However, the relationship between pharmacological effects and log dose is usually sigmoid in shape, and the central proportion is almost linear. The maximal response is represented by the plateau of the curves, and is higher for drug Y than drug X. The EC_{50} value is the concentration of drug which gives rise to 50% of the maximal response. The lower the value, the higher the potency. The value is lower for drug X. Hence, drug X is more potent. It is not possible to deduce the mechanisms of action from the log dose–response curve alone.

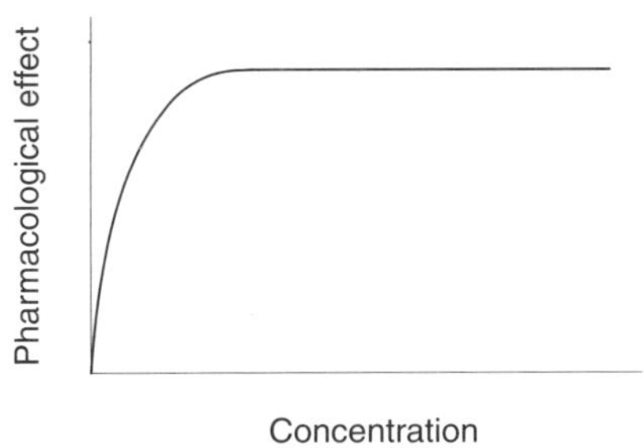

Fig. 2 Pharmacological effects

2.2 **D**

Sensitivity of target tissue reflects the concentration at which it responds to a drug. Loss of sensitivity results in a higher concentration of drug necessary to achieve the same effect. Hence, the EC_{50} value is increased. However, the maximal response is not affected. The log dose–response curve is shifted to the right.

2.3 B D E

A highly selective drug produces one pharmacological effect at a much lower dose than for other pharmacological effects. A formal definition of selectivity is the ratio of its potency for one effect to its potency for another effect. Hence, it has a lower EC_{50} value and a higher potency than for other effects. Selectivity does not compare the effect of one drug with another. The therapeutic index of a drug is its selectivity for its therapeutic effect. For a drug with a high therapeutic index, a wide range of concentrations can be tolerated without side effects. Conversely, for a drug with a low therapeutic index, there is a narrow range of concentrations for which the drug has therapeutic effect without side effects.

2.4 A B

The effects of enzyme inhibitors may be due to either increased concentration of the substrate (e.g. acetylcholinesterase) or to reduced concentration of the products (e.g. angiotensin-converting enzyme inhibitors). Competitive inhibitors bind to the active site, whilst non-competitive inhibitors bind to other sites. Although many competitive enzyme inhibitors are reversible, some are irreversible (e.g. organophosphorus compounds are irreversible competitive inhibitors of actylcholinesterases). This is because they form strong covalent bonds with the enzyme. Whilst the offset of action is longer for irreversible inhibitors, the onset of action depends mainly on the rate of the substrate to product reaction. Hence, the time of onset is independent of whether it is a reversible or irreversible enzyme inhibitor.

2.5 –

An active drug response may be produced by either increasing or decreasing cellular activities. An agonist produces an active response by activating receptors on the cell membrane. It may do so directly by binding to the receptor (e.g. adrenaline binding to adrenergic receptors) or indirectly (e.g. tyramine promotes release of neuronal noradrenaline). An antagonist prevents agonists acting (e.g. by binding to the receptor), but does not produce an effect itself. A partial agonist produces an active response, although the response is less than that from a full agonist even when it occupies all the receptor sites.

2.6 A D E

Plasma membranes consist of a lipid bilayer with polar groups outside and non-polar groups inside. Lipid-soluble drugs (i.e. drugs with high lipid–water partition coefficient) are able to cross the plasma membrane by passive diffusion, and a low molecular weight is associated with more rapid diffusion. Very small water-soluble drugs (e.g. ethanol) can also pass through the membrane via small water-filled pores. Few drugs have specific carrier systems.

2.7 B D

Antagonism between two drugs is said to occur if the effect of the two drugs is smaller than the sum of their individual pharmacological effects. This may occur in many ways. The two drugs may be antagonists of each other at the same receptor (e.g. propranolol and adrenaline), one drug may release a mediator which antagonises the effect of another drug (e.g. tyramine releases noradrenaline, which antagonises the effect of noradrenaline), or the two drugs may act at different receptors which gives rise to opposite effects (functional antagonist, e.g. propranolol, which reduces the heart rate by blocking the β_1 receptor, and atropine, which increases the heart rate by blocking muscarinic acetylcholine receptors in the heart). Potentiation is said to occur if one drug reduces the concentration of another drug necessary to produce a given pharmacological effect (e.g. anticholinesterases potentiate the effect of acetylcholine at the neuromuscular junction).

2.8 E

Modified-release capsules consist of numerous small granules which dissolve at different rates. This results in a smooth sustained release of the drug. If the drug can be activated by acids, enteric-coated tablets are indicated.

2.9 A B C D E

Drugs taken orally are absorbed via the gastrointestinal system. Since the venous drainage is via the hepatic portal system, they may be subjected to significant first-pass metabolism by the liver. Drugs given via other sites (e.g. sublingually via the buccal membrane, by inhalation via the respiratory mucosa, as a skin patch, intramuscularly or intravenously) will avoid first-pass metabolism since venous drainage is via the systemic circulation. Drugs given rectally are less predictable. In general, rectal mucosa of the lower rectum is drained directly to the systemic circulation, but the rest of the rectum is drained via the portal circulation.

2.10 B C D

Systemic bioavailability is the proportion of a drug administered that finally reaches the systemic circulation. For intravenous injection, the systemic bioavailability is 1. Systemic bioavailability for drugs given orally is often small for several reasons. The drug may not dissolve completely; it may be broken down in the gut lumen (e.g. benylpenicillin); the absorption may be poor (e.g. aminoglycosides); it may bind to substances in the gut lumen (e.g. tetracyclines binding to calcium ions); and it may be metabolised either in the gut (e.g. levodopa) or in the liver (e.g. opiates). Hence, the dose of drugs given orally is often greater than that given via the other routes.

2.11 D E

Most drugs bind to plasma proteins (e.g. albumin) reversibly by non-covalent bonds. For lipid-soluble drugs, the proportion of bound drugs remains constant over the therapeutic range of concentrations. This is also true for polar drugs which bind to specific sites of a plasma protein, as there is often an excess of binding sites over drugs. Rarely, the drugs have a very high affinity for the receptors and they become saturated, and the proportion of bound drugs decreases with increasing concentration of drugs. Furthermore, the presence of another drug which competes for the same binding site may increase the free concentration of the first drug. Protein binding often smoothes out the plasma concentration and speeds up distribution of the drug.

2.12 A

The apparent volume of distribution of a drug is a measure of the extent of the drug distribution in the body at equilibrium. It is defined as the ratio of the amount of the drug in the body to the plasma drug concentration at equilibrium. Hence, if the drug distributes equally between all tissues and plasma, the volume of distribution is equivalent to the total body water. However, if the drug binds strongly to tissues, only a small proportion of the drug will be found in plasma, and the apparent volume of distribution can be much higher than the total body volume. Binding to plasma proteins will have no effect on the apparent volume of distribution.

2.13 D E

Lipid-soluble drugs are mostly metabolised by the liver into water-soluble substances. Water-soluble drugs and metabolites are mostly eliminated by the kidney. The clearance of a drug is defined as the rate of elimination of a drug divided by the plasma concentration of the drug. It can be thought of as the volume of blood cleared of the drug per unit time. The production of creatinine in the body is relatively constant, and it distributes throughout the extracellular fluid with minimal protein binding, and there is often no net secretion or reabsorption in the renal tubules. Hence, creatinine clearance is often used as a measure of GFR.

2.14 A B E

Three broad factors determine the rate at which a drug is excreted by the kidneys: its rate of filtration at the glomerulus, rate of reabsorption at the tubules, and the rate of secretion at the tubules. The rate of filtration depends on the proper function of the kidneys and the concentration of the drug in plasma. A high rate of tubular reabsorption reduces the renal clearance of a drug. Tubular reabsorption is usually passive, but may be active for a few drugs (e.g. thyroxine) which resemble physiological metabolites. Passive reabsorption is higher for non-polar, lipid-soluble drugs than highly polar water-soluble drugs. The proportion of non-polarised form of the drug is higher with low urinary pH for acidic drugs, and a high urinary pH for basic drugs. As only the polarised form of the drug is reabsorbed, the reabsorption rate is lower (and the renal clearance is higher) for acidic drugs in the presence of a high urinary pH, and for basic drugs in the presence of a low urinary pH. Active secretion of drugs into the renal tubules (e.g. penicillin, salicylates) decreases the renal clearance.

2.15 B C D

The cytochrome P_{450} system is the most important mixed-function oxidase (MFO) system. This enzyme system is largely located in the smooth endoplasmic reticulum, but may also be present in the mitochondria (e.g. monoamine oxidase). The system is responsible both for the metabolism of endogenous substances (e.g. corticosteroids) and drugs. Most enzymes in the systems are involved in oxidation, although a few are involved in reduction. The system may be induced or inhibited by drugs. This is clinically important, as the therapeutic effects of drugs may be reduced if the enzymes are induced, and side effects may be enhanced if the enzymes are inhibited. Changes in drug doses are necessary to avoid this.

2.16 A B C

The steady-state concentration of a drug when regularly repeated intravenous doses of a drug are given depends mostly on the average rate of the drug given and the clearance rate from the plasma. The clearance rate from the plasma is largely contributed to by clearance from the kidneys and the liver. The volume of distribution of the drug determines the time taken to reach the steady-state concentration. The larger the volume of distribution, the longer is the time taken to reach steady-state concentration. However, the steady-state concentration is not affected. Similarly, an initial large intravenous dose of the drug will reduce the time taken to reach the steady-state concentration without affecting the actual steady-state concentration.

2.17 C

A first-order elimination process is said to occur if the rate of elimination is proportional to the plasma concentration. The elimination half-life (time taken for the plasma concentration to reduce to half) is constant. Since the rate of elimination increases with the concentration, a steady-state concentration will be reached even if the infusion rate is above the current elimination rate. By contrast, a zero-order elimination process is said to occur if the rate of elimination is constant and independent of the plasma concentration. The half-life is shorter for a smaller concentration of the drug. If the infusion rate exceeds the current elimination rate, the plasma concentration will continue to increase to a toxic level, and a steady-state concentration will never be reached.

A zero-order elimination process usually occurs if the elimination is eliminated primarily by metabolism and the enzymes responsible for the metabolism are saturated. This is more likely to occur if the concentration of the drug is high.

2.18 A B D

Monitoring of the plasma concentrations of a drug is useful in ensuring that the drug plasma level is between the therapeutic and the toxic level of the drug. It is particularly valuable if either therapeutic or toxic effects are difficult to monitor over a short period of time. For example, the effect of an anti-epileptic agent is difficult to monitor over a short period of time. Similarly, the toxic effect of aminoglycosides is difficult to monitor clinically. The therapeutic index is the ratio of the minimum therapeutic concentration and the minimum toxic concentration. The therapeutic window is the range of concentrations between the minimum therapeutic and toxic concentrations. Monitoring of plasma concentrations is more important for drugs with a low therapeutic index and a narrow therapeutic window.

2.19 C E

Compared with younger adults, the elderly are more likely to suffer from side effects of drugs. There are many reasons for this. The metabolism of drugs by the liver and the excretion of drugs by the kidneys are lower, which results in higher plasma concentrations. Furthermore, the response of the elderly to a given concentration of a drug is greater. Hence, the doses required for a given drug are generally smaller. As the proportion of body water decreases and that of fats increases in the elderly, the volume of distribution for water-soluble drugs is decreased, but that for lipid-soluble drugs is increased.

2.20 –

Most adverse drug effects can be predicted from the pharmacological properties of the drug. Amongst those adverse effects which are unpredictable, true drug allergy is the commonest. True drug allergy is due to one of the hypersensitivity reactions involving antigen–antibody reactions, and is unrelated to the mechanism of its therapeutic effects. A period of induction is required on primary exposure, but the side effects may be rapid and severe on re-exposure. True drug allergy is often over-diagnosed. However, with a history of true drug allergy, the drug should not be prescribed in future.

2.21 D

Agonists are substances which resemble the natural transmitter and activate the receptors. Antagonists are substances sufficiently similar to the natural transmitter to occupy the receptors without eliciting a response. Inverse agonists are substances which produce effects opposite to those of the agonists. An example is β-carbolines, which act on the benzodiazepine receptors. Benzodiazepines cause muscle relaxation whilst β-carbolines cause convulsions. However, they both act on the same receptors and through modulating the effects of the neurotransmitter GABA.

2.22 C

Partial agonists activate the receptors, but to a lesser extent than the natural transmitter. Hence, they produce maximal responses less than those of full agonists. The partial agonists also prevent the natural transmitters from reaching the receptors. Hence, they also act as antagonists. The effect of a combination of a full and a partial agonist may be less than that of the full agonist alone, as the partial agonists prevent the full agonists from reaching some of the receptors. However, the effect of a full and a partial agonist together is usually greater than that of the partial agonist alone. Partial agonists may be clinically useful. For example, oxyprenolol is a partial agonist whilst propranolol is an antagonist of the β-adrenergic receptors. On its own, oxyprenolol causes less bradycardia and patients on oxyprenolol have a higher resting heart rate than patients on equivalent doses of propranolol. However, oxyprenolol has the same protective effect as propranolol against the natural adrenaline during exercise or under stressful situations. Substances which produce effects that are opposite to those of the full agonists are called inverse agonists.

2.23 B C E

In order for an orally administered drug to reach the systemic circulation, it must pass through the stomach intact, undergo absorption from the small intestine and pass through the liver without being metabolised. If the drug is unstable under low pH, it is liable to be inactivated by gastric acid. Slow gastric emptying, intestinal hurry or binding of the active drugs to food tends to reduce absorption of the drug from the intestinal wall. Lipid-soluble drugs are easier to absorb from the gut. Metabolism through the liver is the single most important reason for the low systemic availability for orally administered drugs.

2.24 A C E

Drugs are usually given by an initial loading dose followed by maintenance doses at regular intervals. The half-life of a drug is the time it takes for the plasma concentration to decline by half. As a rough general principle, intervals between maintenance doses may be approximately equal to the half-life of the drug. If a loading dose is not given (i.e. the loading dose being the same as the maintenance dose), it would take five half-life periods to achieve a steady-state concentration. Hence, for a drug with a half-life of 10 min, it may be acceptable not to give a loading dose as the steady-state concentration will be reached in 50 min. For a drug with a half-life of 2 h, it should be administered roughly every 2 h.

Since this will not be acceptable to the patient, either sustained-release preparations should be given, or the drug should be given as a continuous infusion. A drug with a half-life of 12 h may be given twice daily. A drug with a half-life of 72 h should be given daily with the maintenance dose just sufficient to replace the amount eliminated in 24 h. A drug with a half-life of 120 h should be given a loading dose higher than the maintenance dose, as it would otherwise take 600 h to reach steady-state concentration.

2.25 C E

In general, the effect of the regulation of receptors is to restore the function of cells to its usual state. Hence, prolonged exposure to an agonist results in downregulation of receptors. This may be achieved by a decrease in the number of receptors, a decrease in the capacity of the receptors to respond, or a decrease in the receptor occupancy. Hence, patients can become tolerant or refractory to treatment by agonists. Conversely, prolonged exposure to an antagonist results in upregulation of receptors, which may be achieved by an increase in the number of receptors, an increase in the capacity of the receptors to respond, or an increase in receptor occupancy. Patients may become supersensitive to the effects of agonists.

2.26 A B D

The rebound phenomenon on withdrawal of a drug is due to the up or downregulation of receptors following prolonged use. For example, chronic use of β-blockers may result in upregulation of the adrenergic receptors. When administration of the drug is stopped, the effect of physiological β-adrenaline and noradrenaline on the supersensitive receptors will be enhanced. The likelihood of the phenomenon is greater the longer the drug has been previously administered, the more abrupt the withdrawal, the shorter the half-life of the drug (as the withdrawal from the target organ is more abrupt), and if the drug is a partial agonist rather than if it is either a pure agonist or a pure antagonist. The rebound phenomenon is equally likely for drugs with inhibitory or excitatory effects.

2.27 D E

Drug interactions may occur at any stage from preparation to excretion. A drug which increases bowel motility is likely to reduce the absorption and hence the effects of orally administered drugs. Binding to another drug in the gut lumen will reduce the effect of both drugs. An enzyme inducer may decrease the effect of drugs by increasing the rate of metabolism in the liver, whilst an enzyme inhibitor may increase the effect of drugs by decreasing the rate of metabolism in the liver. Inhibition of the active transport of a drug across the renal tubular epithelium may increase its effect by reducing its rate of elimination.

3. Nutrition and energy
Questions

3.1 The following statements about the conversion of ATP into ADP and inorganic phosphate are true:

A The reaction is endothermic
B Free energy is required for the conversion
C It may be coupled with an anabolic reaction
D It has the highest free energy amongst all important biochemical reactions involving organophosphates
E It occurs during muscle contraction

3.2 Sources of high-energy phosphates in the living cell include:

A The urea cycle
B Glycogenesis
C Oxidative phosphorylation
D Glycolysis
E The citric acid cycle

3.3 The following statements about oxidative phosphorylation are true:

A It occurs in the smooth endoplasmic reticulum
B It may occur anaerobically
C Water is formed as a by-product
D Reducing equivalents (e.g. free electrons) are needed for the process
E It is inhibited by cyanide

3.4 The following statements about the respiratory chain are true:

A It consists of redox carriers which transport the reducing equivalents
B It consists of no more than three components
C The first component is the most electropositive
D The inorganic phosphate to oxygen (P : O) ratio is higher for NAD-linked dehydrogenase than flavoprotein-linked dehydrogenase
E The oxidation and phosphorylation processes occur simultaneously

3.5 Examples of monosaccharides include:

A Glucose
B Glycogen
C Maltose
D Fructose
E Starch

3.6 The citric acid cycle may be involved in the oxidation of:

A Glucose
B Starch
C Fatty acids
D Lipids
E Protein

3.7 The following statements about the citric acid cycle are true:

A It occurs in the mitochondria
B It provides reducing equivalents for oxidative phosphorylation
C It may occur without oxygen
D 12 ATPs are formed every full cycle
E Two carbon dioxide molecules are formed every full cycle

3.8 The activity of the citric acid cycle is increased when energy is required (e.g. during muscular contraction). The following substances are likely to contribute significantly to this regulation of the citric acid cycle:

A NADH
B ADP
C Calcium ions
D Glycogen
E Glucose

3.9 The citric acid cycle plays a role in the following processes:

A Gluconeogenesis
B Nucleic acid synthesis
C Fatty acid synthesis from glucose
D Lactic acid synthesis
E Non-essential amino acid synthesis

3.10 The following statements about the glycolysis pathway are true:

A It is the main mechanism for the metabolism of glucose
B It is the main mechanism for the metabolism of fructose
C ATP is consumed in the process
D It is a more important pathway in the heart than in the brain
E The quantity of lactic acid increases with the concentration of oxygen

3.11 The inability to metabolise pyruvate (into acetyl CoA by pyruvate dehydrogenase):

A May occur with thiamine deficiency
B May be inherited
C Results in hypoxia
D Results in accumulation of lactic acid
E Results in adverse effects particularly on the brain

3.12 The following statements about glycogen are true:

A It is a linear chain of monosaccharides
B It is mainly found in the heart muscle
C Liver glycogen provides an important source of energy for vigorous physical activities
D Disorders of glycogen storage result in muscle weakness
E Muscle glycogen store is usually significantly depleted after about 8 h of fasting

3.13 During starvation, the enzymes which catalyse the following carbohydrate metabolic reactions are inhibited:

A Conversion of glucose to glucose 6-phosphate
B Conversion of fructose 6-phosphate to fructose 1,6-bisphosphate
C Conversion of pyruvate to acetyl CoA
D Conversion of glycogen to glucose
E Conversion of phosphoenolpyruvate to pyruvate

3.14 The following statements about the source of fuel for the body during starvation are true:

A There is a net conversion of fatty acids to glucose
B Oxidation of glucose may be completely eliminated
C Glycogen is converted to glucose in preference to the breakdown of essential amino acids
D Free glucose is used in preference to fatty acids
E Free fatty acids are used in preference to ketone bodies

3.15 The energy expended by an individual is increased:

A By fever
B By high environmental temperature
C In males
D By increased physical activity
E By sleep

3.16 The following minerals must be present in the diet to maintain health:

A Phosphorus
B Magnesium
C Calcium
D Aluminium
E Iodine

3.17 The following statements about dietary proteins are true:

A All 20 types of amino acids must be present in the diet
B About 50% of the energy should be supplied by protein
C The quality of protein is measured by the amount of energy it contains per unit weight
D An adequate intake of carbohydrate and fat minimises the requirements for dietary high-quality protein
E Complementary proteins are defined as the combination of an animal and a plant protein

3.18 The following vitamins are water-soluble:

A Vitamin A
B Vitamin B_{12}
C Vitamin C
D Vitamin D
E Vitamin K

3.19 The following B vitamins are correctly matched to their functions:

A Thiamine (vitamin B_1) – provides one-carbon residues for nucleic acid synthesis
B Riboflavin (vitamin B_2) – prosthetic groups in flavoprotein enzymes in oxidoreduction reactions
C Pyridoxal phosphate (vitamin B_6) – coenzyme for amino acid metabolism
D Cobalamin (vitamin B_{12}) – coenzyme for oxidative carboxylation of α-keto acids and the pentose phosphate pathway
E Niacin (vitamin B_3) – coenzyme for oxidoreduction enzymes

3.20 The following vitamins are correctly matched to the clinical conditions associated with their deficiencies:

A Thiamine (vitamin B_1) – megaloblastic anaemia
B Niacin (vitamin B_3) – beriberi
C Cobalamin (vitamin B_{12}) – pellagra
D Vitamin A – night-blindness
E Vitamin C – scurvy

3.21 Ketone bodies:

A Include acetoacetate
B Are formed when fatty acid oxidation is inhibited
C Are mostly produced in skeletal muscles and kidneys
D Cannot be used as an energy source by any tissues
E Are produced in large quantities in untreated diabetes mellitus

3.22 Brown fat:

A Is mainly located around the buttocks
B Is not present below two years of age
C Is mainly innervated by parasympathetic nervous system

D Is metabolised by strict coupling with oxidative phosphorylation
E Produces more heat per ATP than white fat

3.23 The basal metabolic rate:

A Is determined whilst the subject is asleep
B Is determined whilst the subject is eating
C Is higher in women than in men
D Is higher in children than in adults
E Is increased during starvation

3.24 The respiratory quotient:

A Is the ratio of the steady state of the volume of oxygen produced to the weight of food consumed per unit time
B For carbohydrates is approximately 1
C Is lower for fat than for carbohydrate
D Is higher for protein than for carbohydrate
E Is important in the calculation of heat energy released by combustion of foodstuffs using direct calorimetry

3. Nutrition and energy
Answers

3.1 **C E**

ATP is the most important high-energy carrier compound in the living cell. Energy is given out when it is broken down into ADP and inorganic phosphate, and the reaction is exothermic (i.e. giving out heat or energy). This reaction is usually coupled with essential processes requiring energy, such as muscle contraction, synthesis and active transport. Compared with other important biochemical reactions involving organophosphates, the value of the free energy associated with hydrolysis of ATP occupies an intermediate position between low-energy and high-energy phosphates. This allows the ATP/ADP cycle to play an important role in energy transfer. ATP acts as a donor of high-energy phosphates to form some organophosphate compounds and ADP accepts high-energy phosphates to form ATP from other compounds.

3.2 **C D E**

High-energy phosphates act as the energy currency of the cell. The most important source of high-energy phosphates is respiratory chain oxidation using molecular oxygen within mitochondria. The other two sources are glycolysis (breakdown of glucose into lactic acid or pyruvate) and the citric acid cycle (which also provides reducing equivalents for oxidative phosphorylation). Glycogenesis is the conversion of glucose into glycogen.

3.3 **C D E**

Oxidative phosphorylation occurs in the mitochondria ('the powerhouse of the cell'), and couples respiration to the production of ATP. It makes use of reducing equivalents (e.g. free electrons) derived from the breakdown of food, and is transported through the respiratory chain (a series of catalysts) to combine with oxygen to form water. High-energy phosphates are produced in the process. This energy-producing process is much more efficient than anaerobic processes. This process may be of clinical significance, as it may be inhibited by cyanide or carbon monoxide.

3.4 A D E

The respiratory chain consists of a series of redox carriers arranged in order of increasing redox potential, starting with the most electronegative component. It consists of FAD and/or NAD, iron–sulphur protein, coenzyme Q and several types of cytochromes. The yield via an NAD-linked dehyrogenase is 3 mol of ATP to 1 mol of oxygen atoms, but the corresponding P : O ratio for FAD-linked dehydrogenase is 2. The oxidation and phosphorylation processes are coupled and occur simultaneously. The respiratory chain functions as a proton pump, and the electrochemical potential difference generated is used to drive a membrane-located ATP synthase.

3.5 A D

Monosaccharides are carbohydrates which cannot be broken down into simpler carbohydrates. All carbohydrates need to be broken down into monosaccharides before they may be oxidised to provide energy. Glucose, fructose, galactose, sucrose and ribose are examples of monosaccharides. Maltose is a disaccharide, as it may be broken down into glucose and sucrose. Glycogen and starch are polysaccharides.

3.6 A B C D E

The citric acid cycle acts as the final common pathway for the oxidation of all major foodstuffs including carbohydrates, lipids and protein. Glucose, fatty acids and amino acids are all metabolised to either acetyl CoA or intermediates of the citric acid cycle.

3.7 A B D E

Reducing equivalents in the form of electrons or hydrogen are produced in the citric acid cycle and fed into the respiratory chain to generate ATP. Both these processes are closely linked and occur in the mitochondria. As oxygen is required for oxidative phosphorylation, the citric acid cycle is inhibited in the absence of oxygen. A total of 12 ATP molecules are produced per full cycle (from the oxidation of three NADH, one $FADH_2$ and the release of one ATP molecule in the formation of succinate from succinyl CoA). The first step of the citric acid cycle involves the formation of citrate (a six-carbon atom compound) from oxaloacetate (a four-carbon atom compound) and acetyl CoA (a two-carbon atom compound). This has to be converted back to oxalocacetate at the end of the cycle. Hence, two carbon atoms must be lost by the generation of two carbon dioxide molecules.

3.8 A B C

As the primary function of the citric acid cycle is to provide energy and because it is closely coupled to the oxidative phosphorylation process, oxidative phosphorylation is the most important regulatory mechanism for the citric acid cycle activity. A reduction in energy status indicated by a reduction of ATP/ADP or NADH/NAD levels will result in increased citric acid cycle activity. The biochemical steps for regulation are likely to be at the non-equilibrium reactions catalysed by dehydrogenases (e.g. pyruvate dehydrogenase, citrate synthase, isocitrate dehydrogenase, α-ketoglutarate dehydrogenase). All these enzymes are also activated by calcium ions, which are increased during muscular contraction.

3.9 A C E

Whilst the oxidation of major foodstuffs to produce energy is the primary function of the citric acid cycle, it also plays a role in other metabolic pathways. For example, it may play a role in gluconeogenesis by the conversion of oxaloacetate into phosphoenolpyruvate, and into the main gluconeogensis pathway. Acetyl CoA, an important component of fatty acid synthesis, is formed by the action of pyruvate dehydrogenase, which is a mitochondrial enzyme. Since the enzymes responsible for fatty acid synthesis are outside the mitochondria, the acetyl CoA is converted into citrate via the citric acid cycle, which is then transported out of the mitochondria to be reconverted into acetyl CoA. The citric acid cycle is also important in providing the carbon skeleton in the formation of some non-essential amino acids. Lactic acid may be converted into pyruvate and then enters the citric acid cycle.

3.10 A B

Glycolysis is the main mechanism for the metabolism of monosaccharides such as glucose, fructose and galactose. In the process, glucose is converted into pyruvate and ATP is produced. It may occur either aerobically or anaerobically. In the absence of oxygen, pyruvate is converted into lactic acid (lactate). In the presence of oxygen, pyruvate is converted into acetyl CoA in the mitochondria and enters the citric acid cycle. As it can produce energy rapidly in the absence of oxygen, it is especially important in the brain and in skeletal muscle during vigorous activity. However, only two ATP molecules are generated per glucose molecule. This is much less efficient than if it occurs under aerobic conditions when a total of 38 ATP molecules per glucose molecule are produced.

3.11 A B D E

Normally, pyruvate produced during glycolysis is converted into acetyl CoA by pyruvate dehydrogenase in the mitochondria. However, poisoning by mercuric ions, a deficiency of thiamine (e.g. dietary deficiency) or inherited pyruvate dehydrogenase deficiency may make this impossible. This results in the conversion of pyruvate into lactate (lactic acid). As the brain depends especially on glucose for its energy, neurological disturbances are particularly likely.

3.12 D

Glycogen is a branched polymer of α-D-glucose, and represents the principal store for carbohydrates in animals. It is mainly stored in the liver and muscle. The primary function of liver glycogen is to maintain a stable blood glucose, and fasting depletes liver glycogen. Muscle glycogen is an importance source of energy for vigorous physical activity, and is usually depleted after a period of strenuous exercise. In disorders of glycogen storage diseases, deficiency in enzymes responsible for glycogen metabolism results in either deficient glycogen mobilisation or the deposition of abnormal forms of glycogen. They are usually inherited; muscle weakness is a characteristic symptom due to lack of mobilisation of muscle glycogen.

3.13 A B C E

Glucose is a very important source of energy for the body which the brain depends heavily on. If the glucose level falls below a certain level, brain dysfunction occurs and the patient may lapse into a coma. Hence there are elaborate mechanisms to maintain an adequate glucose concentration during starvation. Ketone bodies and fatty acids are oxidised in preference to glucose. All the principal enzymes responsible for regulating glycolysis (breakdown of glucose to pyruvate) and pyruvate oxidation are inhibited. The regulatory enzymes for glycolysis are glucokinase (which converts glucose to glucose 6-phosphate), phosphofructokinase (which converts fructose 6-phosphate to fructose 1,6-bisphosphate) and pyruvate kinase (which converts phosphoenolpyruvate). Pyruvate dehydrogenase converts pyruvate to acetyl CoA, which is used in the citric acid cycle. The conversion of glycogen to glucose is activated to maintain the level of blood glucose. If a patient lapses into coma due to low blood glucose, one of the treatments is glucagon, which converts glycogen to glucose.

3.14 C

Although carbohydrates can be readily converted into fatty acids via the citric acid cycle, the conversion of pyruvate to acetyl CoA by pyruvate dehydrogenase is essentially irreversible. Hence, there cannot be net conversion of fatty acids to glucose. Since the brain and red blood cells depend on glucose for their energy sources, there is an obligatory rate of oxidation of glucose for the body. During starvation, glycogen stores are mobilised. Ketone bodies are used in preference to fatty acids, which in turn are used in preference to glucose.

3.15 A C D

The basal metabolic rate is the energy expended in maintaining basic physiological functions when a subject is at rest, awake and in a warm environment. The basal metabolic rate is higher in males, with increasing surface area of the body, in fever and in those with hyperthyroidism. Sleep reduces the basal metabolic rate. Physical exercise is the most important factor which increases the energy expended above the basal metabolic rate. Other factors which increase the energy expended above the basal metabolic rate include high environmental temperature and following a meal, due to energy expended on digestion (i.e. its specific dynamic action).

3.16 A B C E

Several minerals are essential for both physiological and biochemical functions. For example, sodium is the principal cation in the extracellular fluid, and potassium is the principal cation in intracellular fluid. Calcium, magnesium and phosphorus are important constituents of bones and teeth. In addition, calcium plays an important part in regulating the function of nerves and muscles, and magnesium is essential for some enzyme cofactors. Iodine is an important constituent of thyroxine. Other important minerals include chloride, copper, iron, manganese, selenium, zinc and fluoride. Aluminium is not an essential mineral, but has been suspected to cause disease (e.g. renal damage and possible links with Alzheimer's dementia).

3.17 D

Dietary proteins are digested into individual amino acids to synthesise specific proteins required by the body. Although there are 20 different types of amino acids, only nine of these (essential amino acids) cannot be synthesised in the body and must be present in the diet. The others (non-essential amino acids) can be formed in the body. High-quality proteins are those with the appropriate proportions of essential amino acids, and include eggs, milk and meat. Proteins which are deficient in some essential amino acids (e.g. wheat) are not of high quality. However, the deficiency may be complemented by other proteins (e.g. beans) to yield a satisfactory protein diet. These proteins are said to be complementary. If the intake of carbohydrates and fat is inadequate, the proteins ingested may be used for gluconeogenesis.

3.18 B C

All the B vitamins and vitamin C are water-soluble. The remaining vitamins (A, D, E, K) are fat-soluble. The importance of classifying vitamins into these two categories is that water-soluble vitamins are excreted in urine and rarely accumulate in toxic concentrations. However, their storage is limited and they must be replenished regularly.

3.19 B C

The B vitamins are generally important coenzymes for important processes in the metabolism of carbohydrates, lipid and proteins. Thiamine (vitamin B_1) is a cofactor in oxidative decarboxylation of α-keto acids and for transketolase in the pentose phosphate pathway. Deficiency in thiamine results in accumulation in the substrates in these reactions (e.g. pyruvate, pentose sugars, leucine, valine) and a clinical picture known as beriberi. It affects the heart muscles, skeletal muscles and nerves, resulting in oedema and heart failure, muscle weakness, peripheral neuropathy and Wernicke's encephalopathy. Riboflavin (vitamin B_2) forms the prosthetic groups in flavoprotein enzymes in oxidoreduction reactions. Surprisingly, in spite of the important role it has in many biochemical reactions, deficiency of riboflavin results in non-life-threatening symptoms such as angular stomatitis, glossitis and photophobia. Pyridoxal phosphate (vitamin B_6) is the coenzyme of several enzymes of amino acid metabolism, and of enzymes for breaking down glycogen. Deficiency states are rare and not well recognised. Cobalamin (vitamin B_{12}) and folate are essential constituents for nucleic acid synthesis. Hence deficiency results in impaired DNA synthesis and prevents cell division and formation of nuclei in new red blood cells. This results in megaloblastic anaemia. Active niacin (vitamin B_3) is NAD, and is a coenzyme to many enzymes for oxidoreduction. Deficiency results in a pellagra syndrome characterised by depression, dementia, diarrhoea and weight loss.

3.20 D E

See question 3.19 above for the B vitamins. Ascorbic acid (vitamin C) is a water-soluble vitamin and an antioxidant that maintains many metal cofactors in the reduced state, and which is required for collagen synthesis. Deficiency results in a clinical syndrome called scurvy. Scurvy is related to defective collagen synthesis, and is characterised by subcutaneous and other haemorrhages, swollen gums and loose teeth, and muscle weakness. Vitamin A is a fat-soluble vitamin and is a component of the visual pigment rhodopsin in the retinal rod cells. Hence, vitamin A deficiency results in night-blindness.

3.21 A E

Ketone bodies are produced in mitochondria in the liver when there is already a high rate of fatty acid oxidation through β-oxidation to acetyl CoA. Ketone bodies include acetoacetate, 3-hydroxybutyrate and acetone, and can be used by tissues outside the liver (e.g. skeletal and heart muscles). Since oxidation of fatty acids occurs during starvation, ketone bodies are mildly elevated. The level of ketone bodies is dramatically raised in untreated diabetes. This is because insulin has antilipolytic and lipogenic effects, and these are lost in untreated diabetes.

3.22 E

Brown fat consists of only a small proportion of total body fat, and is particularly important in regulating heat production. It is more abundant in infancy, and is mainly located in the nape of the neck, between the scapulae, and along the great vessels in the thorax and abdomen. It is extensively innervated by the sympathetic nervous system. Stimulation of the sympathetic nervous system releases noradrenaline, which acts via the β_1-adrengeric receptors. Although the oxidative phosphorylation pathway can be used in the metabolism of brown fat, another pathway which does not generate ATP can also be utilised. Hence, the amount of heat energy per ATP molecule produced is higher than in white fat. Brown fat is an important mechanism in animals and humans for adaptation to the cold.

3.23 D

The basal metabolic rate is the metabolic rate of a subject determined at rest at a temperature within the thermoneutral zone 12–14 h after the last meal. It is slightly higher than when the subject is asleep. The basal metabolic rate is determined 12–14 h after the last meal because energy is required in absorption and digestion of food (the specific dynamic action). The basal metabolic rate is higher in men than in women, and higher in infants than in adults. It is reduced during starvation, due partially to a reduction in the level of circulating catecholamines and thyroid hormones. This explains why the rate of weight reduction for weight-watchers is fast initially but rapidly slows down.

3.24 B C

The respiratory quotient is the ratio in the steady state of the volume of carbon dioxide produced to the volume of oxygen consumed per unit time. It differs according to the type of foodstuff consumed. The respiratory quotient for carbohydrates, fat and protein is approximately 1, 0.70 and 0.82 respectively, although it may rise above 1 for anaerobic respiration. Indirect calorimetry is used to calculate the energy released on combustion of foodstuff by calculating the amount of carbon dioxide produced from the amount of oxygen consumed. Hence, the respiratory quotient of the foodstuff is important. In direct calorimetry, the energy released is measured directly using a bomb calorimeter. Knowledge of the respiratory quotient is not required.

4. General principles of pathological processes
Questions

4.1 Examples of external barriers against infection include:

- **A** Lysozyme in tears
- **B** Lactic acid in sebaceous secretions
- **C** Cilia on respiratory epithelial cells
- **D** Mucus secretion from epithelial cells
- **E** Acid in gastric secretions

4.2 The following are phagocytic cells:

- **A** Lymphocytes
- **B** Eosinophils
- **C** Polymorphonuclear neutrophils
- **D** Macrophages
- **E** Mast cells

4.3 The following statements about acquired immunological memory are true:

- **A** The secondary response is usually slower than the primary response
- **B** It extends to other unrelated antigens
- **C** The memory cells are macrophages
- **D** It forms the basis of vaccination
- **E** The effectiveness of acquired memory remains constant throughout life

4.4 The following protect mainly against extracellular microorganisms:

- **A** Antibodies
- **B** T-helper cells
- **C** Natural Killer (NK) cells
- **D** Complement-mediated system
- **E** Soluble cytokines

4.5 The following statements about immunoglobulin are true:

A It consists of two identical heavy and two identical light chains joined by disulphide links
B All chains on an immunoglobulin molecule are coded for by the same chromosome
C There are about 100 different immunoglobulin molecules in normal human serum
D The variable region is responsible for complement fixation
E The constant region forms the antigen binding site

4.6 The following statements about classes of immunoglobulins are true:

A IgG crosses the placenta and confers passive immunity to the fetus
B IgM is usually produced early in the immune response
C IgD is the most effective class of immunoglobulin for agglutinating bacteria
D IgA exists as a dimer on seromucous surfaces
E IgE is important in cell-mediated immunity

4.7 The following are possible mechanisms for tolerance of T-cells to self-antigens:

A Separation of self-antigen from lymphocytes
B Deletion of self-reactive T-cells in the thymus
C Clonal anergy of T-cells
D Production of antibodies against self-antigens
E Production of autoantibodies

4.8 The following types of hypersensitivity and examples are correctly matched:

A Type 1 hypersensitivity – allergen-induced asthma
B Type 2 hypersensitivity – granulomatous reaction to tuberculosis
C Type 3 hypersensitivity – glomerulonephritis associated with systemic lupus erythematosus
D Type 4 hypersensitivity – rhesus incompatibility resulting in haemolytic disease of the newborn
E Type 5 hypersensitivity – hyperthyroidism caused by thyroid-stimulating autoantibody in Graves' disease

4.9 The following may reduce the risk of graft rejection after transplantation:

A Cross-matching donor and recipient for ABO antigens
B Cross-matching donor and recipient for major histocompatibility complex antigens
C Use of antimitotic drugs (such as azathioprine) after transplantation
D Use of cyclosporin A after transplantation
E Transfusion of blood from the donor before transplantation

4.10 Hyperplasia significantly contributes to the following tissue responses:

- **A** Increase of breast tissue at puberty
- **B** Increase of muscle bulk with exercise
- **C** Enlargement of thyroid gland during pregnancy
- **D** Enlargement of uterus during pregnancy
- **E** Thickening of the left ventricular wall due to narrowing of the aortic valve

4.11 Dysplasia:

- **A** Is associated with an increase in mitotic figures
- **B** May be caused by chronic chemical injury
- **C** Is always irreversible
- **D** Is associated with a reduction in nuclear/cytoplasmic ratio
- **E** Is a pre-malignant condition

4.12 Mechanisms of cellular injury may be mediated by:

- **A** Osmotic pressure
- **B** Glucose deprivation
- **C** Damage to ion pumps
- **D** Interruption of protein synthesis
- **E** Free radicals

4.13 The following types of adult tissues heal by complete restitution:

- **A** The skin epidermis
- **B** Nerve cells
- **C** Intestinal epithelium
- **D** Striated muscles
- **E** The heart

4.14 The following tissues are particularly susceptible to damage by ionising radiation:

- **A** The liver
- **B** The bone marrow
- **C** The ovaries
- **D** The uterus
- **E** The intestinal epithelium

4.15 Necrosis:

- **A** Is the inevitable consequence of any cellular injury
- **B** May be caused by ischaemia
- **C** May be caused by mechanical trauma
- **D** Is often accompanied by inflammation
- **E** Is usually associated with cell shrinkage

4.16 The following statements about apoptosis are true:

- **A** It is usually triggered by cellular injury
- **B** It is associated with leakage of lytic lysosome enzymes
- **C** The dead cells are phagocytosed by macrophages
- **D** Increased apoptosis may result in neoplasia
- **E** Decreased apoptosis may result in tissue atrophy

4.17 The following types of necrosis and their causes are correctly paired:

- **A** Coagulative necrosis – myocardial infarction
- **B** Caseous necrosis – malignant hypertension
- **C** Fibrinoid necrosis – tuberculosis
- **D** Fat necrosis – acute pancreatitis
- **E** Gangrene – *Clostridium perfringens* infection

4.18 Predisposing factors for thrombosis in an artery include:

- **A** Laminar blood flow
- **B** Fibrin deposition on the vessel wall
- **C** Loss of endothelial cells
- **D** Increased blood cholesterol level
- **E** Decreased serum high-density lipoprotein level

4.19 The possible outcomes of thrombi include:

- **A** Dissolution
- **B** Embolism
- **C** Organisation
- **D** Apoptosis
- **E** Recanalisation

4.20 Consequences of systemic emboli include:

- **A** Pulmonary infarction
- **B** A cerebrovascular accident
- **C** Foot gangrene
- **D** Ischaemic bowel
- **E** Pulmonary hypertension

4.21 Possible sources of emboli include:

- **A** Tumour
- **B** Vegetations
- **C** Amniotic fluid
- **D** Gas
- **E** Fat

4.22 Causes of acute inflammation include:

- **A** Bacterial infection
- **B** Acid burn
- **C** Trauma
- **D** Tissue necrosis
- **E** Exotoxins

4.23 Characteristic physical features of acute inflammation include:

A Loss of function
B Pallor
C Coldness
D Swelling
E Pain

4.24 The following processes occur in the early stages of acute inflammation:

A A reduction in vascular permeability
B Persistent arteriolar constriction
C Formation of fluid transudate
D Accumulation of lymphocytes
E A reduction in blood viscosity

4.25 Chemical mediators of acute inflammation include:

A Histamine
B Prostaglandin
C C5a and C3a of the complement system
D Dopamine
E Bradykinin

4.26 In the presence of extensive necrosis, acute inflammation is particularly likely to result in:

A Suppuration
B Formation of granulation tissue
C Chronic inflammation
D Dystrophic calcification
E Fibrosis

4.27 Examples of chronic inflammation include:

A Anaphylactic reactions
B Crohn's disease
C Sarcoidosis
D Hashimoto's thyroiditis
E Pneumococcal pneumonia

4.28 In the presence of chronic inflammation, the following cells are often present in the cellular infiltrate:

A Neutrophils
B Multinucleate giant cells
C Lymphocytes
D Plasma cells
E Macrophages

4.29 The following tumour shapes are associated with malignancy:

- **A** Ulcerated
- **B** Papillary
- **C** Fungating
- **D** Sessile
- **E** Pedunculated

4.30 The following histological features are more characteristic of benign than malignant tumours:

- **A** Endophytic growth for tumours on mucosal surfaces
- **B** Irregular outlines
- **C** Presence of necrosis
- **D** Multiple nucleoli
- **E** Nuclear hyperchromaticism

4.31 Human tumours which may be caused by oncogenic viruses include:

- **A** Cervical carcinoma
- **B** Uterine carcinoma
- **C** Hepatocellular carcinoma
- **D** Nasopharyngeal carcinoma
- **E** Breast cancer

4.32 The following statements about oncogenes and oncoproteins are true:

- **A** Oncogenes may be absent in normal cells
- **B** A larger quantity of oncoproteins may be produced in malignant compared to normal cells
- **C** Oncoproteins produced from malignant cells may be different from those from normal cells
- **D** All oncoproteins stimulate DNA synthesis
- **E** Oncoproteins are important in regulating cellular growth and differentiation

4.33 Frequent sites for blood-borne metastases of common cancers include:

- **A** The spleen
- **B** The lungs
- **C** Bone
- **D** The liver
- **E** The heart

4. General principles of pathological processes
Answers

4.1 A B C D E

External barriers prevent microorganisms from gaining access to the body, and are first-line defences of infections. Two important external barriers are in the skin and in the respiratory epithelial cells. Fatty acids and lactic acid secreted by sebaceous and sweat glands in the skin inhibit bacterial growth. Cough and sneeze reflex, as well as mucus secretion and cilia of respiratory epithelium, form the external barriers against respiratory infection. Other external barriers include lyzozyme in tears, acid in gastric secretions, and commensal bacteria which secrete substances (e.g. lactic acid by vaginal commensals and colicins by gut commensals) preventing opportunistic infections.

4.2 C D

The main phagocytic cells are polymorphonuclear neurtrophils and macrophages. These cells kill microorganisms by engulfing and digesting them. Polymorphonuclear neutrophils are found mainly in the bloodstream and are particularly important in the defence against bacterial infections. Macrophages are larger cells, and are present throughout the connective tissue and around the basement membrane of small blood vessels. They are particularly effective in killing microbacteria, viruses and protozoa.

4.3 D

Exposure to an antigen for the first time induces immunological memory, so that responses to future exposure to the specific antigen are faster and greater. The memory cells are lymphocytes. This forms the basis of vaccination, and explains why some vaccines (e.g. tetanus toxoid) need to be given more than once. The effectiveness of acquired memory declines slowly throughout life, and is only sustained by recurrent stimulation. Hence, booster vaccines are often needed.

4.4 A D

Immunological mechanisms to protect against extracellular organisms include antibodies, the complement-mediated system and neutrophil polymorphs. Intracellular organisms live inside host cells and antibodies cannot reach them. Cell-mediated immunity systems such as T-cells, macrophages and NK cells help to protect against them. Some organisms avoid the killing mechanisms of macrophages and survive inside them. T-helper cells, if primed to the antigen, can recognise and bind to the antigen with class 2 major histocompatibility complex (MHC) molecules on the macrophage surface and produce soluble cytokines, which may trigger intracellular killing of the organisms.

4.5 A

Immunoglobulins consist of four peptides – two identical heavy chains and two identical light chains – joined by disulphide links. Each chain is coded for by a different chromosome. The variable regions form the antigen binding sites, and are specific to a particular antigen. There are over 100 million different immunoglobulin molecules in human serum. The constant region carries out secondary biological functions such as complement fixation or binding to macrophages.

4.6 A B D

Of the five classes of immunoglobulins, IgG are the most abundant, and are especially important in neutralising toxins and fixing complement via the classical pathway in the extracellular fluids. Since IgG molecules are small, they can cross the placenta and provide passive immunity to the fetus. IgM are usually produced early in the immune response. Since they exist as pentamers, they are extremely effective in agglutinating bacteria and mediating complement-dependent cytolysis. IgA usually occur as dimers in seromucous secretions, and are important in the defence of external body surfaces against infections, especially in the gastrointestinal tract. IgD are present largely on lymphocytes. They are susceptible to proteolytic degradation, have a short half-life, and are likely to be cell surface antigen receptors for the control of lymphocyte activation and suppression. IgE bind to mast cells and binding to antigens leads to degranulation of mast cells and release of mediators such as histamine. They are important in allergic reactions.

4.7 A B C

T-cell tolerance to self-antigens is essential to avoid self-reactivity. This may be achieved either by compartmentalisation of self-antigens so that they are not exposed to T-lymphocytes (e.g. lens proteins or sperms), lack of major histocompatibility antigens, deletion of self-reactive T-cells in the thymus (i.e. negative selection process) and clonal anergy (paralysed T-cells) due to lack of stimulatory signals from antigen-presenting cells. Inability of T-cells to achieve tolerance results in the production of autoantibodies and possibly tissue destruction.

4.8 A C E

Type 1 hypersensitivity (anaphylactic hypersensitivity) is due to antigen interacting with specific IgE antibody binding to the mast cells, causing release of mediators such as histamines and leukotrienes. Clinical effects occur shortly after exposure to the antigen. Clinical examples are anaphylactic reactions and atopic allergy. Type 2 hypersensitivity (antibody-dependent cytotoxic hypersensitivity) is due to killing of cells bearing IgG by polymorphs, macrophages or K cells through an extracellular antibody-dependent cell-mediated cytotoxicity mechanisms. Examples are haemolytic disease of the newborn through rhesus or ABO incompatibility. Type 3 hypersensitivity (complex-mediated hypersensitivity) is mainly due to activation of complement and attraction of polymorphonuclear cells due to antigen–antibody complexes. Examples are serum sickness following injection of large quantities of foreign proteins (e.g. antitetanus serum), and glomerulonephritis due to systemic lupus erythematosus. Type 4 hypersensitivity is due to interactions of antigens with primed lymphocytes, resulting in release of soluble cytokines which in turn activate macrophages inappropriately. Clinical effects may occur more than 24 h after exposure to the antigen. Examples are Mantoux reaction to tuberculin and granulomatous reaction to tuberculosis. Type 5 hypersensitivity is due to an antibody which reacts with a surface receptor that activates the cell. An example is thyroid-stimulating antibody stimulating the thyroid gland, causing hyperthyroidism.

4.9 A B C D

Graft rejection after transplantation is mediated by lymphocytes. The major histocompatibility complex (the HLA in humans) antigens are responsible for the most severe graft rejections. Measures that may reduce the risk of graft rejection include matching donor and recipient for ABO and HLA antigens, producing general immunosuppression by drugs (e.g. corticosteroids, antimitotic drugs and cyclosporin A, which targets T-cells specifically). In animals, antigen-specific tolerance may be induced via suppression by regulatory T-cell by injection of donor's bone marrow or dendritic cell precursors, which display little or no MHC antigens.

4.10 A C D

Growth is brought about by either hyperplasia or hypertrophy. Both may occur due to either physiological or pathological conditions. Hyperplasia is growth by an increase in the number of cells. Examples include breast enlargement during puberty and pregnancy, and an increase in the number of bone marrow cells in haemolytic anaemia or at high altitudes. Hypertrophy is growth by an increase in cell size without an increase in the number of cells. Examples are increase in muscle bulk in athletes, and thickening of the left ventricular wall due to narrowing of the aortic valve. Enlargement of the uterus during pregnancy or puberty is caused by a combination of hypertrophy and hyperplasia.

4.11 A B E

Dysplasia is a pre-malignant condition, and may be caused by chronic inflammation or chronic exposure to physical or chemical injuries. It is characterised by increased mitosis, abnormally large nuclei, and increased variations in the size and shape of cells and their nuclei. An important site for dysplasia is the squamous epithelium of the uterine cervix, and the long period of time between the development of dysplasia and neoplasia allows screening for cervical cancer by cervical smears.

4.12 A B C D E

Cellular injury may be mediated by a number of mechanisms. These include mechanical damage to cell membranes or interference with cell function, a deficiency of metabolities, damage to the energy generation process in the mitochondria, and interference to the DNA and protein synthesis process. Mechanical damage may be caused by sudden changes in the osmotic pressure of the intracellular and extracellular fluid. Damage to membrane integrity may be complement-mediated, perforin-mediated, or as a result of alteration to the membrane lipid or proteins, or blockage of the ion channels or ion pumps. Free radicals also damage cell membranes by damaging its fatty acids. Deprivation of essential metabolites such as vitamins, oxygen or glucose results in cellular damage.

4.13 A C

The cells in adult tissues can be classified into three types: labile cells, stable cells and permanent cells. Labile cells, such as the skin epidermis and intestinal epithelium, are constantly lost and replaced under physiological conditions. They heal by complete restitution. By contrast, permanent cells such as nerve cells, striated and cardiac muscle cells, and red blood cells, have no capacity to divide. They heal by forming fibrous tissues. Stable cells, such as the liver and the kidneys, divide at a slow rate physiologically. They have only a very limited capacity to regenerate.

4.14 B C E

All tissues are liable to damage by ionising radiation. However, tissues consisting of rapidly dividing cells are particularly susceptible. Hence the gonads, epidermis, intestinal epithelium and bone marrow are particularly susceptible to damage by ionising radiation.

4.15 B C D

Cellular injuries may result in healing, repair or cellular death. Necrosis is the death of tissues following cellular injury, and is always a pathological process. There are a large number of causes, which include ischaemia, trauma, infection and metabolic disturbances. Characteristically, there is a loss of cell membrane integrity, a leakage of lytic lyzosome enzymes, cell swelling and lysis. Inflammatory responses are usual, and the injured cells are often phagocytosed by neutrophils or macrophages. This contrasts with the process of apoptosis, another mechanism of cell death. Apoptosis is a physiological process to get rid of unwanted or abnormal cells, although it may also be triggered by pathological stimuli. It is initiated by energy-dependent fragmentation of DNA. It is associated with intact cell membrane, cell shrinkage and an absence of inflammatory response. The dead cells are phagocytosed by surrounding cells. Apoptosis is an important physiological process in controlling organ size and removing abnormal cells. Reduced apoptosis may result in inappropriate cell accumulation and neoplasia, whilst increased apoptosis may result in tissue atrophy.

4.16 –

See answer to question 4.15 above. Apoptosis can be a physiological process, is initiated by an energy-dependent fragmentation of DNA, and the dead cells are phagocytosed by surrounding cells. Increased apoptosis may result in tissue atrophy, and decreased apoptosis may result in neoplasia.

4.17 A D E

The type of necrosis is determined by the type of tissue involved and the cause of the cellular injury. Coagulative necrosis is the commonest. The outlines of the cells are preserved as the proteins coagulate. Necrosis following a myocardial infarction is a common example. Coagulative necrosis results from liquefaction of the tissues, and mainly occurs in the brain due to a lack of supporting structure. Fibrinoid necrosis is associated with a deposition of fibrin. It may occur in the smooth muscle walls of the arterioles in malignant hypertension. Fat necrosis results from the inflammatory response to a release of intracellular fat, and may occur after mechanical trauma to adipose tissues or following acute pancreatitis as a result of pancreatic lipase. Caseous necrosis describes a cheesy appearance with no recognisable structure. It commonly occurs in tuberculosis infection. Gangrene is necrosis of putrefaction of the tissues, and may be caused by clostridia. *Clostridium perfringens* is characteristically associated with gas gangrene.

4.18 B C D

Virchow first described the three general predisposing factors for thrombus formation: changes in the intimal surface of the vessel, changes in the pattern of blood flow and changes in blood constituents. In an artery, changes in the intimal surface of the vessel may include loss of endothelial cells, fibrin deposition and platelet clumping. Thrombus formation is more likely with turbulent than laminar blood flow. Changes in blood constituents may include increase in cholesterol and high-density lipoprotein levels and an increase in blood viscosity.

4.19 A B C E

Most thrombi are dissolved and cleared by the physiological fibrinolytic system. When this is unsuccessful, the thrombi are replaced by a scar and fibrous tissue in the process of organisation. Alternatively, the intimal cells within the thrombi may proliferate and new capillaries may grow into the thrombus to form a new channel. This is the process of recanalisation. Unfortunately, these protective mechanisms may fail. The thrombi may break off to form emboli, or the thrombi may cause ischaemia to vital organs, resulting in death.

4.20 B C D

Emboli in the pulmonary circulation (pulmonary emboli) usually arise from venous thrombi in the leg veins. Emboli in the systemic circulation (systemic thrombi) usually arise from the left side of the heart or major arteries. Pulmonary emboli may result in pulmonary hypertension or pulmonary infarction. Systemic emboli may be lodged in any systemic organs and cause ischaemic death (infarction). They may result in gangrene if lodged in the legs, a cerebrovascular accident (a stroke) if lodged in the brain, ischaemic bowel, or renal infarct it lodged in the kidneys.

4.21 A B C D E

Thrombi are by far the commonest source of emboli. Other sources of emboli include vegetations on heart valves, fat (e.g. release of fat into the bloodstream from the bone marrow following fracture of the long bones), gas (e.g. during surgical procedures such as laparoscopy), amniotic fluid (e.g. during delivery), tumour and foreign matter (e.g. contaminated intravenous fluid).

4.22 A B C D E

Acute inflammation describes the initial tissue reaction to injury, and may be caused by a variety of agents. Infection, especially bacterial and viral, is a common cause. Other causes include hypersensitivity reactions (other than type IV), physical injury (e.g. heat or cold injuries, direct trauma, ionising radiation), chemical injury (e.g. acids, alkalis, exo-or endodoxins) and tissue necrosis.

4.23 A D E

Celsus (first century AD) first described heat, redness, swelling and pain as the four characteristic features of acute inflammation. Loss of function is also characteristic.

4.24 –

In the early stages of acute inflammation, a brief and transient arteriolar constriction is followed by a longer period of arteriolar dilatation. This is accompanied by an increase in blood flow. This phase of hyperaemia is followed by a slowing of blood flow due to increased vascular permeability, resulting in a higher proportion of blood cells to plasma in the vessel. The increased vascular permeability causes proteins to escape into the extravascular space, forming a protein-rich fluid exudate. Another component of acute inflammation is the formation of cellular exudate with the accumulation of neutrophil polymorphs.

4.25 A B C E

Chemical mediators play an important role in initiating vasodilatation, increased vascular permeability, and attracting neutrophils to the site of tissue injury. Chemical mediators may be released from the cells (e.g. histamine, prostaglandin, leukotrienes, serotonin and cytokines) or through the major cascade systems in the plasma (complement, kinin, coagulation and fibrinolytic systems). C3a and C5a mediate vascular dilatation and emigration of neutrophils, and are the most important mediators from the complement systems. Bradykinin is an important mediator of pain. Hageman factor (coagulation factor XII) can activate the kinins, coagulation and fibrinolytic systems.

4.26 B E

Acute inflammation usually results in complete resolution. However, in the presence of extensive necrosis, healing by organisation is likely. Hence the formation of granulation tissue and fibrous (scar) tissues is likely. Suppuration is likely if there is excessive exudate. Dystrophic calcification usually results from long-standing abscesses.

4.27 B C D

Chronic inflammation may occur with its characteristic features from the beginning of the course (primary chronic inflammation), or it may progress from acute inflammation. General causes of primary chronic inflammation include failure to eliminate infective agent or foreign body by phagocytosis or intracellular killing (e.g. tuberculosis, leprosy, asbestosis), autoimmune diseases (e.g. Hashimoto's thyroiditis, rheumatoid arthritis), and chronic inflammatory bowel diseases. Anaphylactic reactions are caused by type 1 hypersensitivity reaction, and is an example of acute inflammation. Pneumococcal pneumonia is a bacterial infection, and is a classical example of acute inflammation.

4.28 B C D E

The presence of lymphocytes, plasma cells and macrophages is characteristic of chronic inflammation. Macrophages may form multinucleate giant cells in chronic inflammation. Neutrophils are characteristic of bacterial infection.

4.29 A C

Tumour shapes are often associated with the malignant potential of the tumour. Ulcerated, fungating and annular tumours are more likely to be malignant. Papillary, sessile and pedunculated tumours are more likely to be benign.

4.30 –

Benign tumours are associated with slow growth, infrequent mitotic figures, smooth borders and a histological appearance similar to that of normal tissues. The presence of ulceration, necrosis or invasion into underlying structures indicates possible malignancy. Multiple nucleoli reflect increased DNA synthesis, and nuclear hyperchromaticism reflects an excess of DNA. Both features are characteristic of malignancy. For tumours on the skin or mucosal surfaces, tumours which grow into the underlying structure (endophytic growth) are more likely to be malignant than tumours which grow away from the underlying structure (exophytic growth).

4.31 A C D

DNA viruses may cause cancers by incorporating their viral genome into the host cell DNA. For RNA viruses, the RNA viral genomes have to be transcribed into DNA by reverse transcriptase before incorporation. Viruses which are known to cause cancers include hepatitis B virus (which may cause hepatocellular carcinoma), Epstein–Barr virus (which may cause Burkitt's lymphoma or nasopharyngeal carcinoma) and human papillomavirus (which may cause cervical cancer or warts). Kaposi's sarcoma is associated with HIV infection, although the mechanism is not entirely clear.

4.32 B C E

Oncogenes are DNA sequences controlling tumour growth. They are present in both normal and tumour cells. Oncogenes exert their effect through their gene products, called oncoproteins. Oncoproteins are important in regulating cellular growth and differentiation. Different oncoproteins have different functions. They may be stimulators of DNA synthesis, growth factors, receptors for growth factors, or they may bind to GTP, which has an important role in intracellular signalling. Tumour cells may either produce excessive amounts of normal oncoproteins, or they may produce a abnormal (mutant) form of oncoproteins.

4.33 B C D

Lung, breast and bowel cancers are the most common. Organs which are perfused by blood drained from the tumours are liable to be sites of metastasis. Frequent sites for blood-borne metastases include bone, the liver, the lungs and the brain. It is unclear why tumours rarely metastasise to the spleen.

5. General principles of microbiology
Questions

5.1 The following increase the likelihood of a particular type of bacteria infecting the lungs:

A The ability of the bacteria to attach to a receptor molecule on the epithelial surface
B Prior infection by measles virus
C Suppression of the cough reflex
D Impairment of the ciliary function
E Increased activity of the alveolar macrophages

5.2 Viruses:

A May consist of both RNA and DNA
B May replicate without entering into host cells
C May incorporate their genome information into the host DNA
D Contain Golgi bodies
E Contain mitochondria

5.3 Compared to Gram-positive bacteria, Gram-negative bacteria:

A Have a thicker cell wall
B Contain more lipopolysaccharide
C Are more likely to cause fever and disseminated intravascular coagulation
D Are more susceptible to destruction by penicillin
E Possess an outer membrane

5.4 The following procedures are effective in sterilisation:

A Ultraviolet radiation
B Boiling in water
C Hydrogen peroxide vapour
D Washing in alcohol
E Dry heat

5.5 Important host antibacterial defences include:

A Neutrophils
B Activation of alternative complement pathway
C Non-killer cells
D Antibodies
E Interferon

5.6 Interferon

A Causes non-specific flu-like symptoms
B Enhances T-cell recognition of the infected cells
C Is a protein
D May be released from B-cells, activated T-cells or macrophages
E Increases the rate of protein synthesis

5.7 Important host antiviral defences include:

A Antibodies
B Neutrophils
C Macrophages
D T-cells
E Activation of the classical and alternative complement pathways

5.8 Bacteria may alter their genetic information by:

A Mutation
B Taking up soluble DNA fragments from other species across their cell wall
C Incorporation of human DNA from the host
D Being infected by bacteriophages
E Transfer of nucleic acid via plasmids

5.9 Gram-positive cocci include:

A *Streptococcus pneumoniae* (pneumococcus)
B *Neisseria meningitidis* (meningococcus)
C *Clostridium tetani*
D *Legionella pneumophila*
E *Staphylococcus aureus*

5.10 Acid-fast bacilli:

A Are easily seen after Gram staining
B Include *Mycobacterium tuberculosis*
C Include *Mycobacterium leprae*
D Include *Bordetella pertussis*
E Include *Mycoplasma pneumoniae*

5.11 Unlike *Staphylococcus epidermidis*, *Staphylococcus aureus*:

A Forms white colonies
B Is coagulase-positive
C Does not possess DNase
D Does not produce toxins
E Commonly causes abscesses

5.12 Clostridia:

A Are aerobic
B Usually produce endotoxins
C Seldom form spores
D May be found in soil
E Can be easily identified by Gram staining

5.13 The following types of clostridia and their associated clinical infection are correctly matched:

A *C. tetani* – flaccid paralysis
B *C. perfringens* – pseudomembranous colitis
C *C. botulinum* – gas gangrene
D *C. difficile* – food poisoning
E *C. perfringens* – spastic paralysis

5.14 Diphtheria:

A Is caused by a Gram-negative rod
B May be transmitted via droplets
C Can be prevented by a course of toxoid
D Can be treated by metronidazole
E May be associated with myocardial damage

5.15 *Listeria monocytogenes*:

A Is a Gram-negative bacillus
B May be transmitted via contaminated soft cheeses
C May cause abortion in pregnant mothers
D Particularly affects teenagers
E May cause meningitis in newborn babies

5.16 Meningococci:

A Belong to the genus *Neisseria*
B May be carried in the throat by healthy individuals
C Are often carried by farm animals
D May produce endotoxin
E May cause septicaemia without meningitis

5.17 *Haemophilus influenzae* type b:

A Is a Gram-positive bacillus
B Is capsulated
C Can be vaccinated against
D Infects teenagers more commonly than other age groups
E May cause epiglottitis

5.18 *Legionella pneumophila*:

A May cause atypical pneumonia
B Can be easily cultured
C Can only survive within human cells
D Is usually transmitted via droplets from person to person
E Can be effectively treated with erythromycin

5.19 *Bacteroides*:

A Are obligatory aerobic bacteria
B Should be vigorously treated if found in the stools
C May cause peritonitis
D Are Gram-positive bacilli
E Are most appropriately treated by penicillin

5.20 Bacteriophages:

A Are particular types of bacteria
B Allow accurate typing of some viruses
C May cause lysis of bacteria
D Have a very wide host range
E May be responsible for toxin production by some bacteria

5.21 Antibiotics which act by interfering with the cell walls of bacteria include:

A Penicillin
B Gentamicin
C Tetracycline
D Trimethoprim
E Cephalosporin

5.22 The following viruses and their associated diseases are correctly matched:

A Mumps virus – parotitis
B Respiratory syncytial virus – foot and mouth disease
C Coxsackie A virus – bronchiolitis
D Herpes simplex type 1 virus – shingles
E Herpes zoster virus – chickenpox

5.23 Diseases attributable to the Epstein–Barr virus include:

A Glandular fever
B Measles
C Burkitt's lymphoma
D Nasopharyngeal carcinoma
E Myeloma

5.24 The following viruses and their associated diseases are correctly matched:

A Parvoviruses – rubella
B Rotaviruses – pharyngitis
C Adenovirus – conjunctivitis
D Parainfluenza virus – gastroenteritis
E Small round virus – gastroenteritis

5.25 Human immunodeficiency virus (HIV):

A Contains DNA
B Contains reverse transcriptase
C May infect host T-helper cells (CD4 cells)
D Causes a reduction in host CD4 cells at late stages of the disease
E May be transmitted from mother to fetus during pregnancy

5.26 The following antiviral agents are effective against the corresponding viral infections:

A Amantadine – pneumonia due to cytomegalovirus
B Acyclovir – encephalitis due to herpes simplex
C Zidovudine – human immunodeficiency virus
D Interferon – influenza
E Ribavirin – bronchiolitis caused by respiratory syncytial virus

5.27 The following statements about plasmodia are true:

A They are fungi
B Sexual reproduction occurs in the human liver and red blood cells
C Asexual reproduction occurs in the intestines in mosquitoes
D They may cause anaemia in humans
E They characteristically cause continuous prolonged pyrexia

5.28 The following diagnostic tests are useful for the corresponding purposes:

A Ziehl – Neelsen's (ZN) stain – detection of mycobacteria
B Electron microscopy – identification of fungus
C Immunofluorescence – detection of influenza virus
D Specific IgM antibodies – rubella immune status
E Specific IgM antibodies – detection of acute infections

5.29 The following are examples of passive immunisation:

A Protection against hepatitis A after exposure by administration of pooled human immunoglobulin
B An administration of three doses of hepatitis B vaccine
C Oral polio vaccine
D Mumps, measles and rubella (MMR) vaccine
E Immunity from measles in the first six months of life via maternal antibodies

5.30 Examples of toxoids include:

A Pertussis vaccine
B Cholera vaccine
C Diphtheria vaccine
D Tetanus vaccine
E BCG (bacille Calmette–Guérin) vaccine

5.31 Unlike killed vaccines, live attenuated vaccines:

A Can be given during pregnancy
B Can be given to leukaemic patients
C Usually require three doses
D Rapidly decline in efficacy
E Are usually more expensive

5. General principles of microbiology
Answers

5.1 A B C D

Defences of the respiratory tract against infection include the cough reflex, ciliated cells (which drive foreign particles upwards from the lungs to the back of the throat), mucus-secreting globlet cells, and the alveolar macrophages if microorganisms succeed in reaching the alveoli. Mechanisms which increase the likelihood of bacterial infection of the lungs include depressed cough reflex (e.g. due to stroke or after anaesthesia), the ability of the bacteria to attach to the epithelial cells (e.g. *Bordetella pertussis*), impaired ciliary function (e.g. due to cigarette smoke or atmospheric pollution) or reduced macrophage activity (e.g. concurrent infection by respiratory viruses).

5.2 C

Viruses consist of a genome of either DNA or RNA (but not both) enclosed in a shell of protein and sometimes a lipid membrane. They do not contain protein or energy production machinery (e.g. Golgi bodies and mitochondria) and must depend on the biochemical mechanisms of the host cell for replication by incorporating their genome into the host DNA. (They are obligatory intracellular parasites.) Viruses are reproduced by assembling individual components produced by the host cell biochemical machinery rather than by binary fission.

5.3 B C E

Bacteria may be classified into Gram-positive and Gram-negative depending on their ability to retain Gram stain. An outer membrane is present in a Gram-negative bacterium but not in a Gram-positive bacterium. The cell walls are thinner for Gram-negative bacteria, but are more complicated structurally than Gram-positive bacteria. Gram-negative, but not Gram-positive bacteria, contain lipopolysaccharide (LPS), or endotoxin. Endotoxin activates the immune response and is liable to cause fever and disseminated intravascular coagulation.

5.4 **A C E**

Sterilisation is the total destruction of all microbes, including the more resistant bacteria spores and non-enveloped viruses. This may be achieved by physical means (e.g. dry heat or using steam under pressure, ultraviolet or ionisation radiation), gas vapour sterilisation (e.g. formaldehyde or hydrogen peroxide vapour) or by chemical means (e.g. hydrogen peroxide vapour). Only a maximum temperature of 100°C can be achieved by boiling in water, and is ineffective in destroying bacterial spores. Similarly, washing in alcohol is effective in destroying most, but not all, microbes. It is used as a disinfectant.

5.5 **A B D**

Important antibacterial defences against bacteria include neutrophils and macrophages which phagocytose bacteria by oxygen-dependent or oxygen-independent mechanisms, antibodies which bind to the surface structure of bacteria and facilitate opsonisation of bacteria, activation of the alternative complement pathway initially followed by the classical complement pathway by which chemotactic factors are produced, and enzymes such as lysozyme or lactoferrin. Non-killer cells and interferon are important for antiviral defences.

5.6 **A B C D**

Interferon is the body's first defence against viruses. Production is stimulated by double-stranded RNA. Interferon acts by activating the immune response by enhancing T-cell recognition of the infected cell, and inhibits viral replication by inhibiting protein synthesis in the cell. Interferon consists of a family of proteins produced by different cells (e.g. B-cells, macrophages, fibroblasts and activated T-cells) with different modes of action. It is partially responsible for non-specific flu-like symptoms in the patient.

5.7 **A C D**

Important host antiviral defences include interferon, antibodies (which may neutralise or opsonise viruses), T-cells (e.g. promote antibody and inflammatory responses and kill infected cell by CD8 cells), macrophages (which inactivate opsonised virus particles and present viral antigen to CD4 T-cells) and NK cells (which kill infected cells). Neutrophils and complements are important antibacterial but not antiviral defences.

5.8 **A B D E**

The ability of bacteria to change their genetic information is essential to their adaptation and survival in different environments, and determines their invasiveness and resistance to antibiotics. Bacteria may change their genetic information either through mutation or genetic transfer. Natural selection selects out mutants which have a selective advantage (e.g. increased invasiveness or resistance to certain antibiotics). Genetic transfer may be achieved either through taking up soluble DNA fragments from other species directly across their cell walls (i.e. transformation), through infection by viruses (i.e. bacteriophages) or by transfer of DNA via plasmids. Plasmids are extrachromosomal segments of DNA present in some bacteria which divide independent of the chromosome.

5.9 A E

- *Streptococcus pneumoniae* – Gram-positive coccus
- *Neisseria meningitidis* – Gram-negative coccus
- *Clostridium tetani* – Gram-positive bacillus
- *Legionella pneumophila* – Gram-negative bacillus
- *Staphylococcus aureus* – Gram-positive coccus

5.10 B C

Acid-fast bacilli include all bacteria of the genus *Mycobacterium*. They are characteristically difficult to Gram stain, and resist decolorisation by acid after staining with hot carbol fuchsin. They include *M. tuberculosis* (which causes tuberculosis), *M. leprae* (which causes leprosy) and atypical mycobacteria. Mycoplasmae are bacteria which do not form cell walls.

5.11 B E

S. aureus and *S. epidermidis* are the two main types of staphylococci, and they are different in several aspects. They can be distinguished in the laboratory in several ways. *S. aureus* forms golden-yellow colonies whilst *S. epidermidis* forms white colonies. *S. aureus* possesses the enzymes coagulase (which forms clots in plasma) and DNase, whilst *S. epidermidis* does not. Both exist as skin commensals. However, *S. aureus* may produce different types of toxins, and may cause boils, abscesses, osteomyelitis, septic arthritis and gastroenteritis. Infections by *S. epidermidis* are rarer, and this organisim may infect artificial heart valves and intravenous catheters.

5.12 D E

Clostridia are anaerobic spore-forming Gram-positive bacilli, and the spore can be seen at the one terminal of the bacillus. They can be easily identified by Gram staining as the bacteria take up the stain but the spores do not. They characteristically cause disease by the production of exotoxins.

5.13 –

- *C. tetani* – causes tetanus (spastic paralysis) by a powerful neurotoxin
- *C. perfringens* – may cause gas gangrene, food poisoning or cellulitis by production of α-toxins

- *C. botulinum* – causes botulism (flaccid paralysis) by a powerful neurotoxin
- *C. difficile* – causes pseudomembranous colitis especially in patients on broad-spectrum antibiotics, by the production of two toxins

5.14 B C E

Diphtheria is caused by the Gram-positive bacillus *Corynebacterium diphtheriae*. Symptoms are caused by an exotoxin which destroys epithelial cells. It causes infection in the upper respiratory tract, and affected patients may have pyrexia and acutely inflamed upper respiratory tract. In severe cases, the airway may be compromised, and the toxin may damage myocardial cells and neurones. A course of toxoid may prevent the disease. Patients with suspected diphtheria should be admitted to the intensive care unit and treated with both antibiotics (penicillin or erythromycin) and diphtheria antitoxin.

5.15 B C E

Listeria monocytogenes is a Gram-positive bacillus which occurs naturally in the environment and in the gastrointestinal tract of some animals. It is usually transmitted via contamination of food products, especially soft cheeses. It may cause meningitis and septicaemia in the newborns and in immunocompromised individuals, but very rarely affects previously healthy subjects. However, it may cause abortion and premature labour in pregnant mothers. Hence pregnant mothers are often advised to avoid soft cheese.

5.16 A B D E

The *Neisseria* genus includes two important bacteria: gonococci (which cause gonorrhoea) and meningococci (which cause meningococcal septicaemia and/or meningitis). Humans are the only natural host for meningococci, which may be carried in the upper respiratory tract by up to 20% of the population. It is unclear why some individuals who carry the organisms develop the disease whilst others do not. Meningococcal septicaemia without meningitis often has a worse prognosis than with meningitis. Endotoxins are important in the pathogenesis of some meningococci.

5.17 B C E

Haemophilus influenzae type b is a capsulated Gram-negative bacillus, and the capsule confers its invasive properties. It particularly infects young children under the age of five years. It may cause meningitis, epiglottitis, otitis media and chest infection. However, the incidence has been declining in recent years due to the introduction of a vaccine against type b polysaccharide capsule which is offered to all children in the United Kingdom.

5.18 A E

Legionella pneumophila has been known only since 1976 when an outbreak occurred amongst the delegates at a conference in Philadelphia. This is because it has very particular requirements for its culture. The organism is found in the environment, and especially in water systems, such as fountains, water storage tanks and showers. It usually spreads by water droplets from these water sources, but is seldom transmitted from person to person. Erythromycin is the most appropriate treatment.

5.19 C

Bacteroides is a genus of Gram-negative anaerobic bacilli which form a large proportion of the normal gut flora. *Bacteroides* may protect the gut against colonisation and infection by other more pathogenic bacteria. However, it may cause intra-abdominal sepsis, especially in bowel perforation and after bowel surgery. The most effective treatments are metronidazole and clindamycin.

5.20 C E

Bacteriophages are viruses which infect bacteria. Bacterial lysis may occur. Since the phages (viruses) have a very narrow host range, they allow accurate typing of some types of bacteria by observing which phages lyse the bacteria. The genome of the viruses may be incorporated into the bacteria. Some phages code for the production of toxin (e.g. diphtheria toxin) and cause the disease.

5.21 A E

The mechanisms of action of the antibiotics are as follows:

- Penicillin, cephalosporin – interfere with cell wall
- Aminoglycosides, tetracyclines, chloramphenicol – interfere with protein synthesis
- Sulphonamides and trimethoprim – interfere with DNA synthesis
- Rifampicin – interferes with RNA synthesis

5.22 A E

The correct answers are:

- Mumps virus – mumps (parotitis, meningitis, pancreatitis)
- Respiratory syncytial virus – bronchiolitis in infants
- Coxsackie A virus – hand, foot and mouth disease
- Herpes simplex type 1 virus – cold sores, keratoconjunctivitis
- Herpes zoster – chickenpox and shingles

5.23 A C D

The Epstein–Barr virus is a DNA virus. It commonly causes glandular fever with tonsillitis and lymphadenopathy. It may cause hepatitis and meningoencephalitis in severe cases. It is also implicated in Burkitt's lymphoma and nasopharyngeal carcinoma.

5.24 C E

The correct answers are:
- Parvoviruses – 'slapped cheek disease' in children, abortion in pregnant mothers
- Rotaviruses – gastroenteritis in children,
- Adenovirus – pharyngitis and conjunctivitis
- Parainfluenza virus – tracheitis, bronchiolitis, pneumonia
- Small round virus – gastroenteritis

5.25 B C D E

Human immunodeficiency virus (HIV) is a retrovirus. It contains single-stranded RNA. cDNA is synthesised from the RNA by viral reverse transcriptase. The virus infects mainly the T-helper cells (CD4 cells). The host CD4 cells decline at late stages of the disease, which is useful for monitoring the disease. The virus is transmitted mainly via sexual intercourse (homosexual or heterosexual) and blood products. However, the virus is transmitted from mother to fetus during pregnancy, and rarely through breast milk.

5.26 B C E

The correct answers are:
- Amantadine and rimantadine – influenza
- Acyclovir – herpes simplex and zoster infections
- Zidovudine – human immunodeficiency virus
- Interferon-α – chronic hepatitis B and C
- Ribavirin – bronchiolitis due to respiratory syncytial virus

5.27 D

Plasmodia are protozoa (a type of parasite). Plasmodia cause malaria in humans. The life cycle of plasmodia can be divided into two stages: sexual reproduction occurs in the gut of mosquitoes, and asexual reproduction occurs in the human liver and red blood cells. Patients with malaria characteristically have bouts of pyrexia and sweating. These are due to the release of toxins when schizonts burst and release the merozoites. Anaemia occurs due to haemolysis of red blood cells.

5.28 A C E

The correct answers are:
- ZN stain – detection of mycobacteria
- Electron microscopy – identification of viruses
- Immunofluorescence – detection of viruses and chlamydia
- Specific IgM antibodies – detection of recent infection
- Specific IgG antibodies – detection of past infection or immune status

5.29 A E

Passive immunisation is the protection against infection by antibodies. This usually gives rapid protection, but lasts for only about half a year. Examples are protection against infection in the first six months of life by the transfer of antibodies via the placenta, and post-exposure prophylaxis by the administration of antibodies.

5.30 C D

Pertussis and cholera vaccines are killed vaccines. BCG is a live attenuated vaccine. Diphtheria and tetanus vaccines are inactivated bacterial toxins (toxoids).

5.31 –

Unlike killed vaccines, live attenuated vaccines are live organisms whose virulence has been reduced. Since they replicate in the body in a similar manner to true infections, they are more effective, and usually only require one or two doses. Killed vaccines usually require several doses. Live attenuated vaccines are generally cheaper. However, mutation may occur in live attenuated vaccines and they may regain their virulence. Furthermore, they cannot be given to immunocompromised patients (as this may give rise to disease) or to pregnant mothers (as they may infect the fetus).

6. General principles of histology and embryology Questions

6.1 **The following statements about the epidermis of the skin are correct:**

A It is highly vascular
B The outer layer (stratum corneum) is keratinised
C The germinal layer (stratum germinativum) lies adjacent to the dermis
D Melanocytes are found in the germinal layer (stratum germinativum) of the epidermis
E Cells in the prickle cell layer (stratum spinosum) undergo continuous mitosis

6.2 **The following statements about the dermis of the skin are true:**

A It meets the epidermis at the dermal papillae
B It contains elastin
C The cells of the dermis consist mainly of fibroblasts
D It partly relies on the epidermis for metabolic support
E It provides non-specific defence against infection

6.3 **The following statements about arrector pili muscles are true:**

A Relaxation may cause hair erection
B Contraction may cause 'goose-flesh appearance'
C Contraction may result from an increase in environmental temperature
D Contraction may result from fear
E They are supplied by the parasympathetic nervous system

6.4 **The following changes occur in the skin when the body temperature increases:**

A The hairs become more erect
B The number of melanocytes decreases
C The secretion from sweat glands increases
D Blood flow to the skin decreases
E The secretion from sebaceous glands decreases

6.5 Epithelial basement membranes:

A Are made up of connective tissues
B Provide structural support to the epithelium
C May be breached by physiological epithelial growth
D Are richly vascularised
E May form a selective filter for the passage of substances from one body compartment to another

6.6 The epithelia at the following sites and the associated epithelial types are correctly matched:

A Distal convoluted renal tubule – simple squamous epithelium
B Capillary wall – simple cuboidal epithelium
C Gallbladder lining – simple columnar epithelium (unciliated)
D Bronchial lining – simple columnar ciliated epithelium
E Oviduct lining – pseudostratifed columnar ciliated epithelium

6.7 The following statements about transitional epithelium are true:

A It is a form of simple epithelium
B It can withstand a greater degree of stretch than stratified squamous epithelium
C The apparent number of cell layers decreases when stretched
D The lining of the bladder is an example
E The lining of the uterine cervix is an example

6.8 Intercellular adhering junctions:

A Bind the cells of the epithelium together
B Act as anchorage sites for the cytoskeleton of each cell
C Include desmosomes
D Include occluding junctions
E Contribute to the resistance of the epithelium to mechanical stress

6.9 Communicating junctions:

A Are also known as tight junctions
B Allow electrical impulses to pass directly from one cell to another
C Allow small positively charged ions to pass between epithelial cells
D Are important for transfer of chemical signalling agents
E Can be found in cardiac muscle

6.10 Unlike syneytiotrophoblasts, cytotrophoblasts in the second week of development:

A Constitute the outer layer of the trophoblast
B Are in direct contact with maternal sinusoids
C Are multinucleated
D Never contain mitotic figures
E Produce human chorionic gonadotrophin (hCG)

6.11 Structures developed from the ectoderm include:

A The aorta
B The optic nerve
C The peripheral nerves
D Muscle fibres
E The bladder

6.12 Structures developed from the endoderm include:

A The heart
B The lungs
C Bones
D The stomach
E The liver

6.13 A baby was born with gross structural defects of the heart, gut and brain. The gestational period when these defects are induced may be:

A Two weeks
B Four weeks
C Six weeks
D 16 weeks
E 32 weeks

6.14 The following agents are teratogenic:

A Chickenpox virus
B X-rays
C Lithium
D Alcohol
E Rubella virus

6.15 The following statements about fetal development between the third and ninth month of gestation are true.

A The chambers of the heart are formed during the fifth month
B The rate of increase in fetal length is faster between the sixth and ninth month than between the third and sixth month of gestation
C The rate of increase in fetal weight is faster between the sixth and ninth month than between the third and sixth month of gestation
D Between the sixth and ninth month of gestation, the rate of growth is faster for the fetal head than the body
E The sex of the fetus can be determined by external ultrasound by about 12 weeks

6.16 A pair of twins can be confidently diagnosed to be dizygotic if:

A There are two placentas
B There are two chorionic cavities
C There are two amniotic cavities
D They are of different sex
E One twin is larger than the other

6. General principles of histology and embryology Answers

6.1 B C D

The skin consists of the epidermis (superficial layer) and the dermis (the deeper layer). The epidermis has no blood supply. The cells in the outer layer (corneum) are keratinised, and are continuously shed. They are replaced by cells generated by mitosis in the innermost layer (stratum germinativum) of the epidermis, which lies adjacent to the dermis. Melanocytes, which produce the pigment melanin, are found in the stratum germinativum. The quantity of the pigment melanin determines the skin colour. Stratum germinativum is also known as stratum malpighii. The prickle cell layer (stratum spinosum) lies adjacent and superficial to the stratum germinativum, and is concerned with growth of the cells produced in the germinal layer.

6.2 A B C E

The dermis provides almost all the metabolic demands for the epidermis. It meets the epidermis at the dermal papillae, where the downward folds of epidermal ridges interdigitate with the upward projections of the dermis. This facilitates the adhesion between the epidermis and the dermis. There are two layers in the dermis: a superficial papillary dermis, and a deeper reticular layer. The papillary dermis consists mainly of collagen, and is highly vascular. The reticular layer consists of an interlacing arrangement of collagen fibre. Elastin is found in both layers, and accounts for the elastic property of the skin. The dermis provides non-specific defences against infection both as a physical barrier and via the tissue macrophages, white cells and mast cells.

6.3 B D

The arrector pili muscles originate from the sheath of hair follicles to the dermal papillae. The muscles are supplied by the sympathetic nervous system. Cold and fear cause contractions of the muscles, and results in 'goose-flesh' appearance of the skin as well as hair erection. Hair erection results in increased insulation due to more air being trapped by a thicker layer of hair. However, this effect is much less pronounced in humans than in other furry animals.

6.4 A C

When the temperature increases, heat loss from the skin increases via several mechanisms. Firstly, the sweat production increases, and heat loss via evaporation increases. Secondly, blood flow to the surface of the skin increases. Thirdly, the hairs become less erect, and a thinner layer of air is trapped. An increase in temperature per se does not alter the number of melanocytes, although increased exposure to sunlight may increase the melanocyte count. Sebaceous glands secrete sebum, an oily substance, onto the hair surface. The secretion of sebum varies little with temperature.

6.5 A B E

A basement membrane is a condensed layer of connective tissue at the boundary of epithelia or muscle fibres. The basement membrane is particularly important for the adhesion between cells and the support of epithelia as they are made up of closely packed cells. The basement membrane also acts as a control of epithelial growth, as physiological growth does not breach the basement membrane. Any growth of epithelial tissues which breaches the basement membrane is probably malignant. Basement membranes do not receive a blood supply, and they rely on nutrients diffused from the epithelium. In many tissues (e.g. the glomeruli), the basement membrane forms a highly selective filter for the passage of substances from one body compartment to another.

6.6 C

The correct matching is:

- Distal convoluted renal tubule – simple cuboidal epithelium
- Capillary wall – simple squamous epithelium
- Gallbladder lining – simple columnar epithelium (unciliated)
- Bronchial lining – pseudostratified columnar ciliated epithelium (i.e. one layer of cells, but nuclei are at different levels to give a false impression of more than one layer of cells)
- Oviduct lining – simple columnar ciliated epithelium

6.7 B C D

Transitional epithelium is a form of stratified epithelium, as not all the cells rest on the basement membrane. It is arranged so that the apparent number of cell layers decreases when stretched, although the total number of cells remains constant. Hence, it can withstand a greater degree of stretch. It is found almost exclusively in the urinary tract, where the epithelia also have to withstand the toxicity of urine. The lining of the uterine cervix consists of stratified squamous epithelium.

6.8 A B C E

There are three main types of intracellular junctions: occluding (or tight) junctions, adhering junctions, and communicating (or gap) junctions. The main function of occluding junctions is to prevent passage of substances from one side of the epithelium to the other. The main function of adhering junctions is to link the constituent cells of the epithelium together so that the whole epithelium functions together. This confers resistance to the epithelium against mechanical stress. This is achieved by the adhering junctions binding the constituent cells together, as well as acting as anchorage sites for the cytoskeleton of each cell. They may be of the continuous belt type or the spot type (desmosomes). Desmosomes are small circular patches circumferentially arranged around epithelial cells.

6.9 C D E

Communicating junctions are also known as gap (or nexus) junctions. They consist of numerous tiny pores allowing passage of substances from one cell to another. These substances include small ions or molecules important in the passage of chemical messengers and ions responsible for the depolarisation of cell membranes. Communicating junctions are also important for cell recognition. They also occur in cardiac and visceral muscle.

6.10 –

In the second week of development, the trophoblast differentiates into two layers: an outer layer (syncytiotrophoblast) and an inner layer (cytotrophoblast). The cells in the cytotrophoblast can undergo mitosis and divide, and migrate into the syncytiotrophoblast. The cells in the cytotrophoblast are mononucleated. The syncytiotrophoblast is in direct contact with maternal sinusoids. The cells in the syncytiotrophoblast have fused and lost their individual cell membranes. Hence, they are multinucleated. The two layers also have different functions. The syncytiotrophoblast produces (hCG) to maintain pregnancy. The cytotrophoblast later forms the primary villi.

6.11 B C

Major structures developed from the ectoderm include:
- The central nervous system
- The peripheral nervous system
- Pituitary glands
- Enamel of the teeth
- Sensory organs
- Epidermis

Major structures developed from the mesoderm include:
- The heart and blood vessels
- Muscle fibres
- Bone and cartilage
- Spleen
- Kidneys (not bladder)
- Gonads

6.12 B D E

See question 6.11 above. Structures developed from the endoderm include:

- Gastrointestinal tract and liver (being an outgrowth from the embryological gut)
- Respiratory tract
- Urinary bladder
- Parenchyma of thyroid and parathyroid glands, pancreas

6.13 B C

Gross structural defects of multiple major organs are most likely to be induced during the period of organogenesis, when the main organs in the body are formed. The period of organogenesis is about three to eight weeks of gestation.

6.14 A B C D E

Teratogenic agents include radiation, drugs, hormones and infections. Many drugs are potentially teratogenic, and include alcohol (which results in fetal alcohol syndrome), lithium (which causes specific heart abnormality) and thalidomide (which causes limb defects). Infections causing congenital malformations include the TORCHS infection (toxoplasmosis, rubella, cytomegalovirus, hepatitis B, syphilis), chickenpox virus (which causes limb and brain abnormalities) and HIV.

6.15 C E

Nearly all major organs have been formed by three months gestation, and maturation of these organs and growth occur between the third and ninth months of gestation. The rate of increase in fetal length is faster, but the rate of increase in fetal weight is slower between the third and sixth months than between the sixth and ninth of months of gestation. The rate of fetal head growth declines rapidly after the fifth month. The external genitalia are visible on ultrasound by 12 weeks.

6.16 D

Whether a pair of monozygotic twins share the same placenta, chorionic cavity or amniotic cavity depends on when splitting of the zygote occurred. If it occurred at the two-cell stage, each twin will have its own placenta, amniotic cavity and chorionic cavity. If splitting occurred at a late stage of development, there will be only one placenta, amniotic cavity and chorionic cavity. Monozygotic twins share exactly the same genes, and hence must be of the same sex. In about 10% of monozygotic twins who share the same chorionic cavity, the blood flow to the placenta is such that one twin receives much more blood than the other. This results in one twin being larger than the other.

7. General principles of genetics
Questions

7.1 The following statements about trinucleotide repeat amplification as a mechanism of length mutation are true:

A It is inherited as a chromosome disorder
B Longer trinucloeotide repeats are generally more unstable
C Longer trinucleotide repeats are associated with more severe disease
D Members of the same affected family usually have the same number of repeats
E Dystrophic myotonia results from trinucleotide repeat amplification

7.2 The following are appropriate uses of DNA analysis techniques:

A To exclude or identify suspects in rape offences
B To resolve paternity disputes
C To determine the carrier status of an asymptomatic female with a family history of a sex-linked recessive inherited disorder
D To identify meningococcal antigens in patients with suspected meningococcal disease
E To diagnose an autosomal recessive disease in an asymptomatic individual before symptoms develop

7.3 The following statements about meiosis are true:

A It occurs in all tissues
B It results in the formation of two diploid daughter cells
C It occurs throughout life in the adult male
D It occurs throughout life in the adult female
E Crossover allows wider variation of genetic make-up of the gametes

7.4 The following human karyotypes are examples of trisomy:

A 69, XXY
B 69, XXX
C 47, XX, +21
D 45, XO
E 46, XY

7.5 The following human karyotypes are examples of polyploidy:

A 47, XX, +18
B 46, XX
C 69, XYY
D 92, XXYY
E 47, XXY

7.6 The following statements about a mosaic are true:

A It arises from more than one zygote
B It almost always results in a non-viable fetus
C A gonadal mosaic trisomy has a high risk of producing abnormal children
D A gonadal mosaic trisomy can be easily diagnosed clinically
E It is caused by double fertilisation of the egg

7.7 Jane suffers from a disease. Two of her three sons and one out of her three daughters also have the disease. Three of her seven grandsons and two of her three granddaughters have the disease. Likely modes of inheritance for the disease include:

A Autosomal recessive
B Autosomal dominant
C Sex-linked recessive
D Sex-linked dominant
E Chromosomal disorder

7.8 Compared to autosomal recessive disorders, autosomal dominant disorders:

A Are less severe
B Tend to have a horizontal pedigree pattern
C Have a higher risk of transmission to offspring
D Are more likely to be associated with defective enzymes
E Affect more males than females

7.9 Non-penetrance:

A Usually occurs in autosomal recessive disorders
B May give rise to individuals with a normal genotype but an abnormal phenotype
C May give rise to individuals with an abnormal genotype but a normal phenotype
D Implies that a phenotypically normal individual will not pass on an abnormal autosomal dominant gene to the offspring
E Makes it easier to offer genetic counselling

7.10 The following statements about sex-linked recessive disorders are true:

A They affect males and females with equal frequency
B 50% of the sons of an affected father have the disease

C 50% of the daughters of an affected father have the disease
D 50% of the sons of a carrier mother have the disease
E 50% of the daughters of a carrier mother have the disease

7.11 Amongst the offspring of a normal father and a mother who is a homozygote for a sex-linked recessive disorder:

A 50% of all children have the disease
B 25% of all children have a normal genotype
C 50% of all daughters are carriers
D 50% of all daughters have the disease
E 50% of all sons have the disease

7.12 The following statements about X-linked dominant conditions are true:

A They are commoner than X-linked recessive conditions
B They affect more males than females
C They have a knight's move pedigree pattern
D Females are affected more severely than males
E The severity of the condition is uniform amongst all females

7.13 A newly discovered disease can be shown to be multifactorial in inheritance by:

A Analysis of the pedigree of a single family
B Chromosomal analysis
C Twin concordance study
D Family correlation study
E Biochemical analysis of gene products

7.14 The following relations have a quarter of their genes in common:

A Mother and daughter
B Grandfather and grandson
C Brother and sister
D Uncle and nephew
E First cousins

7.15 The following statements about trisomy 21 are true:

A In over 50% of affected individuals, one of the parents is a carrier of balanced translocation
B The incidence is lower amongst spontaneous abortus than live births
C The incidence is lower amongst stillbirths than live births
D Overall, the risk of recurrence in future pregnancy is 25%
E Carriers of a balanced translocation can usually be diagnosed by physical examination

7.16 The offspring of the following have a significantly increased risk of Down's syndrome compared with the general population:

A A mother with Turner's syndrome
B A 40-year-old mother
C A carrier of balanced translocation involving chromosomes 21 and 22
D Parents with consanguineous relationships
E A father with spina bifida

7.17 The following statements about fragile X syndrome are correct:

A It is the commonest inherited cause of mental handicap in males
B It generally affects males more severely than females
C Prenatal diagnosis is possible
D It results from deletion of part of an X chromosome
E All females of the same family who inherit the condition are affected equally

7.18 Methods of prenatal diagnosis include:

A Fetal DNA analysis
B Amniotic fluid biochemistry
C Ultrasound scan
D Fetal enzyme assay
E Fetal karyotyping

7.19 The prevalence of an autosomal recessive disorder in a population is one in 2500. Assuming heterozygotes do not have selective advantages over normal individuals:

A The carrier frequency is one in 1250
B The risk of disease to the offspring of two carrier parents is one in two
C The risk of disease to the offspring of a carrier parent and a parent randomly chosen from the general population is one in 100
D The risk of disease to the offspring of an affected parent and a parent randomly chosen from the general population is one in four
E The risk of disease to the offspring of two affected parents is one in two

7.20 The ability to roll the tongue is inherited as an autosomal dominant. Assuming that the gene is in genetic equilibrium in a population, and that the current proportion of those who cannot roll their tongue is q^2:

A The current proportion of those who can roll their tongue is $1 - q^2$
B The current proportion of heterozygotes is $q\,(1-q)$
C The current proportion of those who have two tongue-rolling genes is $(1-q)^2$
D The proportion of heterozygotes in the next generation is $2q\,(1-q)$
E The proportion of those who cannot roll their tongue in the next generation is $2q^2$

7. General principles of genetics
Answers

7.1 B C E

Trinucleotide repeat amplification is a type of length mutation. Repeats of trinucleotides normally occur between and within genes. However, if the number of repeats is longer than normal, it may become unstable. Single-gene disorders result if it is associated within a gene. The longer the trinucleotide repeat, the more severe the disease. Different members of an affected family may have different lengths of repeats, and this explains the different degree of severity of the disease within the family. Examples of diseases associated with trinucleotide repeat amplification include dystrophic myotonia and Huntington's chorea.

7.2 A B C D E

DNA analysis techniques have been used for a wide range of purposes such as genetic counselling and research, detection of crime and to resolve paternity disputes. DNA analysis may be used to detect the carrier status of a female in a family with a sex-linked recessive disorder (e.g. haemophilia). It may also be used to diagnose a recessive condition before symptoms develop (e.g. cystic fibrosis).

The two basic DNA analysis techniques are the Southern analysis and polymerase chain reaction (PCR) techniques. In Southern analysis, the DNA under analysis is cleaved into fragments using a specific restriction enzyme the fragments are then separated according to size by electrophoresis. These are transferred to a DNA binding site filter, and the fragments may be identified by autoradiography. PCR analysis is more sensitive and faster. Two oligonucleotide primers complementary to the target segment of DNA are used. The primers initiate repeated DNA replication to produce numerous copies of the target sequence. The amplified DNA fragment can then be cleaved, separated by electrophoresis and directly visualised under ultraviolet light.

7.3 C E

Meiosis is a type of cell division which occurs in the gonads and results in the formation of gametes. It starts with a diploid cell and results in the formation of two daughter haploid gametes. It occurs after puberty in males and continues throughout life, although the rate declines in old age. In females, the maximum number of germ cells is less than 200 000 at puberty, and only about 400 will ovulate (about once a month) in her lifetime. Meiosis ceases after the menopause. Crossover during meiosis is the exchange of genetic material between the two chromosomes. This adds considerably to the variation of the genetic make-up of the resulting gametes.

7.4 C

Trisomy is the presence of an extra copy of a chromosome. Since the normal number of chromosomes in humans is 46, trisomy results in a cell with 47 chromosomes. In 47, XX, +21, an extra number 21 chromosome is present, and is characteristic of Down's syndrome. 69, XXY and 69, XXX result from the presence of a complete extra set of chromosomes, and is known as triploidy. 46, XY is the karyotype of a normal male. 45, XO results from the loss of an X chromosome from the normal female, and is characteristic of Turner's syndrome.

7.5 C D

Polyploidy results from complete extra sets of chromosomes. 69, XYY is an example of triploidy with an extra set of chromosomes. The exact sex chromosome constitution depends on whether they are of maternal or paternal origin. 92, XXYY is an example of tetraploidy with two extra sets of chromosomes. 47, XX, +18 results from an extra number 18 chromosome, and is known as Edwards' syndrome. It is an example of trisomy. 47, XXY results from an extra X chromosome, and is known as Klinefelter's syndrome. 46, XX is the karyotype of a normal female.

7.6 C

A mosaic is an individual with two or more cell lines derived from a single zygote. It arises after fertilisation. A chimera is an individual with two cell lines derived from two separate zygotes, and could be caused by double fertilisation of the egg. A mosaic trisomy usually has a normal cell line and a trisomy cell line. The clinical features are usually less marked than a pure trisomy. A gonadal trisomy has trisomy cell lines confined to the gonads. Whilst they appear outwardly normal, they have a high risk of producing abnormal children.

7.7 B

In sex-linked recessive disorders, females who carry the affected gene in one of the chromosomes are carriers, and only males are affected. Sex-linked dominant disorders are rare. A father never transmits the disease to his sons. Autosomal recessive disorder is usually characterised by a horizontal pedigree pattern, and the risk of transmission to offspring is small. In autosomal dominant disorder, approximately half of the offspring are affected, and it occurs equally in each sex. Chromosomal disorder may occasionally transmit from parent to child (e.g. balanced translocation of trisomy). However, usually less than half of the children are affected.

7.8 **A C**

Autosomal dominant disorders are usually less severe than autosomal recessive disorders. Reproduction may not be possible in severe autosomal dominant disorders (e.g. Apert's syndrome), and new cases arise by mutation. Autosomal dominant disorders have a 50% risk of passing on to the offspring, and usually have a vertical pedigree pattern. It is usually associated with disorders of structural or receptor proteins, whereas autosomal recessive disorders are generally associated with defective enzymes. Both autosomal dominant and recessive disorders affect each sex equally.

7.9 **C**

Non-penetrance occurs in autosomal dominant disorders, when a person with the abnormal gene has the normal phenotype and appears clinically normal. Hence, a phenotypically normal but genetically affected individual has a 50% chance of transmitting the disease to his or her offspring. An example is the autosomal dominant inherited colonic cancer. Non-penetrance makes it difficult to offer genetic counselling, as affected individuals are difficult to distinguish from genetically normal individuals.

7.10 **D**

In sex-linked recessive disorders, a male with an abnormal gene in his X chromosome has the disease, where as a female with an abnormal gene in her X chromosome is a carrier. Hence, it occurs much more frequently in males than females. A father transmits his X chromosome to his daughters and his Y chromosome to his sons. Hence, none of his sons are affected, and all his daughters are carriers. A carrier mother has a 50% chance of transmitting her abnormal gene to both her sons and daughters. The sons with the abnormal gene will have the disease, whilst her daughters with the abnormal gene are carriers.

7.11 **A**

A mother who is a homozygote for a sex-linked recessive disorder has diseased genes on both her X chromosomes. Hence, one of the genes will be passed to all her children. All her daughters are carriers, and all her sons have the disease. Assuming half of her children are daughters, 50% of her children will have the disease.

7.12 **–**

X-linked dominant conditions are extremely rare. Examples are Xg blood groups and vitamin D-resistant rickets. A female has the disease if one or both of her X chromosomes contain the defective genes. Hence, the sex ratio is two females to one male. The pedigree pattern is vertical. It is similar to the autosomal dominant pattern except that there is no male-to-male transmission. Males are more severely affected than females. The severity of affected females is variable due to the process of inactivation of one of the X chromosomes in somatic cells in females (the process of lyonisation).

7.13 C D

Multifactorial disorders are determined by a number of genes at different loci as well as environmental factors. Each gene only has a small effect on the development of the disease. Hence, multifactorial disorders cannot be proved by analysis of the pedigree of a single family. Chromosomal analysis is also not helpful, as the genes involved are often unidentified. Twin concordance study compares the concordance rates between monozygotic and dizygotic twins in a large number of twins. Family correlation study compares the concordance amongst family members with the proportion of genes shared by them. Twin concordance and family correlation studies are the best tools to show multifactorial disorders.

7.14 B D

Monozygotic (identical) twins have 100% of their genes in common. First-degree relations (e.g. parents and child; siblings) have half of their genes in common. Second-degree relations (e.g. grandparent and grandchild; uncle/aunt and nephew/niece) have a quarter of their genes in common. Third-degree relations (e.g. first cousins) have an eighth of their genes in common.

7.15 –

About 95% of trisomy 21 cases result from non-disjunction at meiosis, most commonly at the first meiotic division. Both parents are normal in these cases. As chromosomal abnormalities often result in either spontaneous abortion or stillbirth, the incidence of all trisomies is higher amongst the spontaneous abortus than live births. For young parents who are not carriers of balanced translocations, the risk of recurrence is about 1%, although the risk is higher for older parents. Carriers of a balanced translocation are phenotypically normal, and cannot be diagnosed by physical examination. Chromosomal analysis is necessary.

7.16 B C

The incidence of Down's syndrome increases steeply with maternal age. The incidence is slightly higher in offspring of older fathers. A translocation refers to the transfer of chromosomal material between chromosomes. If the transfer results in no overall increase or reduction of chromosomal material, it is said to be a balanced translocation. The person appears normal. About 0.2% of the general population has balanced translocation. The offspring of carriers of a balanced translocation have a significantly increased risk of Down's syndrome. The risk depends on the type of balanced translocation. For example, the risk to the offspring of a parent with centric fusion of the chromosomes 13;14 is only 1%, whereas the corresponding risk for centric fusion 21;21 has a 100% risk.

7.17 A B C

Fragile X syndrome results from an unstable mutation of a trinucleotide CGG repeat in the X chromosome. In the pre-mutation condition, there are less than about 200 trinucleotide repeats. In the full mutation condition, there are over 200 repeats. Fragile X syndrome is the commonest inherited cause of mental handicap. The full mutation condition occurs in about one in every 1250 males, and the pre-mutation condition occurs in about one in 750 males. Males with the full mutation are mentally handicapped. Females with the full mutation may range from being normal to moderately mentally handicapped. This variability is partly due to lyonisation (inactivation of one X chromosome in the female), and partly due to different lengths mutation. Prenatal diagnosis is possible by DNA analysis of samples taken by chorionic villous biopsy.

7.18 A B C D E

Methods of prenatal diagnosis include fetal DNA analysis (e.g. for single-gene disorders such as cystic fibrosis), fetal karyotyping (e.g. for chromosomal disorders), fetal enzyme assay (e.g. for inborn errors of metabolism), amniotic fluid biochemistry (e.g. AFP level for increased risk of neural tube defect) and ultrasound scan (e.g. for structural abnormalities).

7.19 C

For autosomal disorders, the risk of the disease to the offspring from two carrier parents is one in four. If the carrier frequency is x, the expected prevalence of disease would be $1/4\ x^2$. Putting $1/4x^2 = 1/2500$ gives the carrier frequency of one in 25. The same answer can be obtained using the Hardy–Weinberg law.

The risk of disease to the offspring of a carrier parent and a parent from the general population would be $1/4 \times 1/25 = 1/100$. The risk of disease to the offspring of an affected parent and a parent from the general population is $1/2 \times 1/25 = 1/50$.

The risk of disease to the offspring of two affected parents is 100%.

7.20 A C D

If the proportion of those with homozygous recessive gene is q^2, the proportion of those who can roll their tongue is $1 - q^2$. According to the Hardy–Weinberg law, the proportion of those with the two dominant genes is p^2 (where $p = 1 - q$), and the proportion of heterozygotes is $2pq$. (NB: the total is $p^2 + 2pq + q^2 = 1$.) If the population is in genetic equilibrium, these proportions do not change in subsequent generations.

8. General principles of psychological and sociological processes
by Dr Susan Laidlaw
Questions

8.1 The Registrar General's classification of social classes:

- **A** Includes a category for unskilled non-manual workers
- **B** Is based on income or salary
- **C** Would place an unemployed man in social class V
- **D** Can classify retired men and women
- **E** Would place a single woman in the same class as her father

8.2 Social mobility:

- **A** Is an example of impression management
- **B** Can be influenced by luck
- **C** Is not influenced by marriage
- **D** Refers to the movement of people within a social stratification system
- **E** May be achieved through political means

8.3 The Black Report suggests the following explanations for the association between social class and health:

- **A** Social class may determine health because there may be differences in the health-related behaviour of people in different classes
- **B** The associations may be due to artefact
- **C** Health may determine social class because unhealthy people may move into lower social classes
- **D** There are differences in material circumstances between different social classes
- **E** People in higher social classes become ill more often

8.4 The National Health Service:

- **A** Employs more women than men
- **B** Was established in 1946, following the Beveridge Report
- **C** Is an example of a health insurance system of health care
- **D** Was reorganised in 1974, resulting in the development of the internal market
- **E** Is funded through taxation

8.5 The behavioural approach to health promotion:

- **A** Is concerned with the behaviour of the individual
- **B** Seeks to modify the socio-economic constraints on health
- **C** Cannot be applied to primary prevention
- **D** Can be used alongside a medical model
- **E** Is concerned with environmental determinants of ill health

8.6 Characteristics of a profession include:

- **A** A code of ethics
- **B** A monopoly
- **C** Merit awards
- **D** Autonomy
- **E** Specialised knowledge

8.7 According to Parson's model of the sick role:

- **A** It is a role given by doctors to the individual
- **B** The individual is exempted from responsibilities whilst sick
- **C** The individual has an obligation to want to get better
- **D** The sick role is permanent
- **E** The sick individual is not obliged to co-operate with medical interventions

8.8 Illness behaviour:

- **A** Is that demonstrated by a nurse towards a patient
- **B** May be influenced by the accessibility of resources
- **C** Can be influenced by the patient's family
- **D** Does not show any cultural variation
- **E** Can depend on the type of symptoms experienced

8.9 Communication techniques which may be used by a doctor to improve the patient's recall of a discussion include:

- **A** The use of short sentences
- **B** Giving non-specific advice (e.g. 'you should exercise more') rather than specific advice (e.g. 'you should exercise for 20 minutes three times a week')
- **C** Avoidance of the use of written material
- **D** The primacy effect
- **E** Asking the patient to repeat the information

8.10 According to Kubler-Ross, people who know they are dying:

- **A** Usually go through five stages
- **B** Initially become depressed
- **C** Sometimes try to bargain with medical staff in an attempt to postpone their death
- **D** Eventually reach a stage of acceptance
- **E** Become angry before going into denial

8.11 According to the World Health Organization:

A Disability is the 'loss of, or restriction in, functional ability or activity as a result of impairment'
B Health is 'simply the absence of disease'
C A disease always leads to impairment
D Handicap is the same as disability
E Impairment may be temporary

8.12 Consequences of deindividuation include:

A Increased ability to plan rationally as part of a team
B Possible increase in impulsive behaviour
C Tighter regulation of one's own behaviour
D Increased sensitivity to immediate cues
E Anonymity

8.13 Regarding Piaget's Stages of Cognitive Development:

A The formal operational stage precedes the concrete operational stage
B Conservation of weight occurs after conservation of number
C Object permanence is achieved during the sensorimotor stage
D A four-year-old child cannot classify objects according to several features
E Autonomy and doubt characterise the pre-operational stage

8.14 Attachment behaviour:

A Is not seen in animals
B Can be assessed using the Strange Situation
C Is the same as bonding
D Takes an average of six months to become fully established
E Has been observed in adults

8.15 Cognitive learning:

A Is an active form of learning
B Involves a reinforcer
C Involves cognitive maps
D May occur apparently spontaneously
E Includes insight and latent learning

8.16 The following are features of classical conditioning:

A An unconditioned stimulus
B Delayed conditioning
C Law of effect
D Generalisation
E Discrimination

8.17 Regarding operant conditioning:

A Extinction and partial recovery may be observed
B Trial and error learning is involved
C An electric shock may be used as a positive reinforcer

D Punishment is a negative reinforcer
E A variable interval schedule of reinforcement can be used to maintain a conditioned response

8.18 According to Erikson:

A There are eight stages of psychosocial development in children
B At each stage there is a developmental crisis which the individual has to negotiate
C The first stage deals with basic trust versus mistrust
D Ego identity does not occur until adolescence
E Authoritarian morality characterises the final childhood stage

8.19 Factors which influence childhood gender role development include:

A Observation of adults
B Television
C Influence of other children
D Stranger anxiety
E Children's stories

8.20 According to Freud's theory of personality development:

A Inadequate resolution of the Oedipal conflict can lead to difficulties relating to authority in adult life
B The phallic stage precedes the anal stage
C Children resolve the Oedipal conflict during the latency stage
D The anal stage follows the oral stage
E The phallic stage occurs sometime during the genital stage

8.21 People may overeat because:

A There is a breakdown in conscious restraints
B They are emotionally aroused
C They have heightened sensitivity to external cues
D When they were young, their mother interpreted all their distress signals, such as crying, as hunger
E They have difficulty in distinguishing hunger from other feelings

8.22 Memory can generally be improved by:

A Increasing the number of chunks in the memory span
B Increasing the amount of information in each chunk
C Recreating the situation in which the original learning took place
D Using the method of loci
E Semantic encoding

8.23 Regarding memory:

A Implicit memory refers to that which is concerned largely with the recall of facts
B A photographic memory is also known as a flashbulb memory
C The sensory memory holds information for longer than the short-term memory

D The primacy effect explains why it is easier to remember the first item on a list than one in the middle
E It is often necessary to rehearse information in order to retain it in the short-term memory for longer than a few seconds

8.24 The following theories and theoretical models are associated with motivation:

A James Lang theory
B Drive reduction theory
C Maslow's Hierarchy of Needs
D Psychoanalytic theory
E Social learning theory

8.25 Factors predicting a health behaviour include:

A Social norms
B Inherited tendency
C Previous learning
D Levels of anxiety and fear
E The beliefs of the health professionals

8.26 The chance of an individual adopting a health behaviour will be increased if they believe:

A Their health is determined by fate
B Their health is entirely controlled by doctors
C Health problems are infrequent
D They can do little themselves to affect their health
E The behaviour is associated with personal costs

8.27 According to the theory of reasoned action:

A Social values are unimportant in determining an individual's behaviour
B The behaviour contributes to the attitude of the individual
C The motivation to comply with the values of an individual's 'important others' contributes to the behaviour
D An individual's evaluation of the outcomes contributes to the behaviour
E An individual's behaviour contributes to his or her belief

8.28 Factors associated with high patient compliance include:

A Adequate explanation by the health professionals about the illness
B Good emotional support in the consultation from the health professionals
C A clear diagnosis communicated by the health professionals even if the condition is serious
D High patient recall of information given in the consultation
E Good understanding of the causality of the illness by the patient

8.29 The following measures are likely to improve patient compliance:

A Leave the important message towards the end of the consultation
B Make the message simple
C Provide written information to supplement oral information
D Give general rather than specific instructions
E Inform the patient that the treatment may or may not work

8.30 The following are examples of operant conditioning:

A In-patients with anorexia nervosa have their privileges given or withdrawn according to weight gain
B Children with bed-wetting are rewarded with 'stars' in the star chart if they are dry for two consecutive nights
C Individuals with spider phobia become extremely anxious when they visit a room where they had previously seen spiders
D A six-year-old boy follows his mother's example of placing rubbish in the waste basket
E A teenage girl starts smoking, following her parents' example

8.31 Placebo effects have been observed in the treatment of the following conditions:

A Skin rash
B Asthma
C Insomnia
D Allergies
E Numbness

8.32 The following theories may explain placebo effects on chronic pain:

A Classical conditioning
B Anxiety reduction
C Expectancy theory
D Cognitive dissonance theory
E Reduction in endorphin release

8.33 Factors which may affect the retrieval of memories from the long-term memory store include:

A The mood at the time of learning
B The circumstances in which information was originally learnt
C The current mood
D Whether the task involves recognition or recall
E The way the information was originally encoded

8. General principles of psychological and sociological processes Answers

8.1 **D**

The Registrar General's classification of social classes is widely used in medical research. It is based on occupation and consists of the following classes:

I Professional
II Intermediate
III Skilled, which is further divided into III N (skilled non-manual) and III M (skilled manual)
IV Semi-skilled manual
V Unskilled manual

Men are classified according to their occupation, married women according to their husband's occupation, single women according to their own occupation and the retired and unemployed according to their last significant period of employment.

8.2 **B D E**

Social mobility describes the movement of people within a social stratification system, which may be up or down. The following can influence social mobility: education, marriage, change in finances, and politics (which is particularly important for groups of people). *Impression management* is a term developed by Goffman to describe social mobility due to the personal attraction of an individual and use of status symbols.

8.3 **A B C D**

The Black Report (Report of the Department of Health's Research Working Group on Inequalities in Health, 1980) suggested four explanations for the differences in health between social classes. These were social selection (health determines social class through health-related social mobility); behavioural/cultural (social class determines health through differences in health-related behaviours); materialistic (social class determines health through material differences between classes) and artefact.

8.4 **A E**

The Beveridge Report was published in 1942 and the National Health Service was formed in 1948. It was reorganised in 1974, but the internal market was not developed until the reforms in the early 1990s which followed the publication of the White Paper *Working for Patients* in 1989.

8.5 A D

Approaches to health promotion include medical, behavioural and socio-environmental. The behavioural approach seeks to change the unhealthy behaviour of individuals by informing them of the risks of their behaviour, e.g. smoking. It does not take into account why people behave as they do. The socio-environmental approach is concerned with the social, economic and environmental influences on health, which may be outside the individual's control. These models can be used in conjunction with each other. Primary prevention aims to prevent the onset of a disease, secondary prevention to detect and treat the disease early and tertiary prevention to minimise disability and handicap due to the disease.

8.6 A B D E

Merit (distinction) awards may be given to hospital consultants in addition to their salary.

8.7 B C

According to Parson, *the sick role* is given by society to the individual and involves two privileges or rights and two obligations. The sick person is allowed to give up some of their usual responsibilities and activities and is regarded as being in need of help. However, they should want to get better and give up the sick role as quickly as possible and they should obtain the appropriate help.

8.8 B C E

Illness behaviour describes how people behave when they are unwell and is largely concerned with consulting behaviour. There are various influences on consulting behaviour, many of which are related to external factors, personal beliefs and the nature of any symptoms rather than the illness itself. There are cultural differences.

8.9 A D E

Other techniques include emphasising important information and categorising information. Specific information is more helpful than non-specific and written materials are useful. See also questions 8.28 and 8.29.

8.10 A C D

The stages are (in order) denial and isolation, anger, bargaining, depression and acceptance.

8.11 A E

WHO defined impairment, disability and handicap. *Impairment* is 'a disturbance of the normal structure or functioning of the body, which

may be temporary or permanent'. *Handicap* is 'a disadvantage for a given individual resulting from an impairment or a disability that limits or prevents his or her fulfilment of a role that would be expected for a group of which that individual is a member'.
WHO produced a formal definition of health in 1946: 'Health is a state of complete physical, psychological and social well-being and not simply the absence of disease or infirmity.'

8.12 B D

Deindividuation is a psychological state sometimes experienced when an individual loses his or her personal identity and become anonymous within a group. The consequences of this are decreased ability to make rational plans: a lack of restraint against impulsive behaviour and ability to monitor one's own behaviour; less concern about what others might think; heightened sensitivity to immediate cues.

8.13 B C D

Piaget's four stages are the *sensorimotor stage* (0–2 years), the *pre-operational stage* (2–7), *the concrete operational stage* (7–11 or 12) and *the formal operational stage* (11+ or 12+). Object permanence is achieved in the sensorimotor stage, which is also associated with circular reactions. The next stage is associated with egocentrism, animism and precausal reasoning. An understanding of the laws of conservation is normally achieved during the concrete operational stage (number, volume, then weight). Autonomy and doubt are terms used by Erikson in his classification of psychosocial development.

8.14 B D E

Attachment describes the tendency for human infants and young mammals to seek closeness to other individuals (usually the mother or caregiver) with whom they have an emotional tie, especially in a fear-inducing situation. Bonding takes place in the opposite direction, between the mother and child. The security of a child's attachment can be assessed in the Strange Situation (Ainsworth) and will influence later adult behaviour. Bowlby is associated with attachment theory.

8.15 A C D E

Cognitive learning involves forming cognitive maps which allow mental images to be formed.

8.16 A B D E

The law of effect was described by Thondike on the basis of operant conditioning. See also 8.30.

8.17 A B E

An electric shock is an example of a negative reinforcer because it causes the subject to perform an action or behaviour in order to avoid the electric shock (aversive stimulus). See also 8.30.

8.18 B C D

Erikson described four stages occurring up to the age of 12 and a further four throughout later life. The final crisis of the childhood stage is described as industry versus inferiority.

8.19 A B C E

8.20 A D

According to Freud the stages of personality development in children are the oral stage, the anal stage, the phallic stage, a latency period, then the genital stage during adolescence. If a child has problems at a particular stage, this may halt development and lead to a particular personality type in adulthood. The Oedipal conflict is described in a boy as sexual feeling towards his mother, followed by a perception that his father is a rival for his mother's affection. He then develops a fear that his father will retaliate by castrating him (castration anxiety). The only way the boy can cope with this is to identify with his father and internalise an idealised perception of his father.

8.21 A B C D E

8.22 B C D E

The number of items which can be held in the memory span is usually 7 ± 2. It is difficult to increase this figure, but it is possible to split up a lot of information into a small number of chunks of information. The amount of information in each chunk can then be increased. See also question 8.33.

8.23 D E

Implicit memory is concerned with remembering skills; explicit memory is concerned with facts and recognition. A flashbulb memory is a vivid memory of the circumstances when someone learnt of a particularly emotionally charged, significant event. The sensory memory only holds information for a very short time: less than a second.

8.24 B C D E

James Lang theory is concerned with emotion.

8.25 A B C D E

A health behaviour is a behaviour aimed at preventing disease (e.g. refraining from smoking, eating a healthy diet), whereas an illness behaviour is a behaviour aimed at curing or alleviation of an illness (e.g. seeking treatment from a doctor). It has been estimated that more than half of all deaths are attributable to behaviour. Factors which predict health behaviour are complex, and include genetic factors, previous learning, social factors (e.g. social norms and modelling others' behaviour), level of anxiety and fear, symptoms perceived by the patient, health beliefs of the patients and the professionals.

8.26 –

According to the attribution theory, people are more likely to attribute an action to a cause rather than to a consequence if it has high distinctiveness (i.e. it is specific to that particular action), high consensus (i.e. everyone believes it), high consistency over time (i.e. the same action at another time will also be regarded as the cause), and high consistency over modality (i.e. that the same action in another situation will also be regarded as the cause). This is incorporated into the health locus of control theory. People are more likely to adopt health behaviour if they regard their health as controllable by themselves and not by others. According to the health belief model, the chance of adopting health behaviour increases if people believe that the behaviour will bring benefits, the personal costs of carrying out the behaviour are not excessive, and if they are exposed to either internal or external cues for action.

8.27 **C D**

The theory of reasoned action is concerned with the relationship between attitude and behaviour. The behaviour of people is determined by their attitude towards the behaviour (e.g. their beliefs and evaluations about the outcome), and their beliefs concerning the social norm (e.g. their beliefs regarding the attitude of their 'important others' to the behaviour and their motivation to comply with their beliefs). This model therefore incorporates the individual's belief about the social values.

8.28 **A B C D E**

Factors associated with high patient compliance include high patient satisfaction, good patient understanding and high patient recall of information given at the consultation. Patient satisfaction is generally improved if there is adequate emotional support and explanation by the health professionals, and if the patient perceives the health professionals' behaviour as appropriate (e.g. in prescribing and referral).

8.29 **B C**

In order to improve patients' understanding and recall of information, the information should be simple and specific to the patient. The first message is often remembered best (i.e. the primacy effect). Repeating the information and supplementing oral information with written information are effective. Compliance is improved if the health professional is perceived to be enthusiastic and confident about the treatment given.

8.30 A B

Classical conditioning is an example of associative learning. Initially an unconditioned stimulus (e.g. the sight of food) leads to an unconditioned response (e.g. a dog salivating). If the unconditioned stimulus is paired with a second stimulus (e.g. a bell), then eventually the response can be elicited by the second stimulus (the bell) alone, which is then know as the conditioned stimulus. Salivation on hearing a bell has become a conditioned response. In operant conditioning, the chance of a conditioned response (e.g. a guinea-pig pressing a button) is increased if positive reinforcement (e.g. food) is given after a conditioned response, or if negative reinforcement (e.g. electric shock, withdrawal of food) is given for non-performance of the conditioned response. Examples of in-patient treatment of anorexia nervosa patients include giving privileges for weight gain, and rewarding a child who wets the bed with stars for star charts for having been dry for two consecutive nights. Behaviours learnt by observing significant others are examples of social modelling.

8.31 A B C D E

Placebo effects have been observed in the treatment of a wide variety of conditions. Placebo effects in the treatment of chronic pain have been observed most frequently. Other conditions include insomnia, allergy, other skin rashes, depression, numbness and weakness.

8.32 A B C D

There are many plausible physiological and psychological explanations for placebo effects. Physiologically, placebos have been shown to release endorphins, which reduce the pain level. According to classical conditioning theory, doctors or hospitals (an unconditioned stimulus) may be paired with reduction of chronic pain (an unconditioned response). Placebos have also been shown to reduce anxiety, and this may reduce the level of perceived pain. In the expectancy theory, patients expect to experience less pain after taking medication because of past experience. As most illnesses go through periods of change, they may attribute periods of less pain to the effects of the placebo. The cognitive dissonance theory states that if an individual holds two or more beliefs or attitudes which are conflicting or inconsistent (or behaves in a way that is inconsistent with cognitions) then cognitive dissonance (discomfort) will occur. In order to reduce this discomfort, the individual will subconsciously change the cognitions or behaviour to make them consistent with each other. When a patient takes medication they invest time and money and experience inconvenience, if they perceive no benefit from the medication they will experience a high level of dissonance or discomfort. The placebo effect can be explained by the patient subconsciouly altering perceptions to believe that the medication has worked and thus reduce dissonance.

8.33 A B C D E

It is thought that there are three memory stores: the working memory, the short-term, and the long-term memory stores. Information from the working memory is transferred to the short-term memory if sufficient attention is paid to it. Short-term memory lasts for less than half a minute if the information is not continuously rehearsed. If it is rehearsed, it may be transferred to the long-term memory stores. This has a much larger capacity than short-term memory, and loss of information from this stores is much slower. However, not all information from the long-term store can be retrieved. There are many factors which affect the ease of retrieval. The way the information was originally encoded is important. It has been found that organising information in a meaningful way facilitates retrieval. The circumstances in which information was originally learnt are important, and retrieval may be facilitated if the circumstances under which the information was first acquired are similar to when the information is retrieved. Hence, a patient may recall information given by a health care professional better in the clinic than in a pub. Similarly, retrieval may be facilitated if the mood at the time of retrieval is similar to the mood when the information was first learnt. Retrieval by recognition (e.g. if a choice is given) is easier than retrieval by recall. Hence, the same information may be retrieved by a multiple-choice question but not by an essay question.

9. General principles of public health and statistics
Questions

Public health

9.1 Applying the concept of triangle of causation of diseases (i.e. agent, host and environment) to explain the probability of catching influenza, examples of host factors include:

- **A** The emergence of a new type of Asian influenza through antigenic shift
- **B** Old age
- **C** Previous lung diseases
- **D** Overcrowded living conditions
- **E** Living in a nursing home with other infected residents

9.2 According to the 'iceberg concept of health care':

- **A** A proportion of patients' requests for consultation from health professionals are unnecessary
- **B** Some ill people do not seek help from health professionals
- **C** Some ill people who seek help nevertheless do not manage to see the health professionals
- **D** Some medical interventions suggested by the health professionals are actually unnecessary
- **E** Some people deemed to require health care are still waiting for it

9.3 A large number of people within a town develop a mysterious diarrhoeal illness over a seven-day period, which was suspected to be caused by contamination of the water supplied by a reservoir. Of 100 000 people who consume water supplied by the reservoir concerned, 80 people developed diarrhoea. Of 500 000 people who consume water not supplied by other sources, 100 people developed diarrhoea. Which of the following statements are true?

- **A** The contamination of the reservoir is not a cause of the disease as there are people who develop the disease without consuming water from the reservoir
- **B** The contamination of the reservoir is not a cause of the disease as there are people who consume water from the reservoir without developing the disease
- **C** Since there were more people amongst those who fell ill who did not consume water from the reservoir than those who did, it is safer to consume water from the reservoir
- **D** The risk amongst those who consume water from the reservoir for developing diarrhoeal illness is four times that of those who consume water from other sources
- **E** The data proves conclusively that contamination of the reservoir causes the diarrhoeal illness

9.4 The population of a town was 5 million. On 1 January 1997, 50 000 people were hepatitis B carriers, and none of the population were immunised. During the period 1 January 1997 to 1 January 1999, 500 of these 50 000 hepatitis B carriers died due to the disease, and none lost their carrier status. On 1 January 1999, the population was still 5 million, and the number of hepatitis B carriers was 54 500. There was no immigration into or emigration out of the town. Which of the following statements are true?

- **A** The prevalence of hepatitis B carriers on 1 January 1997 was 1%
- **B** The prevalence of hepatitis B carriers on 1 January 1999 was 2%
- **C** The incidence rate for becoming a hepatitis B carrier was about 500 per million population per year
- **D** The risk of developing hepatitis B carrier state was about 0.2% between 1997 and 1999
- **E** The crude mortality rate for hepatitis B carriers between 1997 and 1999 was about 1%

9.5 In a nursery with 200 pre-school children, 160 children had been previously immunised and were proven serologically to be immune from measles on 1 April 1998. An outbreak of measles occurred in the nursery between 1 April and 15 April 1998, during which 20 children caught measles, two of whom died. There were no further cases of measles by 1 October 1998:

- **A** The prevalence of measles on 31 March 1998 was 80%

- **B** The incidence of measles during the period 1 April 1998 to 1 October 1998 was 1000 per 1000 children-years
- **C** The risk of contracting measles from 1 April to 1 October 1998 was 50%
- **D** The crude mortality rate for measles from 1 April to 1 October 1998 was about 1%
- **E** The case mortality rate for measles from 1 April to 1 October 1998 was 10%

9.6 Factors which increase the prevalence of a disease within a population include:

- **A** Increase in the incidence of the disease
- **B** Improved curative treatment for the disease
- **C** Increased immigration of healthy individuals into the population
- **D** Increased immigration of diseased individuals into the population
- **E** Increased case mortality rate from the disease

9.7 The following features may explain why a disease has a low prevalence and a high incidence:

- **A** A poor recovery rate from the disease
- **B** A rare disease
- **C** Improved primary preventive measures (e.g. vaccines)
- **D** Rapid transmission of disease from one person to another
- **E** A high mortality rate from the disease

9.8 Fifty children within a health district were noted to have developed leukaemia within the last year:

- **A** A study of the characteristics of these 50 children from their medical records forms a case series
- **B** If the outcomes of these 50 children are followed up for the next three years, it may form a cross-sectional study
- **C** If we select another 100 healthy children in the health district carefully matched to the 50 leukaemic children in age, sex and social class, and compare their exposure to irradiation with the 50 leukaemic children, it forms a case – control study
- **D** If we conduct a survey amongst a randomly selected sample of children in the health district on their dietary habit within the previous week, it forms a cohort study
- **E** If we conduct two surveys amongst two different samples of randomly selected children two years apart, this forms a cohort study

9.9 The incidence of a disease can be deduced from the following types of studies:

- **A** Case series
- **B** Case – control study
- **C** Cohort study
- **D** Cross-sectional study
- **E** Repeated cross-sectional study

9.10 10 000 subjects were involved in a randomised controlled trial to investigate the effect of a drug in the prevention of hypertension. 5000 patients were allocated to each of the treatment and control group. 250 patients in the treatment group and 500 patients in the control group develop hypertension within three years:

A The absolute risk of developing hypertension amongst the treatment group in three years is 2.5%
B The absolute risk of developing hypertension amongst the control group in three years is 10%
C The relative risk of hypertension amongst treatment group is 0.5 compared to controls
D The attributable risk of developing hypertension due to drug X is –5%
E The result of the trial suggests that drug X is effective in preventing hypertension

9.11 A case – control study within a health district found that people working in factories manufacturing certain chemicals have a higher rate of respiratory diseases. The controls were taken from a random sample from the electoral roll within the same geographical area. Data was collected by postal questionnaires, and the response rate was 48% from the subjects and 52% from the controls:

A The study proves that the chemicals caused respiratory diseases
B As long as the numbers of subjects and controls are sufficiently large for statistical analysis to be applied, the relatively low response rates do not affect the validity of the results
C Sex may be a confounding variable
C Smoking may be a confounding variable
D Exposure to the relevant chemicals may be a confounding variable

9.12 A study found that people who had consumed a substance X in their diet were more likely to develop a neurological disease than those who had not. The aetiology of the neurological disease was not clear. The following evidence supports the hypothesis that X caused the neurological disease:

A People who had consumed higher quantities of X had a higher risk of developing the disease
B Similar results were obtained in studies performed in other countries
C It was found that many people started to consume the substance X after they developed the disease
D Substance X was found to inhibit protein synthesis in neurones in vitro
E The probability of recovery was higher after removal of substance X from the diet

9.13 The following are criteria for a good screening programme:

- **A** The disease is an important health problem
- **B** The symptoms appear at a very early stage of the disease
- **C** There is no effective treatment for the condition
- **D** The screening test is simple and acceptable to patients
- **E** The screening programme shows good value for money

9.14 1000 subjects were screened for a certain disease. There were 240 true positives, 630 true negatives, and 60 false negatives. The following values (correct to the nearest per cent) are true:

- **A** The prevalence was 30%
- **B** The sensitivity was 90%
- **C** The specificity was 80%
- **D** The positive predictive value (PPV) was 77%
- **E** The negative predictive value (NPV) was 91%

9.15 1000 subjects were screened for a certain disease. The prevalence of the disease was 10%; the sensitivity and the specificity of the test were 80% and 70% respectively. The following statements are true:

- **A** 20 subjects had a false negative test
- **B** 270 subjects had a false positive test
- **C** 350 out of the 1000 tests were positive
- **D** The PPV was 23% (to the nearest per cent)
- **E** The NPV was 70% (to the nearest per cent)

9.16 A metabolic disease is much more prevalent in country A than in country B. When used in country B, a screening test for the disease had a sensitivity of 80%, a specificity of 90%, a positive predictive value of 8% and a negative predictive value of 99.8%. If the test is used in country A:

- **A** The sensitivity is over 80%
- **B** The specificity is 90%
- **C** The PPV is below 8%
- **D** The NPV is below 99.8%
- **E** It is likely to be less cost-effective than in country B

9.17 Implementation of population screening tests is advisable for the following diseases in developed countries:

- **A** Prostate cancer
- **B** Neonatal hearing test
- **C** Breast cancer
- **D** Ovarian cancer
- **E** Congenital hypothyroidism

9.18 Advantages of population screening strategy over high-risk screening strategy include:

A Lower cost per case detected
B Higher overall benefit to the population
C Lower overall cost
D Increased sensitivity of the screening test
E Higher motivation from those screened

9.19 Examples of primary prevention include:

A Screening for phenylketonuria using Guthrie's test
B Smoking cessation to prevent carcinoma of the lung
C Fluoridation of water to prevent dental decay
D Administering regular inhaled steroid to patients with asthma
E Amniocentesis for older pregnant women to detect fetus with Down's syndrome

9.20 According to one model of health promotion, health promotion includes health education, prevention and health protection. Examples of health protection include:

A Prosecuting shopkeepers who sell cigarettes to children
B Informing young people in secondary education about the adverse health effects of illicit drugs
C Maintaining high quality of drinking water provided by private water companies through regulations
D Increasing the taxation on cigarettes
E Setting up a Food Standards Agency with legal power to enforce good quality of food hygiene amongst food retailers

9.21 In which of the following countries is the percentage of health care costs funded direct by central government higher than in the United Kingdom?

A Japan
B Germany
C Russia
D China
E United States of America

9.22 Rationing of health care for the population can be avoided altogether if the following health care systems are adopted:

A A government-funded national health system
B An internal market system with purchaser – provider split
C A private fee-paying system
D An employer insurance system
E A mixture of private fee-paying and government-funded national health system

9.23 Outcome measures of health care include:

A The number of in-patient beds per million population
B The number of dermatological out-patient consultations per million population per year
C The increase in physical independence after a hip replacement operation
D Improvement in visual acuity after cataract extraction
E The number of surgical consultants per million population

9.24 Quality-adjusted life years (QALY):

A Can be used as a measure of outcome
B Can be used as a measure of cost
C Is easier to measure than the length of life gained
D Is a completely objective measurement
E Can be negative

9.25 Drugs A and B are both used for treating a particular skin infection. After one standard application, drug A eradicates the infection in 95% of both adults and children. Drug B eradicates the infection in 47% of adults and 90% of children. There are otherwise no significant pharmacological differences between the two drugs, and there are no significant side effects. However, the cost of drug A is twice that of drug B. Dr X, a general practitioner, always uses drug B for the first treatment, and resorts to drug A if the infection persists. Dr Y, another general practitioner, always uses drug A for adults and drug B for children. Ignoring indirect costs:

A Drug A is more effective than drug B for treating children
B Drug A is more cost-effective than drug B for treating children
C Drug A is more cost-effective than drug B for treating adults
D Dr Y's regime achieves a higher level of cost-effectiveness than Dr X's
E Dr Y's regime achieves a higher level of equity of access between adults and children than Dr X's

9.26 Students X and Y were living in the same hall of residence of a university. Student X was diagnosed to have meningococcal disease due to meningococcus Group B. Three days later, student Y was diagnosed to have meningococcal disease due to meningococcus Group C. There had been no other cases of meningococcal disease. Recognised appropriate public health measures include:

A Reminding all students in the university about the symptoms of meningitis through the computer network
B Offering chemoprophylaxis to the close contacts of students X and Y
C Offering meningococcal vaccination to the close contacts of student X
D Offering meningococcal vaccination to the close contacts of student Y
E Offering meningococcal vaccination to the students living in the hall of residence

9.27 It is important to trace the contacts of a patient who has been diagnosed with the following diseases:

A Measles
B Tuberculosis
C Pneumococcal pneumonia
D Meningococcal meningitis
E Chlamydia

9.28 Vaccinations are available for the following infections:

A Parvovirus
B Measles
C Influenza
D Human immunodeficiency virus (HIV)
E Malaria

9.29 Clinical governance includes the following key concepts:

A Hospital managers should ensure that the volume of health services commissioned is delivered
B The senior clinician is accountable for improving the quality of the health services provided
C The Chief Executive of a health organisation is accountable for improving the quality of services provided
D Patient satisfaction should be taken into consideration in assessing the quality of services
E The clinicians should govern how the health services will be delivered

9.30 The use of costs per QALY by health service managers in commissioning health services ensures the following criteria are optimised:

A Effectiveness

B Cost-effectiveness
C Efficiency
D Equity
E Value for money

9.31 The following are examples of health demands which are not health needs:

A A patient was admitted compulsorily for treatment of acute schizophrenia under a section of the Mental Health Act
B Antibiotics were prescribed for viral sore throat at the patient's insistence
C An appendicectomy was performed on a patient for acute appendicitis
D A mother did not bring her infant child for vaccination due to lack of transport
E A patient was referred at his insistence to a plastic surgeon for a perceived deformed nose although no objective deformity was detected

Statistics

9.32 The following are examples of continuous data:

A The number of patients in a hospital ward
B Age of patients attending an out-patient clinic
C The ethnic group of patients in a hospital group
D The cholesterol level of patients attending an out-patient clinic
E The gender of patients attending an out-patient clinic

9.33 The following measures of central tendency can be determined from the corresponding type of data:

A Arithmetic mean – discrete data
B Arithmetic mean – categorical data
C Median – continuous data
D Median – categorical data
E Mode – discrete data

9.34 The ages of nine patients (to the nearest year) with a certain disease in a clinic are 25, 29, 38, 45, 48, 56, 56, 61 and 92:

A The mean is 50 years
B The mode is 50 years
C The median is 56 years
D The range is 67 years
E The mode is the most informative

9.35 Ten patients are randomly chosen, and the number of times they consulted their general practitioners within the last two years was 0, 0, 0, 0, 1, 2, 2, 3, 5 and 7:

- **A** The mode is 0
- **B** The median is 1
- **C** The mean is 2
- **D** The variance is 4.6 (to one decimal place)
- **E** The standard deviation is 2.3 (to one decimal place)

9.36 The length of survival after the diagnosis of colonic carcinoma was compared between two groups of six patients who received different treatments. The lengths of survival (in months) were:

Group A: – 6, 14, 18, 22, 27, 33

Group B: – 14, 16, 20, 22, 23, 25:

- **A** The means of the two groups are equal
- **B** In group A, the mean is greater than the median
- **C** The variance in group B is 15
- **D** The standard deviation in group B is 3.9 (to one decimal place)
- **E** The standard deviation is higher for group B than group A

9.37 In order to estimate the age distribution of the patients registered with a general practitioner, a researcher randomly sampled 10 patients for analysis:

- **A** The mean age of the sample is likely to underestimate the mean age of all the patients
- **B** The 95% confidence interval of the mean age can be increased by sampling more patients
- **C** The variance of the sample is likely to underestimate the variance of all patients
- **D** The standard deviation of the ages of the sample is likely to understimate that of all patients
- **E** The standard error of the mean can be halved by increasing the sample size from 10 to 40

9.38 A general practitioner issues a prescription in two out of every five patients who consult her. One out of every four patients never collects their medication from the pharmacy. Of those who obtain the medication, three out of every five patients do not take them. Of those who took them, one out of three do not benefit from them. For a patient who consults the doctor, the probability that he:

- **A** Gets a prescription is 60%
- **B** Obtains medication from the pharmacy is 30%
- **C** Takes the medication is 12%
- **D** Benefits from the medication is 4%
- **E** Does not benefit from medication is 92%

9.39 A general practitioner gave telephone advice to three patients one evening, and offered to see them the next morning if necessary. By previous experience, the probability of a patient consulting the next morning is 2/3. The doctor has reserved sufficient time to see only one patient the next morning. The probability that:

- **A** A consultation is required by none of the three patients is 8/27
- **B** A consultation is required by exactly one of the three patients is 2/9
- **C** A consultation is required by exactly two of the three patients is 4/9
- **D** A consultation is required by all three patients is 1/9
- **E** He would not have sufficient time to see all the patients is 20/27

9.40 The following statements about the normal distribution are true:

- **A** Exactly 50% of the distribution is below the mean
- **B** About 90% of the data lies within 2 standard deviations from the mean
- **C** The shape of the distribution is altered by the mean
- **D** The shape of the distribution is altered by the standard deviation
- **E** The distribution can be determined if both the mean and standard deviation are known

9.41 To test for whether a vaccine prevents infection, a study compared the proportions amongst the unvaccinated and the vaccinated who subsequently contracted the infection. The proportions of those contracting the disease were 0.2 and 0.1 amongst the unvaccinated and the vaccinated respectively:

- **A** The null hypothesis is that the vaccine is effective in preventing infection
- **B** The alternative hypothesis is that the vaccine does not alter the probability of contracting infection
- **C** The data given shows that the unvaccinated were significantly more likely than the vaccinated to contract the disease
- **D** The number of people in the study does not alter the conclusion
- **E** The design of the study was inappropriate to draw any valid conclusion about the efficacy of the vaccine

9.42 A study found $p < 0.05$ with the null hypothesis that there is no association between smoking and bladder cancer:

- **A** Less than one out of every 20 people smoked
- **B** Less than one out of every 20 people had bladder cancer
- **C** The probability of the observations of the study to have occurred, assuming the null hypothesis, is less than one in 20
- **D** The null hypothesis was rejected at the $p = 0.05$ level
- **E** The results suggest that there is no association between smoking and bladder cancer

9.43 A study found that $p = 0.007$ with the null hypothesis that paracetamol has no effect on fever. The null hypothesis was rejected at:

A 90% significance level
B 95% significance level
C 99% significance level
D 99.5% significance level
E 99.9% significance level

9.44 A study found that the relative risk for deep vein thrombosis after an abdominal operation was 1.8 (95% confidence interval 0.9–2.9):

A The risk of deep vein thrombosis after an abdominal operation was estimated to be 1.8 times that at other times
B The relative risk cannot possibly be above 2.9
C If the study were to be repeated 100 times, the relative risk would be estimated to be between 0.9 and 2.9 on about 95 occasions
D p is greater than 0.05 for the null hypothesis that the risk of deep vein thrombosis is unchanged after an abdominal operation
E The results show that abdominal operations were associated with an increased risk of deep vein thrombosis at the 95% confidence level

9.45 A case – control study was carried out to investigate an outbreak of food poisoning. People who attended a banquet were asked whether they consumed certain food, and whether they had diarrhoeal symptoms. The chi-square test was used to investigate whether having consumed chicken was associated with subsequently developing diarrhoeal symptoms:

A Discrete data was collected
B The data can be displayed in a 2×2 table
C The chi-square test was inappropriate
D Calculations are needed to make up a 2×2 table of the expected frequencies
E The analysis depends on the assumption that the data approximates the normal distribution

9. General principles of public health and statistics
Answers

Public health

9.1 B C

The concept of triangle of causation of disease is that causation of disease is multifactorial, and the factors can be grouped under agent, host or environment. Agent factors include the virulence of a microorganism, and the properties of a physical agent or a chemical toxin. For example, a new strain of influenza may be more virulent than the usual strains. Host factors include the genetic, physiological and psychological make-up of the individual. For example, an older person with previous lung disease may be more susceptible to infection by influenza. Environmental factors include the physical, social and cultural environment. Living in overcrowded conditions is an example of an adverse physical environment.

9.2 B C E

The iceberg concept of health care is that only a very small proportion of ill patients are receiving health care. This may be because some ill people do not seek help from health professionals; that some ill people who seek help from health professionals are not seen; and that some people who have been seen by health professionals are still waiting for their care. Whilst items **A** and **D** may be true, they are not related to the iceberg concept of health care.

9.3 D

Items **A** and **B** are false because of the multifactorial causation of disease. Hence, the differences in host factors (e.g. the immune systems of some people are better than others) may explain why some people develop diarrhoea without consuming water from the reservoir, and why some people who consume water from the reservoir nevertheless remain healthy.

The data in the question is from a case – control study, and the key is to compare the rates of disease amongst those who consume water from the reservoir and from other sources.

Risk of disease amongst reservoir water consumer = 80 per 100 000 population. Risk of disease amongst consumer of water from other sources = 100 per 500 000 population = 20 per 100 000 population. Hence the risk amongst those who consume reservoir water is four times that of those who consume water from other sources.

Although the case – control study shows an association between the consumption of reservoir water and disease, it does not show causation. For example, the food supply by a certain wholesaler to the local butcher may be contaminated, and the geographical area of the wholesaler food supply may have coincided with the geographical distribution of the reservoir water supply.

9.4 A C E

The prevalence of a disease is the proportion of the population with the disease at a particular time. Hence, the prevalence of hepatitis B carrier in 1997 was (50 000/5 000 000) × 100% = 1%. The prevalence of hepatitis B carrier in 1999 was (54 500/5 000 000) × 100% = 1.1%.

The incidence rate of a disease is the rate of new cases of the disease arising from a population at risk per unit time period. The population at risk was (5 000 000 – 50 000) = 4 950 000. The number of new cases over a two-year period was (54 500 – 50 000 + 500) = 5000. Hence the incidence was (5000/4.95)/2 = 500 per million population per year.

The risk of a disease is the proportion of the population at risk who developed the disease over a given time period. In the two years between 1997 and 1999, 5000 people became hepatitis B carriers, and the population at risk was 4 950 000. Hence the risk was (5000/4 950 000) × 100% = 0.1%.

The crude mortality rate is the percentage of deaths in a given period amongst the average population within that period. Hence the crude mortality rate for hepatitis B carriers between 1997 and 1999 was (500/50 000) × 100% = 1%.

9.5 B C D E

The prevalence of a disease is the proportion of the population with the disease at a particular time. Since there were no children with measles on 31 March 1998, the prevalence was 0%.

The incidence rate of a disease is the rate of new cases of the disease arising from a population at risk per unit time period. The number of children at risk of developing measles between 1 April to 1 October 1998 was (200 – 160) = 40. Twenty children caught measles during this six-month period. Hence, the incidence rate was 20 children per (40 × 0.5) = 20 children-years. This can be expressed as 1000 children per 1000 children-years.

The risk of a disease is the proportion of the population at risk who developed the disease over a given time period. Between

1 April and 1 October 1998, 20 children developed measles out of 40 susceptible children. Hence the risk was (20/40) × 100% = 50%.

The crude mortality rate is the proportion of the average population within a given period who died of the disease. The average population within the given period was (200 + 198)/2 = 199. Two children died. Hence the crude mortality rate was (2/199) × 100% = 1%.

The case mortality rate is the proportion of the diagnosed cases within a period of time who died from the disease. Two out of 20 children who developed measles died. Hence the case mortality rate was 10%.

9.6 A D

The prevalence of a disease within a population is the proportion of the population having the disease at a given time. Hence factors which increase the prevalence include an increase in the number of new cases (increased incidence), a reduction in the disease duration (either through more rapid recovery or death), increased immigration of diseased individuals or increased emigration of healthy individuals.

9.7 E

The duration of a disease with a low prevalence (i.e. few people have the disease at a given time) and a high incidence (i.e. a large number of new cases) must be very short. This may be because the disease recovers rapidly (e.g. a common cold), or because the disease is rapidly fatal (e.g. cholera during an epidemic in developing countries). A rare disease would have both a low prevalence and a low incidence. Improved primary preventive measures would reduce both prevalence and incidence. Rapid transmission of disease from one person to another would increase both prevalence and incidence.

9.8 A C

A case series describes the characteristics of a group of patients with the same disease. Hence the study of the characteristics of the 50 consecutive leukaemic children form a case series. If the outcomes of these 50 children are followed up for the next three years, it may form a cohort study. For example, the outcomes of different types of leukaemia may be compared. If we select another 100 district healthy children in the health district carefully matched to the 50 leukaemic children in age, sex and social class, and compare their exposure to irradiation with the 50 leukaemic children, it forms a case – control study to investigate whether the level of exposure to irradiation was associated with the development of leukaemia. If we conduct a survey amongst a randomly selected sample of children in the health district of their diet in the previous week, it forms a cross-sectional study as it describes the population at a point in time. If we conduct two surveys amongst two different samples of randomly selected sample of children two years apart, it forms a repeated cross-sectional study. It is not a cohort study as different children are studied in the two surveys.

9.9 C

In order to calculate the incidence, we need to know both the number of new cases and the number of people at risk in the population during a given time period. In a cohort study, a group of people at risk of a disease is followed up, and the number of new cases over a given time period is determined. Hence, the incidence can be calculated. In a case series, we can deduce the number of new cases over a given time period, but not the number of people at risk. This also applies for case–control studies. In a cross-sectional study, we can calculate the proportion of a population who have the disease in question (i.e. prevalence), but we do not know the number of new cases within a given period of time. In a repeated cross-sectional study, we can calculate the prevalence of the disease at two given points in time. However, we do not know the number of new cases which arise for a given time interval, as the two cross-sectional studies were conducted on different subjects.

9.10 B C D E

The absolute risk is the proportion of the population at risk who develop a condition over a given period of time.

Hence the absolute risk amongst the treatment group = (250/5000) × 100% = 5%. The absolute risk amongst the control group = (500/5000) × 100% = 10%.

The attributable risk (or risk difference) is the difference between the risk in the exposed (treatment) group and the unexposed (control) group. Hence attributable risk = 5% – 10% = –5%. (The negative sign signifies that the risk is less with treatment.)

The relative risk is the ratio of the risk of disease in the exposed (treatment) group to the risk of disease in the unexposed (control) group. Hence relative risk = 5%/10% = 0.5. (A relative risk less than 1 signifies that the risk is less with treatment.)

Hence the results of the trial suggest that treatment with drug X reduces the risk of developing hypertension by half.

9.11 C D

The low response rates from both subjects and controls may give rise to systematic bias, as the prevalence of respiratory diseases amongst those who did not respond to questionnaires may differ significantly from those who did. For example, those who had respiratory diseases may regard the questionnaires as more relevant, and might be more motivated to return the questionnaires. The controls in a case–control study must be chosen so they are similar to the cases apart from the factor being studied (i.e.

exposure to certain chemicals). For example, smoking amongst factory staff might be more prevalent than the normal population. Since smoking is strongly associated with respiratory disease, this alone might explain why factory workers have a higher prevalence of respiratory diseases. Smoking is therefore known as a confounding variable, as it is associated with both the putative risk factor (i.e. working in the factory and exposure to chemical) and the outcome (i.e. respiratory diseases). Similarly, sex may be a confounding variable if the proportion of men and women in the case and control groups is different. Exposure to the chemicals is the putative risk factor, and cannot be a confounding variable.

9.12 A B D E

The finding that a putative risk factor (i.e. substance X in diet) is associated with an outcome (i.e. neurological disease) does not necessarily prove that substance X causes the disease. Other alternative explanations may include spurious associations due to methodological limitations of the study and the presence of confounding variables.

Evidence which tends to support causality include:

(*i*) *Dose–response relationship between the putative risk factor and outcome*
If people who consumed higher quantities of X had higher risk of developing the disease, it would satisfy this criterion.

(*ii*) *Consistency of the results*
If similar results were obtained from other studies, this would tend to support causality.

(*iii*) *The putative risk factor precedes the outcome*
If it can be shown that the consumption of X precedes the development of the neurological disease, this criterion would be satisfied.

(*iv*) *Plausibility*
If there is a plausible biological explanation for the effect, it would tend to support causality. For example, in vitro demonstration that substance X is neurotoxic may provide such an explanation.

(*v*) *Reversibility*
If the outcome disappears after the putative risk factor is removed, this tends to support causality. For example, if it can be shown that removing X from the diet improves the outcome of the disease, this tends to support causality.

(*vi*) *Strong association*
A strong association between the putative risk factor and the outcome makes causation more likely.

9.13 A D E

Criteria for a good screening test (Wilson's criteria) include the following:

- The disease is an important health problem
- The natural history of the disease is well understood
- There is a considerable time lag between the onset of disease and the appearance of symptoms
- Diagnostic tests are available
- Effective treatments are available
- The screening test is simple and acceptable to the subjects
- The screening test is reliable (repeatable) and valid (high sensitivity and specificity)
- The screening programme is cost-effective

9.14 A D E

The information can be summarised in a 2 × 2 table as shown in Table 1.

		Disease		Total
		+ve	–ve	
Test	+ve	240	70	**310**
	–ve	60	630	**690**
Total		300	700	**1000**

Prevalence = number with disease/total population = 300/1000 = 30%.
Sensitivity is the proportion of subjects with the disease who were correctly predicted by the test. Hence sensitivity = (240/300) × 100% = 80%
Specificity is the proportion of subjects without the disease who were correctly predicted by the test. Hence specificity = (630/700) × 100% = 90%.
The PPV is the proportion of subjects with a positive test who were correctly predicted by the test. Hence PPV = (240/310) × 100% = 77%
The NPV is the proportion of subjects with a negative test who were correctly predicted by the test. Hence NPV = (630/690) × 100% = 91%.

9.15 A B C D

The information can be summarised in a 2 × 2 table as shown in Table 2.

		Disease		Total
		+ve	–ve	
Test	+ve	80	270	**350**
	–ve	20	630	**650**
Total		100	900	**1000**

The PPV = (80/350) × 100% = 23%.
The NPV = (630/650) × 100% = 97%.

9.16 B D

Sensitivity and specificity of a screening tests are characteristics of the test and do not change with the prevalence of the condition being screened. Hence the sensitivity and specificity of the test remain constant irrespective of the countries where it is being used. On the other hand, positive and negative predictive values of a screening test change with prevalence. If the condition becomes more prevalent, the PPV increases. In fact, the PPV is always 100% if all subjects in the population have the condition (i.e. the prevalence of the condition is 100%). If the condition becomes more prevalent, the NPV decreases. In fact, the NPV is always 0% if none of the subjects in the population have the condition (i.e. prevalence is 0%). A screening programme is likely to be more cost-effective in a country where the disease is more prevalent, as the number of subjects screened for one case to be detected is smaller.

9.17 B C E

Screening programmes have recently been subjected to vigorous systematic reviews (evaluations based on published studies). Neonatal screening for congenital hypothyroidism and phenylketonuria has been found to satisfy most of Wilson's criteria for screening. In a systematic review published in 1998, the neonatal screening test was found to be effective. In 1987, the Forrest report recommended that a national screening programme for breast cancer screening by mammography should be established. Prostate cancer screening by prostatic specific antigen (PSA) was found to be ineffective. The main reasons include imperfect screening tests, lack of effective treatment, and that the natural history of subtypes of prostate cancer is still not well understood. Similarly, ovarian cancer screening (by ultrasound and serum CA125) was found to be ineffective. The main reasons include imperfect screening tests, lack of non-invasive diagnostic tests and lack of effective treatment for cases other than those presenting at a very early stage.

9.18 B

The difference between the two screening strategies is that everyone at risk of the disease is screened in the population screening strategy whilst only those identified to be at high risk are screened in the high-risk screening strategy. The main advantage of the population strategy is that the overall benefit would be higher, as more cases will be detected. It also has the advantage of avoiding the difficulties of identifying high-risk groups for the disease. The main advantages of the high-risk strategy are that the prevalence of the condition is higher amongst those screened, and hence the cost per case detected is lower. Also, the overall cost is lower, as fewer subjects are screened. Furthermore, the motivation for both staff and subjects is likely to be higher. The high-risk subjects tend to regard screening as more relevant to them.

9.19 B C

In primary prevention, action is taken to prevent the development of the disease in the first place. Examples include smoking cessation to prevent carcinoma of the lung and fluoridation of water to prevent dental decay. In secondary prevention, action is taken to detect disease at a stage before symptoms appear, so that effective treatment may be given. Almost all screening procedures are examples of secondary prevention. In tertiary prevention, action is taken to prevent complications of a disease after the symptoms have appeared. Examples include control of diabetes with insulin and treatment of asthma with bronchodilators and steroids.

9.20 A C D E

Health protection is usually achieved by the introduction of legislation or regulations to improve the health of the population. One difference from health education is that subjects who benefit from such measures may not even be aware of them. Examples include the introduction of seat belts, prosecuting shopkeepers who sell cigarettes to children and young people below 16 years of age, fiscal measures (e.g. increased taxation on cigarettes or alcohol), and regulations to maintain good-quality food and water standards.

9.21 C D

The different health care systems in the world form a continuum according to the percentage of health care costs funded by central government. At one end, the health care system in the United States of America is mainly funded by users' fees, and the percentage of health care costs funded by central government is only about 40%. In Japan, Australia, Germany and France, the health care system is selective welfare-oriented, and much use is made of insurance cover. Just over 60% of health care costs are funded directly by government. In the United Kingdom, Norway and Sweden, the health care system is comprehensively welfare-oriented. Over 80% of the health care costs are funded by central government. In Russia and China, the health care system is centrally planned and administered, and the percentage of health care costs funded directly by central government is over 95%.

9.22 –

Rationing of health care is inevitable irrespective of the type of health care system. Rationing can be either implicit or explicit. Rationing in a private fee-paying system is by wealth. Rationing in an employer insurance system is by employment status. Rationing in a government-funded national health system or in an internal market system may be either by explicit criteria or simply by waiting lists.

9.23 C D

To monitor the health services, three types of measures may be used: structure, process and outcome. Structural measures are concerned with the number and nature of the buildings, staff and equipment available. Examples include the number of consultants per million population or the number of in-patient beds per million population. Accurate data for such measures is easily available. However, the structural measures do not necessarily correlate with how good or bad the services provided are. Process measures include data on what has been done to the patients, as well as how much and how well it has been done. Examples include the number of dermatological out-patient consultations per million population per year, and the number of skin biopsies performed. Compared to structural measures, the process measures contain more information about how good or bad the health services provided are. Outcome measures measure the results of the health services provided, and the extent to which the objectives of the health care have been achieved. Examples include reduction in death rates, functional improvements, reduction in pain and discomfort, and improvement in patients' satisfaction. These measures directly measure the results, but accurate data is more difficult to obtain.

9.24 A E

QALY is a measure of the outcome of an intervention. It measures the length of life gained (in years), but adjusts for the quality of life during this time. Hence it is a measure of outcome. In order to measure QALY, both the length of life gained and the quality of life must be measured. The quality of life is usually obtained by the ratings given by the patients or the health professionals, either through an interview or by questionnaire. The ratings usually range between 0 (death) and 1 (full health). However, if the condition entails so much disability and suffering that the patient considers it worse than death, the quality of life may be negative. Measurement of the quality of life is necessarily subjective.

9.25 A C D

Effectiveness is the extent a health intervention achieves the end-result desired. The outcome is eradication of the infection. Since drug A eradicates the infection in a higher proportion of both children and adults than drug B, drug A is more effective than drug B for treating both children and adults.

The cost-effectiveness of the drugs might be compared by measuring the cost incurred per case of infection treated. In children, an application of drug A eradicates infection only by a slightly higher proportion than drug B (95% vs 90%), but the cost of drug A is twice that of drug B. Hence, ignoring indirect costs, the cost-effectiveness of drug B is higher than drug A in children. However, in adults, an application of drug A eradicates infection more than twice as often as drug B (95% vs 47%). Hence drug A is more cost-effective than drug B for adults. Dr Y uses the most cost-effective drug for both children and adults, and therefore achieves a higher level of cost-effectiveness overall. However, one may argue that Dr Y's regime discriminates against children, as children are always given the inferior drug. Dr X's regime is more equitable, but is less cost-effective overall. This demonstrates that striving for cost-effectiveness may sometimes conflict with striving for equity.

9.26 A B D

Whenever a case of meningococcal disease occurs amongst a student population in a university, it is wise to raise the awareness of students to this disease so that they seek medical advice early. Meningococcus is often carried in the nasopharynx by healthy individuals, and close contacts of meningococcal cases have a much higher risk of developing the disease within the next 30 days. Hence, chemoprophylaxis (i.e. either rifampicin or ciprofloxacin) should be given to close contacts. Meningococcal vaccines are available for Group C organism, but it is not currently available for Group B organism. Hence, vaccines should be given to close contacts of an index case of meningococcal disease caused by Group C meningococcus. In deciding whether chemoprophylaxis or vaccines should be extended to other students in the hall of residence who are not close contacts of the index cases, it is important to consider whether the two cases are related or whether they are isolated cases. The fact that the two cases were caused by meningococci of different groups show that the cases were unrelated. Hence wider public health action was not indicated.

9.27 B D E

There are two situations when contacts of an index case of an infection should be traced. The first situation is if the contacts of an index case have a much increased risk for contracting the infection; the infection may result in a serious clinical condition; and that immediate prevention measures are available. Hence, contacts of meningococcal disease and tuberculosis should be traced. The second situation is if the contacts of an index case have an increased risk for contracting the infection; they may become infectious without necessarily having symptoms; and that effective measures are available to stop further spread of the disease. Hence, contacts for both tuberculosis and chlamydia should be traced.

9.28 B C

Measles, mumps and rubella (MMR) vaccines are usually given to children at the age of one year and before school entry in the United Kingdom. Influenza vaccines are indicated for older people aged over 75, those living in nursing homes and those with certain chronic conditions. Parvovirus usually causes 'slapped cheek disease' in children. This is usually mild. However, it may cause abortion in pregnant women. No vaccines are currently available. No vaccines are currently available for HIV and malaria, although chemoprophylaxis is available for malaria.

9.29 B C D

Clinical governance is a system through which NHS organisations are accountable for continuously improving the quality of their services by creating an environment to allow excellence in clinical care to develop. This concept was given special emphasis in the NHS White Paper published in 1998 in the UK. All clinicians, senior managers, and the Chief Executive are accountable for the quality of the health care delivered. According to the World Health Organization, the assessment of quality should include the following areas: the professional's technical quality, efficiency in the use of resources, management of the risk of injury associated with clinical treatment, and the patients' satisfaction with the services.

9.30 B C E

The cost per QALY is a measure of the cost per unit health gain. Hence it is a measure of efficiency, cost-effectiveness or value for money. Effectiveness is the extent to which a health intervention achieves its desired outcome, and is not measured by cost per QALY. Equity is concerned with 'fairness' of access between different subgroups of the population.

9.31 B E

Health demands are health care requested by patients. Health needs are health care deemed to be necessary by health professionals. Some health demands are also health needs. Examples include an appendicetomy being performed on a patient with acute appendicitis. However, some health demands are not health needs. Examples include antibiotics being prescribed for viral sore throat at the patient's insistence, and a patient being referred at his insistence to a plastic surgeon for a perceived deformed nose although no objective deformity was detected. On the other hand, some health needs are never demanded. Examples include a patient being admitted compulsorily for treatment of acute schizophrenia under a section of the Mental Health Act, and a mother who did not bring her infant child for vaccination due to lack of transport.

Statistics

9.32 B D

There are three major types of data: categorical, discrete and continuous. If the data is gathered by classifying subjects into one of several categories, categorical data is collected. Examples include the ethnic group of a patient, the colour of a patient's eyes and country of residence. If there are only two categories (e.g. gender), it is also known as binary data. If the categories can be ranked (e.g. a patient's social class), it is also called ordinal (ranked) data. Discrete data has meaningful numerical values, but can only take certain values (e.g. integers). Discrete data is usually collected by counting (e.g. the number of patients in a ward, the number of consultations conducted in a year) Continuous data has meaningful numerical values and can usually take all values. It is usually collected by some type of measurement. Examples are the cholesterol or haemoglobin concentrations of a patient, and the duration of a consultation.

9.33 A C E

The mode is the category or value which occurs with the highest frequency. (Mode means fashion, i.e. most fashionable.) The mode can be determined for all types of data.

The median is the result which occurs exactly half way through the data if we arrange the data in ascending (or descending) order. As we can arrange discrete and continuous data in ascending data, it is possible to determine the median from this data. However, as we cannot arrange categorical data (which is not ordinal data) into ascending order, it is not possible to determine the median generally for categorical data.

The mean is what is meant by 'average' in everyday language. It is equal to the sum of all the data divided by the number of items. As only discrete and continuous variables have meaningful values, the mean can be determined only for this data.

9.34 A D

- The mean is 50 years (mean = sum of data/number = 450/9 = 50)
- The mode is 56 years, as it occurs more frequently than other values
- The median is 48 years, the fifth (central) item in the data
- The range is the difference between the maximum and the minimum = 92 – 25 = 67 years

The mode is the least informative for continuous data. The relative usefulness of the median and the mean depends on the purpose.

If the data is not skewed (e.g. in a normal distribution), the mean would be close to the median.

9.35 A C E

- mode (most frequent value) = 0
- median = (1+2)/2 = 1.5 (the fifth and the sixth items are the central items. The median is the sum of these two items divided by 2)
- The mean = sum of data/number = 20/10 = 2
- The variance can be calculated in either by:

$$\text{Var (X)} = \frac{\Sigma\,(x - \bar{x}\,)^2}{n}$$

where $\bar{x}$ is the mean, or by

$$\text{Var (X)} = \frac{\Sigma x^2}{n} - \bar{x}^2$$

Using the second method, Var (X) $= \frac{92}{10}\, 2^2 = 5.2$

- The standard deviation = √[Var (X)] = 2.3 (to one decimal place)

9.36 A C D

- The means of both groups A and B are 20
- In group A, median = (18+22)/2 = 20. Hence the means and the median are equal
- In group B,

$$\text{Var (X)} = \frac{2490}{6} - 20^2 = 15$$

- The standard deviation = √15 = 3.9 (to one decimal place)

It is clear from inspecting the data that group B has a narrower spread than group A. Since the standard deviation is a measure of spread of the data, the standard deviation in group B must be smaller than group A. In fact, the standard deviation for group A = 8.7 (to one decimal place).

9.37 E

The mean of a sample is as equally likely to underestimate as to overestimate the mean of the population. (i.e. sample means are unbiased.) However, the 95% confidence interval of the mean can be reduced (i.e. more certain of the value of the mean) by increasing the sample size. On the other hand, the standard deviation and variance are more likely to underestimate than overestimate the population standard deviation and variance. To understand this, consider a sample size of 1: the variance and standard deviation must be zero. The standard error of the mean can be thought of as follows. Several random samples of size n are selected, and the means of these samples are calculated. The standard error of the mean is the standard deviation of these means. The larger the sample size n, the smaller the standard error. In fact, they are related by the equation

$$\text{SE} = \frac{\sigma}{\sqrt{n}}$$

where σ is the standard deviation in the population.

9.38 B C E

The probability that two independent events would both occur is the product of the probability for each event, p (A and B) = p(A) × p(B).

The probability of an event not occurring = 1 – probability of event occurring, p (not A) = 1 – p(A)

For a patient who consults the doctor:

- Probability of receiving a prescription = 1 – 3/5 = 40%
- Probability of obtaining medication = 40% × (1 – 1/4) = 30%
- Probability of taking medication = 30% × (1 – 3/5) = 12%
- Probability of benefit from medication = 12% × (1 – 1/3) = 8%
- Probability of not benefiting from medication = 1 – 8% = 92%

9.39 B C E

For any one patient, the probability of consulting = 2/3, and the probability of not consulting = 1 – 2/3 = 1/3.

The probability that:

- None of the patients requires consultation = 1/3 × 1/3 × 1/3 = 1/27
- Exactly one of the three patients requires consultation = 3 × (2/3 × 1/3 × 1/3) = 6/27 = 2/9
- Exactly two of the three patients require consultation = 3 × (2/3 × 2/3 × 1/3) = 12/27 = 4/9
- All three patients require consultation = (2/3 × 2/3 × 2/3) = 8/27
- The doctor does not have sufficient time to see all the patients = 12/27 + 8/27 = 20/27

9.40 A D E

The normal distribution (or Gaussian distribution) is bell-shaped, and approximates most biological parameters such as height, weight and intelligence. The distribution is symmetrical about the mean, and the median and the mean coincide. Hence, exactly half of the distribution is below the mean. About 68% of the distribution is within 1 standard deviation from the mean, and 95% of the distribution is within 2 standard deviations from the mean. The normal distribution has two parameters: the mean and the standard deviation. Increasing the mean would shift the distribution to the right, but has no effect on its shape. Increasing the standard deviation would increase the 'spread' of the distribution, and hence alters its shape.

9.41 –

The objective of the study was to show that the vaccine is effective. The null hypothesis was that the vaccine has no effect on the probability of contracting infection, whilst the alternative hypothesis is that the vaccine has an effect. If it is shown that the probability for the observation in the study to have occurred assuming the null hypothesis is very small (less than 0.05, say), then the alternative hypothesis is shown. In the study, a higher proportion amongst the unvaccinated contracted the disease. However, it is necessary to show that this is not due to random variation. It is not possible to calculate this probability as the number of subjects in the study is not given. The probability would be smaller if the number of subjects is larger.

9.42 C D

$p < 0.05$ means that the chance of the observations of the study occurring if the null hypothesis were true is less than one in 20. This is very unlikely, and hence the null hypothesis is rejected. This tends to support the alternative hypothesis that there is an association between smoking and bladder cancer.

9.43 A B C

To reject the null hypothesis at 90% significance level means that the probability for the results to have occurred assuming the null hypothesis must be less than (1–90%) = 0.1. Since 0.007 < 0.01, the null hypothesis is rejected at 90% significance level. Similarly:

- Since 0.007 < 0.05, the null hypothesis is rejected at 95% significance level
- Since 0.007 < 0.01, the null hypothesis is rejected at 90% significance level
- Since 0.007 > 0.005, the null hypothesis is *not* rejected at 99.5% significance level
- Since 0.007 >0.001, the null hypothesis is *not* rejected at 99.9% confidence level

9.44 A C D

A relative risk of 1 means that the risk of deep vein thrombosis is unrelated to abdominal operation. A relative risk of over 1 means that the risk increases, whilst a relative risk of below 1 means that the risk decreases after an abdominal operation.

The relative risk was quoted as 1.8 (95% confidence internal 0.9–2.9). This means the estimated relative risk was 1.8, and that there is 95% probability that the real relative risk lies between 0.9 and 2.9. In other words, if the study were to be repeated 100 times, the relative risk would be estimated to be between 0.9 and 2.9 on 95 occasions. Since the interval of 0.9 to 2.9 includes values less than 1, it cannot be concluded with 95% confidence that the relative risk is above 1. Hence *p* is greater than 0.05 for the null hypothesis that the risk of deep vein thrombosis is unchanged after abdominal operation. The null hypothesis cannot be rejected, and the results did not show at 95% confidence level that abdominal operations were associated with an increased risk of deep vein thrombosis.

9.45 B D

The parameters of the study were whether chicken was consumed, and whether diarrhoeal symptoms developed. Both were categorical (binary) variables. Hence there could not have been assumptions about the relationship between the data and the normal distribution. The data is best displayed in a 2 × 2 table. The chi-square test is the most appropriate, although alternative analytical techniques to compare the proportion of people who develop diarrhoea amongst those who ate and those who did not eat chicken are available. In order to perform the chi-square test, calculations are necessary to make up a second 2 × 2 table showing the expected frequencies assuming the null hypothesis. The chi-square value can then be calculated from the two tables showing observed and expected frequency, and the significance level can be looked up in a statistical table.

Part II
System-based basic medical sciences

10. Blood and bone marrow
Questions

10.1 Significant quantities of red blood cells are normally produced at the following sites in the fetus:

- **A** Bone marrow in tibia
- **B** Bone marrow in sternum
- **C** Bone marrow in vertebra
- **D** Liver
- **E** Spleen

10.2 Significant quantities of red blood cells are normally produced at the following sites in adulthood:

- **A** Bone marrow in tibia
- **B** Bone marrow in radius
- **C** Bone marrow in vertebra
- **D** Liver
- **E** Spleen

10.3 The following statements about normal blood cell formation are true:

- **A** Pluripotent stem cells which are capable of differentiating into red blood cells, white blood cells or platelets exist in the bone marrow
- **B** Once the bone marrow becomes depleted of functioning cells, it cannot produce blood cells even after the transfusion of functioning bone marrow cells
- **C** Megalokaryoblasts are the precursor cells for red blood cells
- **D** Lymphocytes and neutrophils share the same committed stem cells
- **E** Reticulocytes are the precursor cells for platelets

10.4 The following statements about blood cells are true:

- **A** There are more white blood cells than red blood cells in the circulation
- **B** There are more white cell precursors than red cell precursors in the bone marrow
- **C** The average lifetime for red blood cells in the circulation is about three years
- **D** The average lifetime for platelets in the circulation is about 200 days
- **E** The average lifetime for white blood cells in the circulation is about 120 days

10.5 The following cells contain a nucleus:

- **A** Erythrocyte
- **B** Megalokaryocyte
- **C** Platelet
- **D** T-lymphocyte
- **E** Neutrophil

10.6 The following features of red cells are characteristic of impaired splenic function:

- **A** Polycythaemia
- **B** Howell–Jolly bodies
- **C** Spherocytes
- **D** Target cells
- **E** Microcytes

10.7 The following red cell indices are generally higher in normal males than normal females:

- **A** Haemoglobin
- **B** Mean corpuscular volume
- **C** Mean corpuscular haemoglobin
- **D** Red cell count
- **E** Haematrocrit

10.8 The following statements about haemoglobin are true:

- **A** It is a globular molecule
- **B** There are two subunits in each molecule
- **C** The subunits share the same haem group
- **D** The globulin chains contain iron
- **E** The globulin portions consist of polypeptides

10.9 The haemoglobin in the fetus:

- **A** Is mainly haemoglobin A
- **B** Contains two β chains in each molecule
- **C** Contains two α chains in each molecule
- **D** Binds more tightly to 2,3-diphosphoglycerate (2,3-DPG) than adult haemoglobin

E Contains more oxygen than adult haemoglobin given the same partial pressure of oxygen

10.10 Abnormally small red blood cells (microcytes) characteristically occur in:

A Vitamin B_{12} deficiency
B Drug-induced haemolysis
C Iron deficiency
D Bone marrow failure
E Thalassaemia

10.11 The following statements about iron metabolism are true:

A Over 95% of body iron is stored in the liver
B Over 90% of the iron is normally stored as haemosiderin
C The serum ferritin level is an accurate measure of total body iron stores
D The terminal ileum is the main site for iron absorption
E The total iron store is controlled mainly via the rate of urinary excretion

10.12 Recognised haematological findings in iron deficiency include:

A Hypochromic red cells
B Grossly increased reticulocyte count
C Reduced mean cell volume (MCV) index
D Increased mean corpuscular haemoglobin (MCH) index
E Increased total iron-binding capacity

10.13 The following statements about vitamin B_{12} are true:

A It is essential for DNA synthesis
B It is available from most vegetables
C Vitamin B_{12} absorption is not possible in the absence of intrinsic factor
D Symptoms of vitamin B_{12} deficiency develop within a month of defective dietary intake
E Milk can provide sufficient dietary vitamin B_{12} to prevent anaemia

10.14 Causes of vitamin B_{12} deficiency include:

A Crohn's disease
B Gastrectomy
C Pernicious anaemia
D Chronic gastrointestinal bleeding
E Pregnancy

10.15 The following are recognised indications for iron therapy:

A Iron deficiency due to heavy menstrual blood loss
B Pregnant woman with a normal haemoglobin level
C Anaemia due to increased haemolysis
D Thalassaemia
E Iron deficiency due to dietary deficiency

10.16 The following are valid indications for intramuscular rather than oral iron therapy:

- **A** Iron deficiency of nutritional deficiency origin
- **B** Past history of severe intolerable gastrointestinal side effects due to oral iron
- **C** Consistent lack of patient compliance
- **D** A quick response is desired
- **E** A haemoglobin level of below 9 g/dl

10.17 Recognised haematological findings in vitamin B_{12} deficiency include:

- **A** Reduced platelet count
- **B** Reduced white cell count
- **C** Multilobed nucleus in neutrophils
- **D** Low MCV index
- **E** Hypocellular bone marrow

10.18 The following conditions are associated with pancytopenia (anaemia, neutropenia and thrombocytopenia):

- **A** Anti-neoplastic chemotherapy
- **B** Ionising radiation to the bone marrow
- **C** Drug-induced haemolysis
- **D** Bone marrow infiltration by carcinoma
- **E** Folate deficiency

10.19 Causes of haemolytic anaemia include:

- **A** Spherocytosis
- **B** Thalassaemia
- **C** Iron deficiency
- **D** Sickle-cell disease
- **E** Mismatched blood transfusion

10.20 Features associated with abnormally excessive haemolysis include:

- **A** Increased conjugated serum bilirubin
- **B** Increased urine urobilinogen
- **C** Increased reticulocytes in peripheral blood film
- **D** Increased serum haptoglobin
- **E** Small spleen

10.21 Which of the following types of white blood cells and their associated features are correctly matched?

- **A** Monocytes – the commonest type of white cells
- **B** Mast cells – the largest type of white cells
- **C** Eosinophils – important for combating parasite infection
- **D** Basophils – histamine and heparin-containing
- **E** T-lymphocytes – precursor of plasma cells

10.22 In acute leukaemia:

T **A** Neoplastic proliferation of the precursors of white cells occurs
B Anaemia is common
C Reduced platelet levels rarely occur
D Infiltration of the liver rarely occurs
E Abnormal cells are almost always found in the peripheral blood

10.23 Known predisposing factors for leukaemic transformation include:

A Irradiation
B Exposure to certain viruses
C Exposure to certain bacteria
D Down's syndrome
E Air pollution with sulphur dioxide

10.24 Multiple myelomas:

A Are a malignant proliferation of T-cells in the bone marrow
B Usually result in the accumulation of several different types of immunoglobulin chains
C May result in increased urinary excretion of free light immunoglobulin chains
D Are associated with greatly elevated erythrocyte sedimentation rate
E Often result in anaemia

10.25 The following statements about lymph nodes are true:

A Lymph enters the lymph nodes in the medullary area
B The germinal centres contain mainly T-lymphocytes
C The follicles are responsible for humoral response
D The paracortex is responsible for cell-mediated immunity
E Lymph leaves the lymph node via the efferent lymphatic at the hilum

10.26 The following statements about the circulation of lymph are true:

A The total volume of lymph circulated is approximately 30 litres per day
B Fluid enters the lymphatics from the interstitial space
C Fluid drains into the aorta via the thoracic and right lymphatic ducts
D All lymphatics have valves in their walls
E The drainage of lymphatics in the collecting lymphatics is facilitated by contraction of the muscles associated with the organ

10.27 Causes of an enlarged lymph node include:

- **A** Epstein–Barr virus infection
- **B** Mycobacterial infection
- **C** Metastatic spread of leukaemia
- **D** Human immunodeficiency virus infection
- **E** Sarcoidosis

10.28 Hodgkin's disease:

- **A** Is a type of leukaemia
- **B** Spreads predominantly via the bloodstream
- **C** Occurs predominantly amongst those over 70 years of age
- **D** Is characterised by the presence of Reed–Sternberg cells
- **E** Is almost always associated with systemic symptoms such as weight loss or night sweats

10.29 The following statements about the thymus gland are true:

- **A** It develops from the sixth pharanygeal pouch
- **B** It is larger in the elderly than in adolescents
- **C** It contains mostly B-lymphocytes
- **D** Underdevelopment is associated with immunodeficiency disorders
- **E** Thymic hyperplasia or neoplasia is associated with autoimmune disorders

10.30 The rate of platelet production is controlled by:

- **A** A type of colony-stimulating factor
- **B** Erythropoietin
- **C** A type of interleukin
- **D** A type of prostaglandin
- **E** von Willebrand factor

10.31 The following statements about platelet aggregation following injury to a small blood vessel are true:

- **A** Thrombin is essential for platelet adhesion
- **B** Platelet activation is enhanced by von Willebrand factor
- **C** Platelets are activated by contact with collagen
- **D** Platelets produce ADP
- **E** Platelet-activating factor (PAF) is secreted by platelets

10.32 Drugs which inhibit platelet activity include:

- **A** Aspirin
- **B** Warfarin
- **C** Dipyridamole
- **D** Disopyramide
- **E** Ticlopidine

10.33 Recognised indications for anti-platelet agents include:

- **A** Myocardial infarction
- **B** von Willebrand disease

C Transient ischaemic attacks
D Unstable angina
E Post-arterial graft surgery for peripheral vascular disease

10.34 The following statements about the clotting mechanisms are true:

A A secure clot can be formed in the absence of platelets
B The essential final step is the formation of fibrin
C The intrinsic system is triggered by tissue damage
D The extrinsic system is triggered by contact with collagen
E Thrombin catalyses the conversion of fibrinogen into fibrin

10.35 The following statements about vitamin K are true:

A The natural vitamin K is fat-soluble
B It is converted into factor IX and X in the liver
C Bile is necessary for its absorption
D Gastrointestinal haemorrhage may occur in deficiency state
E Prothrombin time is characteristically prolonged in deficiency state

10.36 Warfarin:

A Acts within 24 h of oral administration
B Is a non-competitive inhibitor of vitamin K
C Characteristically causes a high international normalised ratio (INR)
D Characteristically causes a prolonged activated partial thromboplastin time (APTT)
E May be used in the treatment of pulmonary embolism

10.37 The following are components of the fibrinolytic system:

A Binding of thrombomodulin to thrombin
B Inactivation of protein C
C Increase in the serum level of tissue plasminogen activator (t-PA)
D Conversion of plasmin into plasminogen
E Conversion of fibrinogen into fibrin

10.38 The following statements about heparin are true:

A Its effect may be reversed by protamine
B It is a competitive antagonist of antithrombin III
C It causes prolonged APTT
D It may be given orally
E It has a half-life of about 48 h

10.39 Which of the following drugs may remove thrombi?

A Streptokinase
B Tranexamic acid
C Aprotinin
D Tissue plasminogen activator (t-PA, such as alteplase)
E Urokinase

10.40 The following drugs may be useful in the management of haemophilia A (classical haemophilia):

A Factor IX concentrate
B Tranexamic acid
C Warfarin
D Desmopressin (DDAVP)
E Streptokinase

10. Blood and bone marrow Answers

10.1 A B C D E

In the fetus, blood cells are normally produced in all bone marrow cavities, the liver and the spleen. In childhood, blood cells are normally produced in all bone marrow cavities, but not in the liver and spleen. In adulthood, the marrow cavities of most long bones (except the femur and upper part of the humerus) become inactive, and become infiltrated with fat (yellow marrow). The marrow in the vertebrae, sternum, ribs, skull and pelvis are active, and is known as red marrow. This is important clinically. If the liver and spleen become active in producing blood cells in adulthood (extramedullary haematopoiesis), a disease affecting the function of the bone marrow (e.g. fibrosis of the bone marrow) is likely to be present.

10.2 C

See answer to question 10.1 above.

10.3 A

Red blood cells, white blood cells and platelets are derived from a common undifferentiated precursor cell (pluripotent stem cell). This explains why bone marrow transplantation is effective, where blood cell production resumes after infusion of normal bone marrow cells into a subject without functioning bone marrow. The pluripotent stem cell differentiates into differentiated lymphoid or myeloid stem cells. The lymphoid stem cells can differentiate further into B- or T-lymphocytes, whereas myeloid stem cells may differentiate into all other types of cells. Megalokaryocytes are differentiated precursors for platelets found in the bloodstream. In diseases with rapid destruction of platelets in the blood (e.g. idiopathic thrombocytopenic purpura), the number of megalokaryoblasts increases in the bone marrow. Reticulocytes are the precursors of red blood cells. In anaemia due to rapid destruction of red cells, reticulocyte count increases in an attempt to compensate for the anaemia.

10.4 B

Although there are about 500 times more red blood cells than white blood cells in the circulation, about three-quarters of the cellular components of bone marrow are white cell precursors. This is because the bone marrow acts as a reserve store for white blood cells, and respond rapidly to infection or tissue injury by the release of white cells. The white cells usually remain in the circulation for only a few hours. In contrast, there is almost no storage pool for red blood cells, and the average lifetime for red blood cells is about 120 days. This is important clinically, as diseases affecting the bone marrow may cause neutropenia very quickly, whereas it might take over a month before anaemia becomes apparent. The average lifetime for platelets is about 4 –10 days.

10.5 B D E

All stem cells and precursor cells contain a nucleus. For red blood cells, the nucleus is lost in the final step in the maturation of reticulocyte into erythrocyte. Similarly, the nucleus is lost in the maturation of the megalokaryocyte into the platelet cell. Once the nucleus is lost in the erythrocyte and platelet cells, further division of the cell cannot take place, and their lifespan is limited. All white cells contain a nucleus.

10.6 B D

The erythrocytes are usually processed by the spleen before they are released into the circulation. Abnormal red cells may be destroyed by the spleen. For example, remnants of nuclear materials are removed, and red cells of abnormal shapes are removed. In the presence of impaired splenic function Howell–Jolly bodies which are remnants of nuclear materials may be present. Target cells with lack of central pallor may also be present. Impaired splenic function does not affect the size of the red cells. The haemoglobin concentration is also unaffected.

10.7 A D E

The proportion of cells in the blood is higher in men than women. Hence, the packed cell volume (haematocrit) and red cell count are higher in men than women. Since haemoglobin is found in red blood cells, the haemoglobin concentration is higher in men than in women. The normal haemoglobin level is between 13 and 16.5 g/dl for men, and between 11.5 and 15.5 g/dl for women. The mean corpuscular volume is a measure of the red cell size, and is obtained by dividing the haematocrit by the red cell concentration. The mean corpuscular haemoglobin is a measure of the amount of haemoglobin in a red blood cell, and is obtained by dividing the haemoglobin concentration by the red cell concentration. Both these values are the same in men and in women.

10.8 A E

Haemoglobin is the molecule responsible for carrying oxygen in the red blood cells. It is a globular molecule consisting of four subunits. Each subunit consists of a globulin chain (a polypeptide) and a haem group (which contains iron). There are two pairs of globulin chains in each haemoglobin molecule, each containing a different type of polypeptide. In normal adults, most of the haemoglobin is haemoglobin A, consisting of two α chains and two β chains.

10.9 C E

Haemoglobin in the fetus consists mainly of haemoglobin F. Each molecule of haemoglobin F contains two α chains and two γ chains. It binds less tightly to 2,3-DPG than adult haemoglobin. As a result, it holds on to oxygen more tightly, and facilitates the transfer of oxygen from mother to fetus via the placenta. Haemoglobin F level normally declines rapidly after birth, and almost disappears by three months of age. It may persist in certain types of haemoglobinopathies.

10.10 C E

Microcytes result from extra cell division during red cell production. Cell division is usually inhibited by the haemoglobin concentration in the cytoplasm. Hence iron deficiency and thalassaemia result in extra cell division and micocytes. Vitamin B_{12} or folate and folate are essential for nucleic acid synthesis. Hence, in vitamin B_{12} or folate deficiency, mitosis is defective. This gives rise to large red cells (macrocytes). Bone marrow failure results in normal-sized red cells (normocytic anaemia). In haemolysis, the rate of red cell destruction is increased, but the red cell size is usually normal.

10.11 C

Iron absorption takes place mainly in the duodenum and upper jejunum, whereas vitamin B_{12} is mostly absorbed in the terminal ileum. It is excreted both in the urinary and the gastrointestinal tract as desquamated cells. Over half of the body iron exists in the form of haemoglobin in red cells, and less than a third is stored in liver, spleen and bone marrow. Iron is normally stored mainly as ferritin (a water-soluble protein–iron complex), and only a small proportion as haemosiderin (an insoluble aggregate). When there is iron overload, a higher proportion is stored as haemosiderin. The control of total body iron is important. On the one hand, iron is essential for the production of red blood cells; on the other hand, excess iron in tissues may cause damage to the heart, liver and pancreas (as in haemochromatosis). However, the body has little control over its excretion of iron, and its control on absorption is limited. Hence the body is vulnerable to iron deficiency whenever there is increased loss of iron.

10.12 A C E

In iron deficiency anaemia, the blood picture is typically microcytic and hypochromic. The microcytic picture reflects a low MCV whilst the hypochromic picture reflects a low MCH level. The reticulocyte count is usually low for the level of anaemia. This is because the bone marrow does not have sufficient iron to synthesise haemoglobin. The serum iron and ferritin level are usually low, but the total iron-binding capacity is high. Normally, the transferrin is about a third saturated. In iron deficiency anaemia, the total iron-binding capacity increases due to a compensatory increase in transferrin concentration.

10.13 A C E

Vitamin B_{12} is essential for DNA synthesis, and deficiency may cause anaemia and neurological dysfunction (e.g. subacute combined degeneration of the spinal cord, dementia). Vitamin B_{12} is found mainly in food of animal origin, and is absent in fruit and vegetables. However, eggs and milk provide sufficient vitamin B_{12} to prevent deficiency state. Hence only strict vegetarians are at risk of dietary vitamin B_{12} deficiency. The liver normally stores sufficient vitamin B_{12} for several years. Hence symptoms of deficiency do not occur for several years. Vitamin B_{12} is absorbed in the terminal ileum, but it must be bound to intrinsic factor before it can be absorbed. Intrinsic factor is produced by parietal cells in the stomach.

10.14 A B C

Causes of vitamin B_{12} deficiency include lack of intrinsic factor, malabsorption from the terminal ileum and dietary deficiency in strict vegetarians. The causes for lack of intrinsic factor include Addisonian pernicious anaemia, congenital lack of intrinsic factor, and after surgical removal of the stomach (gastrectomy). Causes of malabsorption from the terminal ileum include ileal resection and Crohn's disease. Chronic gastrointestinal bleeding and pregnancy do not give rise to vitamin B_{12} deficiency because the diet usually contains many times the body daily requirements, and the body stores for vitamin B_{12} are extremely large.

10.15 A B E

Recognised indications for iron therapy include iron deficiency and anticipated increased demand for iron (e.g. during pregnancy or in premature babies). Iron should not be avoided in patients with haemolytic anaemia unless there is associated blood loss. This is because iron from the lysed red blood cells is still available and excess iron may result in haemosiderosis. This is especially true in thalassaemia, as patients often require blood transfusion and the risk of iron overload is high.

10.16 B C

Valid indications for intramuscular rather than oral iron therapy include consistent lack of patient compliance, past history of severe intolerable gastrointestinal side effects due to oral iron, and if iron cannot be absorbed from the gastrointestinal tract (e.g. after extensive small bowel resection). The response to intramuscular iron is not faster than that of oral iron. A haemoglobin level of 9 g/dl can usually be treated with oral iron. If the iron deficiency is severe or the patient develops serious symptoms due to anaemia, a blood transfusion should be given.

10.17 A B C

Vitamin B_{12} deficiency results in impaired DNA synthesis. This results in a reduction in mitosis, and affects all three cell lines. Anaemia, reduced white cell count and low platelets may all occur to some extent (i.e. pancytopenia). The red cells are typically large (i.e. high MCV index) due to lack of mitosis, and the neutrophils characteristically show nuclear hypersegmentation (multilobed nucleus). In an attempt to compensate for the pancytopenia, the bone marrow is hypercellular. The developing red cells in the bone marrow are large (megaloblastic).

10.18 A B D E

In pancytopenia, all three cell lines are involved. This may be due either to bone marrow failure or to impaired DNA synthesis. Causes of bone marrow failure include anti-neoplastic chemotherapy, ionising radiation to the bone marrow or bone marrow infiltration by carcinoma or leukaemia. Causes of impaired DNA synthesis include vitamin B_{12} or folate deficiency. Drug-induced haemolysis usually causes anaemia only.

10.19 A B D E

Red cell destruction is increased in haemolytic anaemia, and the red cell lifespan is reduced. Increased destruction may be due either to abnormalities of the red cells or to factors external to the red cells. Abnormalities of red cells which may lead to haemolysis include haemoglobinopathies (e.g. thalassaemia, sickle cell disease), enzyme defects (e.g. G6PD deficiency) and membrane defects (e.g. spherocytosis, elliptocytosis). Factors external to the red cells include antibodies (e.g. rhesus incompatibility, mismatched blood transfusion, drugs or toxins).

10.20 B C

In the presence of excessive red cell destruction, haemoglobin is broken down in the spleen to form haem and globin chains. The spleen therefore enlarges in haemolytic diseases. The haem is then broken down into unconjugated bilirubin. It circulates in the blood, and is then conjugated in the liver, and is excreted in the liver as urobilinogen. Serum haptoglobin binds to haemoglobin, and is therefore absent in the presence of excessive haemolysis. Red cell formation is increased in the bone marrow to compensate for the excessive destruction of red blood cells, and hence the number of reticulocytes increases.

10.21 C D

The commonest type of white cells are neutrophils, which normally constitute about 60% of white cells, and are essential for combating bacterial infections. Monocytes are the largest type of white cells, and are precursors of macrophages. Eosinophils combat parasite infections by producing leukotriene C_4 and platelet-activating factor. Both mast cells and basophils contain histamine and heparin. Mast cells have IgE receptors on their cell membranes, and are important in producing an immediate allergic response. T-lymphocytes are important for cellular immunity, whilst B-lymphocytes are important for humoral immunity. Plasma cells produce antibodies, and are developed from B-lymphocytes.

10.22 A B

In most types of leukaemia, neoplastic proliferation of the white blood cells precursors occurs. However, the precursors of platelets and red cells are also affected in some types of leukaemia (e.g. chronic granulocytic leukaemia). The normal cells in the bone marrow are replaced by leukaemic cells, and hence bone marrow failure occurs. This may give rise to pancytopenia. Infiltration of the liver, spleen and lymph nodes is common, and invasion of meninges and the gonads may also occur. In the early stages of leukaemia, the abnormal cells may remain in the bone marrow and may not be found in the peripheral blood.

10.23 A B D

Known predisposing factors for leukaemia include both genetic and environmental factors. Patients with Down's syndrome have an increased risk of acute leukaemia. Reciprocal translocation between chromosomes 22 and 9 (Philadelphia chromosome) occurs in 95% of cases of chronic granulocytic leukaemia. Known environmental predisposing factors include irradiation, alkylating agents, some chemicals (e.g. benzene) and certain viruses (e.g. human T-leukaemia virus). There is as yet no proven association between leukaemia and bacteria or air pollution.

10.24 C D E

Multiple myelomas are a malignant proliferation of plasma cells in the bone marrow. Plasma cells are developed from B-cells. In most cases, only a single clone of cells is involved, which results in the accumulation of a single type of immunoglobulin. The whole immunoglobulin cannot be excreted in urine as the molecule is too large to be filtered at the glomerulus. However, the light chain can pass through the glomerulus. The high concentration of immunoglobulin increases the blood viscosity, and the red blood cells often have a tendency to adhere to each other. Anaemia is common as a result of interference with the bone marrow function.

10.25 C D E

The lymph node is a kidney-shaped structure. Lymph enters the node via afferent lymphatics to enter the marginal sinus. Beneath the marginal sinus lies the cortex. The cortex contains follicles which are packed with B-lymphocytes. The paracortex lies deep to the cortex, and contains large T-cells responsible for cell-mediated immunity. Towards the hilum of the node are medullary cords which are rich in plasma cells and lymphocytes. The associated sinuses are lined by histiocytes. The lymph leaves the node via the efferent lymphatic at the hilum of the node.

10.26 B E

The main function of the lymphatic circulation is to return excess fluid in the interstitial space back to the systemic circulation. The normal volume of lymph circulated is about 3 litres per day. There are two types of lymphatic vessels. There are no valves or smooth muscles in the walls of the initial lymphatics. The initial lymphatics drain into collecting lymphatics which have valves and smooth muscles in their walls. Hence contraction of the muscles associated with the organ may facilitate its drainage in the collecting lymphatics. The fluid is finally returned to the venous system via the thoracic and right lymphatic ducts.

10.27 A B C D E

The lymph node reacts to a large variety of stimuli (e.g. infecting agents, foreign bodies, neoplasia) by node enlargement. Lymph node enlargement may be a localised response (e.g. to local infection) or a generalised response (e.g. autoimmune disorders, sarcoidosis, HIV infection or Epstein–Barr virus infection). In order to diagnose the precise cause for the enlargement, a lymph node biopsy is needed, and the histological features in different parts of the lymph nodes may give valuable information about the aetiology.

10.28 D

Hodgkin's disease is a type of lymphoma – malignancies arising from cells in the lymph nodes. There are two main types of lymphoma: Hodgkin's disease and non-Hodgkin's disease. Unlike non-Hodgkin's disease, Hodgkin's disease occurs more commonly between 30 and 50 years old and is rare in childhood or in old age. Hodgkin's disease is characterised by a large, pale, multilobed nucleus known as Reed–Sternberg cells. In Hodgkin's disease, the lymph node capsule is very seldom breached. Hence only a third of patients suffer from systemic symptoms, and the disease spreads predominantly via the lymphatics.

10.29 D E

The thymus gland is developed from the third and fourth pharyngeal pouches. Its absolute weight increases after birth until puberty, and then gradually atrophies. The thymus is important for the maturation of T-cells and induction of the cell-mediated immune response. In the congenital DiGeorge syndrome, there is defective development of the third and fourth pharyngeal pouches. As a result, immunodeficiency and absent parathyroid glands (which also develop from the third and fourth pharyngeal pouches) occur. Thymus abnormalities are also found in other forms of immunodeficiency.

Thymic hyperplasia is strongly associated with autoimmune thyroid disease, and thymoma (thymic neoplasia) is associated with a range of autoimmune diseases, including myasthenia gravis.

10.30 A C

The rate of platelet production is controlled by a type of colony-stimulating factor (granulocyte–macrophage colony-stimulating factor, or GM-CSF). Interleukin types 1, 3 and 6 (IL-1, IL-3, IL-6) increase the rate of conversion of uncommitted stem cells to committed platelet precursor. Thrombopoietin, which has recently been isolated, facilitates maturation of megakaryocytes. Erythropoietin increases the rate of red cell production. Platelets contain von Willebrand factor, which regulates the circulating levels of factor VIII.

10.31 B C D E

In response to small vessel injury, there are several intermediate steps of platelet aggregation. Firstly, platelets adhere to the exposed vessel wall. This initial step does not require any specific chemical activity. Platelets are then activated and produce ADP and thrombin. Activation may be brought about by binding to collagen or von Willebrand factor on the vessel wall. This causes release of platelet granules, which aggregate with other platelets. PAF is one of the many substances found in the platelets. It has inflammatory properties, and may increase platelet aggregation. This leads to a series of reactions resulting in the production of thromboxane A_2, which promotes vasoconstriction and further platelet aggregation.

10.32 A C E

Aspirin inhibits platelet function by inhibiting the synthesis of thromboxane and promoting the synthesis of prostacyclin. Dipyridamole inhibits the effect of platelets by reversibly inhibiting platelet phosphodiesterase, which in turn causes an increase in cAMP level. Ticlopidine acts by inhibiting the binding of fibrinogen to platelets. Warfarin interferes with the clotting mechanisms but has no effect on platelets. Disopyramide is an anti-arrhythmic agent.

10.33 A C D E

Anti-platelet agents are used to prevent further thrombi formation. Hence they are used in myocardial infarction, transient ischaemic attacks, unstable angina and peripheral vascular disease, especially following arterial graft surgery. There is a combination of clotting and platelet abnormalities in von Willebrand disease.

10.34 B E

The main function of the clotting mechanism is to convert the temporary clots formed by platelet aggregates into secure clots. There are two clotting systems (the intrinsic and extrinsic systems); both result in the conversion of soluble fibrinogen into insoluble fibrin with thrombin, and stabilised by cross-linkages to a tight aggregate. The conversion of fibrinogen into fibrin is catalysed by thrombin. The intrinsic system is activated when blood comes into contact with collagen fibres, or by the release of active factor XII. The extrinsic system is triggered by tissue thromboplastin, which is released in the presence of tissue damage.

10.35 A C D E

Natural vitamin K (K_1 and K_2) is fat-soluble, and bile is necessary for its absorption. Hence vitamin K deficiency may occur in long-standing obstructive jaundice or biliary fistula. Synthetic vitamin K (K_3) is water-soluble. Vitamin K is a cofactor for an enzyme responsible for metabolising glutamic acid residues in six of the clotting factors. Hence these clotting factors cannot be manufactured in the liver in the absence of vitamin K. Vitamin K deficiency may result in haemorrhage, especially in the gut. As the extrinsic system is mostly affected, the prothrombin time is characteristically prolonged in vitamin K deficiency.

10.36 C E

Warfarin is a competitive inhibitor of vitamin K. Since the synthesis of six of the clotting factors requires vitamin K, warfarin has anticoagulant properties which may be reversed by vitamin K. As warfarin affects mainly the extrinsic system, the prothrombin time is characteristically prolonged whilst the APTT is usually normal. The INR expresses the prothrombin time as a ratio of the control, and is usually used to monitor warfarin therapy. Warfarin is used to treat deep vein thrombosis, systemic or pulmonary embolism, and is occasionally used to prevent thrombosis in atrial fibrillation, transient ischaemic attack or valvular heart disease.

10.37 A C

To balance the clotting mechanism, there are in vivo body mechanisms to dissolve clots. The final pathway is to lyse fibrin. Several mechanisms are involved. Prostacyclin has an anti-aggregating effect which opposes the action of thromboxane A_2. Antithrombin III blocks the activity of clotting factors IX, X, XI and XII. Endothelial cells produce thrombomodulin. When thrombomodulin binds to thrombin, it activates protein C. This results in inactivation of factors VII and V, as well as increasing the effective concentration of t-PA. t-PA promotes the conversion of plasminogen into plasmin, which has the effect of lysing fibrin.

10.38 A C

Heparin acts mainly by making antithrombin III in the plasma more active. Antithrombin III acts as an inhibitor of thrombin and activated factor X. Heparin also acts by inhibiting platelet aggregation. As it affects the intrinsic system mostly, it is monitored by the APTT (or kaolin–cephalin clotting time). Heparin cannot be given orally as it is poorly absorbed from the gut. Its half-life is between 1 and 3 h, depending on the dose given. Hence the effect of heparin wears off rapidly. This may be an advantage over warfarin when the dose required is uncertain, or if anticoagulation is required before an operation, but is undesirable during surgery. In the unlikely event that the effect of heparin needs to be reversed quickly, protamine may be used.

10.39 A D E

Plasmin destroys fibrin. Hence drugs which promote the formation of plasmin will remove thrombi (i.e. fibrinolytics). Plasmin is converted from plasminogen in the blood. Drugs such as streptokinase and urokinase are plaminogen activators, and hence tend to remove thrombi. Alteplase is a tissue type plasminogen activator and favours binding of plasminogen to fibrin. Hence it also tends to remove thrombi. By contrast, tranexamic acid blocks the binding of plasminogen to fibrin, and aprotinin is an inhibitor of plasmin. Hence they tend to favour formation of clots (antifibrinolytics), and are used in the treatment of severe haemorrhage.

10.40 B D

Haemophilia A (classical haemophilia) is a sex-linked inherited disorder caused by factor VIII deficiency, whilst haemophilia B (Christmas disease) is due to factor IX deficiency. Hence, moderate or major bleeding in haemophilia should be treated with injection of factor VIII concentrate. In the past, patients receiving factor VIII ran the risk of contracting hepatitis B or HIV infection. This should no longer be the case as factor VIII is now synthesised using recombinant DNA technique. Tranexamic acid stabilises any temporary clots formed by platelet reactions, and may be a useful adjunct. DDAVP is given intravenously, and it increases factor VIII activity by about five times. It is useful in patients with mild or moderate deficiency of factor VIII.

11. The cardiovascular system
Questions

11.1 The following statements about cardiac muscle are correct:
- **A** There are no banding patterns in the sarcomere
- **B** The cardiac muscle fibres branch irregularly
- **C** T tubules are not present
- **D** Calcium ions are efficiently removed from the cytoplasm into the sarcoplasmic reticulum between contractions
- **E** The function of the intercalated discs includes rapid spread of contractile stimuli between cardiac muscle cells

11.2 The following statements about cardiac muscle are true:
- **A** Striations are absent
- **B** The muscle fibres branch and interdigitate
- **C** Gap junctions exist to allow impulses to travel from one cardiac fibre to another
- **D** It contains actin, myosin, troponin and tropomyosin
- **E** Over 25% of the energy is derived from anaerobic respiration

11.3 The sino-atrial (SA) node:
- **A** Is located at the junction of the superior vena cava and the right atrium
- **B** Contains the pacemaker cells
- **C** Is developed from the left side of the embryo
- **D** Is supplied by both the sympathetic and parasympathetic nervous system
- **E** Largely depends on influx of sodium ions for its action potential

11.4 The following statements about the SA node are true:
- **A** The cells in the SA node discharge spontaneously
- **B** Its impulse is slower than that of the atrioventricular (AV) node
- **C** Stimulation of the vagus nerve increases the rate of conduction through the SA node
- **D** Depolarisation spreads through the atria and converges directly on the Purkinje system
- **E** Disease affecting the SA node may lead to marked bradycardia

11.5 The following statements about the conduction of impulses from the SA node to the ventricles are true:

A The time taken is represented by the PR interval on the ECG
B It is slowed by adenosine
C Stimulation of the vagus nerve increases the rate of conduction
D Increased rate of conduction may result in supraventricular tachycardia
E Complete interruption of the conduction results in first-degree heart block

11.6 The following statements about atrial fibrillation are true:

A It may be due to multiple re-entrant excitation waves in the atria
B There are multiple P waves on the ECG
C The ventricular rate exceeds the atrial rate
D The ventricular rhythm is irregular
E The cause may be myocardial ischaemia

11.7 Cardiac actions of calcium channel blockers may include:

A Increased contractility
B Positive chronotropic effect
C Prolonging conduction in the AV node
D Reducing the refractory period in the AV node
E Terminating an attack of supraventricular tachycardia

11.8 Cardiac actions of cardiac glycosides (e.g. digoxin) may include:

A Stimulation of membrane adenosine triphosphatase (ATPase)
B Influx of calcium ions into cardiac cells
C Negative inotropic effect
D Enhancing vagal activity on the conducting system
E Abolishing atrial fibrillation

11.9 The following increase the heart rate in sinus rhythm:

A Atropine
B Propranolol
C Exercise
D Expiration
E Sleep

11.10 The following statements about ventricular systole are true:

A The tricuspid valve is closed during a large part of this cardiac cycle
B The pulmonary valve is closed during a large part of this cardic cycle
C It is followed by atrial systole
D It is indicated by the interval between the P and R waves on the ECG
E The left ventricular pressure remains below 50 mmHg

11.11 The following statements about the mitral valve are true:

A It is bicuspid
B It regulates the flow of blood from the right atrium to the right ventricle
C It lies posterior to the sternum at the level of the fourth left costal cartilage
D The associated papillary muscles are smaller than those of the tricuspid valves
E Its closure is associated with the second heart sound

11.12 The following statements about the left atrium are true:

A It forms the base of the heart
B It receives blood from the superior vena cava
C The pressure is significantly lower than that in the right atrium
D The blood is desaturated with oxygen
E A significant portion of the interior wall is smooth

11.13 Cardiac output:

A Is the amount pumped out of the left ventricle per unit time
B Is numerically the same as the stroke volume
C Can be calculated from the amount of oxygen consumed per unit time and the arteriovenous difference in oxygen level
D Can be estimated clinically using echocardiography and Doppler techniques
E May be increased by more than three-fold on exercise

11.14 The following increases cardiac output in a normal heart:

A Decrease in heart rate
B Increase in stroke volume
C Stimulation of the sympathetic nervous system
D Increase in end-diastolic volume
E Standing motionless

11.15 The following significant changes occur during exercise in a physically fit individual:

A Cardiac output increases
B Peripheral resistance increases
C Diastolic pressure increases
D The blood arterioles in the muscles dilate
E The venous return increases

11.16 Cardiac failure:

A Cannot occur if the cardiac output is over 5 litres per minute
B May be compensated for in the early stages by increased ventricular end-diastolic volume
C May be precipitated by severe anaemia
D May be associated with a decrease in cardiac output on exercise
E Often results in ventricular hypertrophy

11.17 Causes of predominantly left heart failure include:

A Acute myocardial infarct
B Severe aortic stenosis
C Systemic hypertension
D Chronic obstructive airway disease
E Cardiomyopathy

11.18 The following classes of drugs used in the treatment of cardiac failure and their mechanisms are correctly matched:

A Diuretics – reduction of afterload
B Nitrates – reduction in afterload
C Hydralazine – reduction of preload
D Cardiac glycosides – increased contractility of myocardium
E Angiotensin-converting enzyme (ACE) inhibitor – reduction of both preload and afterload

11.19 Consequences of cardiac failure include:

A Pulmonary oedema
B Enlarged liver
C Increased loss of sodium and water from the kidneys
D Increased pulmonary venous pressure
E Dilatation of left ventricle

11.20 The following statements about the arch of the aorta are true:

A It develops from the embryological sixth aortic arch on the left side
B The left recurrent laryngeal nerve hooks around it
C It is linked to the root of the left pulmonary artery by the ligamentum arteriosum
D It gives off the left coronary artery
E It gives off the left common carotid artery

11.21 The following statements about the pericardium are true:

A It encloses the heart and the roots of the great vessels
B The pericardial cavity is the space between the fibrous and serous pericardium
C The pericardial cavity normally contains a small quantity of clear fluid
D Inflammation of the pericardium may cause chest pain
E Extensive fluid in the pericardial cavity may restrict the movement of the heart and cause circulation failure

11.22 The arterioles:

A Contain a higher proportion of elastic tissue in their walls than the arteries
B Contain a higher proportion of smooth muscle in their walls than the arteries
C Contribute significantly to the total peripheral resistance

D Contribute significantly to the total blood capacitance
E Are constricted by noradrenaline

11.23 When other factors are kept constant, the arterial pressure increases with:
A An increase in cardiac output
B A decrease in peripheral resistance
C An increase in heart rate
D An increase in stroke volume
E Peripheral vasodilatation

11.24 The arterial blood pressure recorded is higher:
A In the arms than in the legs in the standing position on direct cannulation of the arteries
B The narrower the cuff used over the arm with the sphygmomanometer method
C In the arms than in the legs if the same cuff is used with the sphygmomanometer method in the lying position
D Using the auscultation rather than the palpation method with the sphygmomanometer
E If the mercury column is raised with the sphygmomanometer method

11.25 Clinical hypertension:
A Is universally defined as a blood pressure of 160/100 mmHg or above
B May be diagnosed with a single blood pressure reading of 160/100 mmHg
C Is more common with increasing age
D Is often caused by abnormally high peripheral resistance
E Is often caused by abnormally high cardiac output

11.26 Causes of secondary hypertension include:
A Chronic renal failure
B Addison's disease
C Aortic stenosis
D Corticosteroid therapy
E Acute glomerulonephritis

11.27 Patients with benign hypertension have increased risk for:
A Atherosclerosis
B Intracerebral haemorrhage
C Aortic dissection
D Subarachnoid haemorrhage
E Ischaemic heart disease

11.28 The following classes of antihypertensive drugs and their main mechanisms of action are appropriately matched:

A Calcium blockers – depletion of body sodium and reduction in plasma volume
B ACE inhibitors – reduction in peripheral resistance
C Nitrates – dilatation of capacitance vessels
D β-Adrenoceptor blockers – reduction in heart rate and myocardial contractility
E α-Adrenoceptor blockers – reduction in myocardial contractility

11.29 Atherosclerosis:

A Mainly affects arterioles
B Often begins as fatty streaks
C Is a major predisposing factor for ischaemic heart disease
D Predisposes to thrombi
E Predisposes to aneurysms

11.30 Factors associated with an increased risk of atherosclerosis include:

A Cigarette smoking
B Hypertension
C Female sex
D Raised HDL-cholesterol level
E Diabetes mellitus

11.31 The oxygen consumed by the heart per unit time decreases with increasing:

A Stroke volume
B Heart rate
C Arterial pressure (with constant cardiac output)
D Dilatation of the ventricles
E Sympathetic stimulation

11.32 Coronary blood flow normally increases with:

A Hypoxia
B Increased adenosine concentration
C Stimulation of α-adrenergic receptors
D Stimulation of β-adrenergic receptors
E Rising pH

11.33 Significant myocardial infarction is commonly caused by sudden obstruction of the following arteries:

A Right coronary artery
B Right marginal artery
C Diagonal artery
D Circumflex artery
E Left anterior descending artery

11.34 Causes of ischaemic symptoms of the heart include:

A Stenosis of the coronary artery
B Coronary artery thrombi
C Severe aortic stenosis
D Coronary artery spasm
E Pericarditis

11.35 In the presence of a thrombus in a branch of the coronary artery, the following increases the size of a myocardial infarct:

A The involvement of a major branch of the coronary artery
B The presence of extensive anastomosis within the coronary arterial circulation
C Administration of intravenous streptokinase within an hour of obstruction
D Immediate administration of oral aspirin
E Continuous exercise in spite of ischaemic symptoms

11.36 The following anti-anginal drugs act at least partially via the corresponding mechanism:

A Nitrates – dilatation of the venules
B Nitrates – dilatation of the coronary arteries
C β-Adrenergic blockers – dilatation of capacitance veins
D Calcium channel blockers – dilatation of the venules
E Calcium channel blockers – dilatation of the coronary arteries

11.37 The following changes may occur within 24–48 h of acute complete obstruction of the right coronary artery:

A Pallor and oedema of the right ventricle
B Increased white cell count
C ST elevation in leads II, III, and aVF in the ECG
D Q waves in leads II, III, and aVF in the ECG
E Development of granulation tissue in the right ventricle

11.38 The following statements about the capillary circulation are true:

A About 20% of the circulating blood is in the capillaries
B There is a net movement of fluid from the capillary circulation to the interstitial fluid in the intestines
C The hydrostatic pressure gradient across the arteriole end is higher than the venule end
D Over 80% of the filtered fluid in the capillaries is returned to the circulation via the lymphatic system
E The net pressure gradient across the wall of a capillary is similar at the arteriole and the venule end

11.39 There is a net diffusion of the following substances from the capillaries into the interstitial fluid:

A Oxygen
B Carbon dioxide
C Glucose
D Lactic acid
E Albumin

11.40 The following statements about the circulation of blood in the adult heart are true:

A Deoxygenated blood enters the right atrium via the superior vena cava
B Deoxygenated blood enters the left atrium via the inferior vena cava
C Deoxygenated blood is ejected into the lungs by the right ventricle via the pulmonary veins
D Deoxygenated blood enters the left atrium via the pulmonary veins
E Oxygenated blood is ejected into the aorta by the left ventricle

11.41 The following sites contain well-oxygenated blood in the normal adult:

A Pulmonary arteries
B Pulmonary veins
C Inferior vena cava
D Left atrium
E Right atrium

11.42 The following statements about the fate of most of the blood entering the fetal circulation from the placenta are true:

A It enters the fetus via the umbilical arteries
B It passes through the right atrium
C It passes through the right ventricle
D It passes through the pulmonary arteries
E It supplies the heart and the brain via the ascending aorta

11.43 The following statements about the fate of most of the deoxygenated blood returning from the head and neck of the fetus in the fetal circulation are true:

A It enters the right atrium via the inferior vena cava
B It passes through the right ventricle
C It passes through the pulmonary circulation
D It passes through the left ventricle
E It is returned to the placenta via the umbilical veins

11.44 Blood at the following sites is mostly well oxygenated in the fetal circulation:

A Superior vena cava
B Inferior vena cava

C Ascending aorta
D Descending aorta
E Pulmonary veins

11.45 The following sites in the adult cardiovascular system and their approximate normal systolic pressures are correctly matched:

A Right atrium – 50 mmHg
B Left atrium – 10 mmHg
C Right ventricle – 70 mmHg
D Left ventricle – 120 mmHg
E Pulmonary artery – 50 mmHg

11.46 The following events occur in congestive cardiac failure:

A The sympathetic nervous system is stimulated
B Aldosterone secretion is increased
C Reabsorption of sodium in renal tubules is reduced
D Glomerular filtration rate is increased
E Total body sodium is increased

11.47 Pulse character can be accurately and reliably assessed at the following sites:

A Radial pulse
B Brachial pulse
C Carotid pulse
D Femoral pulse
E Tibial pulse

11.48 A patient's hands are blue, but the lips and tongue are of normal colour. Possible causes include:

A Chronic obstructive airway disease
B Right-to-left shunting of blood
C Cold hands
D Raynaud's phenomenon
E Cyanotic congenital heart disease

11.49 The internal jugular vein:

A Is separated from the right atrium by one or more valves
B Is less reliable than the external jugular vein in assessing a patient's venous pressure
C Lies superficial to the clavicular head of the sternomastoid muscle
D Lies deep to the sternal head of the sternomastoid muscle
E Can be palpated with the patient lying at 45° to the horizontal

11.50 The following statements about the jugular venous pulse are true:

A It can be seen when a healthy subject is sitting upright
B It can be seen when a healthy subject lies horizontally
C Examination is made easier if the subject turns the head as far left as possible
D It may be undetected if the jugular venous pressure is extremely high
E The jugular venous pressure is proportional to the distance between the jugular venous pulse and the sternal angle

11.51 The following phases of the jugular venous pulse and their causes are correctly matched:

A 'a' wave – onset of ventricular systole
B 'c' wave – onset of atrial systole
C 'a–x' descent – atrial relaxation
D 'v–y' descent – emptying of blood from right atrium into right ventricle
C 'y–a' ascent – filling of the right atrium from the venae cavae

11.52 The following heart conditions and their associated jugular venous pulse abnormalities are correctly paired:

A Atrial fibrillation – prominent 'a' waves
B Complete heart block – cannon waves
C Superior vena caval obstruction – raised venous pressure with exaggerated pulsation
D Tricuspid stenosis – giant 'v' wave
E Tricuspid incompetence – slow 'v–y' descent

11.53 The apex beat:

A Is the point on the precordium where the cardiac impulse appears strongest
B Normally lies near the fifth left intercostal space
C Normally lies near the anterior axillary line
D Is detected by auscultation with the stethoscope
E May be displaced laterally in left ventricular enlargement

11.54 Cardiac thrills:

A Do not occur during diastole
B May occur in the absence of a cardiac murmur
C Are vibrations synchronous with certain phases of the cardiac cycle
D May occur in normal subject
E Indicate the presence of turbulent blood flow

11.55 The first heart sound:

A Is partly caused by the closure of the tricuspid valve
B Is partly caused by the closure of the pulmonary valve

C Is louder at the base than the apex of the heart
D Signals the end of ventricular systole
E Has a higher pitch than the second heart sound

11.56 The second heart sound:

A Is best heard with the bell than the diaphragm of the stethoscope
B Is louder at the base than the apex of the heart
C Is normally single on inspiration
D Occurs at the beginning of ventricular diastole
E Usually begins with the aortic component in physiological splitting

11.57 The following conditions and their associated abnormalities of the second heart sound are true:

A Aortic stenosis – soft aortic component
B Pulmonary hypertension – loud aortic component
C Right bundle branch block – wide splitting
D Left ventricular outflow obstruction – fixed splitting
E Pulmonary stenosis – reverse splitting

11.58 The cardiac murmurs due to the following cardiac lesions and their sites of radiation are correctly paired:

A Aortic stenosis – neck
B Aortic regurgitation – neck
C Mitral stenosis – apex of the heart
D Pulmonary regurgitation – right sternal border
E Ventricular septal defect – upper sternal edge

11. The cardiovascular system Answers

11.1 B E

Cardiac muscle fibres are similar to those of skeletal muscle in many ways. The arrangement of the contractile proteins is similar, and there are cross-striations in the cardiac muscle fibres. However, as the cardiac muscle fibres branch irregularly, the banding pattern is also irregular. T tubules and sarcoplasmic reticulum are present in cardiac muscle fibres. However, there is a slow leakage of calcium ions from the sarcoplasmic reticulum into the cytoplasm between contractions, and this accounts for the automaticity of cardiac contractions, and the inherent rhythm of the pacemaker tissues. Intercalated discs are specialised intercellular junctions between the ends of adjacent cardiac muscle cells. They allow rapid spread of contractile stimuli from one cardiac muscle cell to another, so that the cardiac muscle fibre functions as a syncytium.

11.2 B C D

Cardiac muscles are similar to skeletal muscles in many ways. Striations and Z lines are present. Although each fibre is enclosed in a cell membrane, the muscle fibres branch and interdigitate. The cell membranes at the ends of the muscle fibres form intercalated discs to maintain strong cell-to-cell cohesion, and gap junctions are formed in the cell membranes of adjacent fibres to allow electrical impulses to travel from one fibre to another. Like skeletal muscles, cardiac muscles contain actin, myosin, troponin and tropomyosin. The heart relies almost exclusively on oxidative phosphorylation for its energy supply, and the cardiac cells contain numerous mitochondria.

11.3 A B D

The SA node is located at the junction of the superior vena cava and the right atrium, and is developed from the right side of the embryo. Consequently, it is innervated by the right vagus nerve and the right side of the sympathetic innervation. The SA node contains the actual pacemaker cells (P cells). The pacemaking cells have membrane potentials which slowly drift to the threshold level after each impulse. The action potentials are largely due to influx of calcium ions through the slower-opening calcium channels, with little contribution from sodium ion influx.

11.4 A E

See also question 11.1. Due to the slow drift of the membrane potential to the firing level after each impulse, the cells in the SA node discharge spontaneously. Stimulation of the vagus nerve releases acetylcholine, which acts via the muscarinic receptors to slow the opening of the calcium channels, and hence to decrease the firing rate and slow its conduction rate. Conversely, noradrenaline stimulates the β_1-adrenergic receptors, increases the firing rate and speeds up its conduction rate. The depolarisation initiated from the SA node spreads through the atria and converges on the AV node, before it is conducted through the bundle of His to the Purkinje system. The spontaneous rate of conduction in the SA node is about 70 beats per minute, and is faster than any other location in the heart. Otherwise, the other locations may take over as pacemakers. Diseases affecting the SA node may lead to marked bradycardia as the rate of spontaneous discharge from the AV node is slower (about 45 beats per minute). This is known as the sick sinus syndrome, and patients may complain of dizziness and fainting.

11.5 A B D

The P and QRS complexes are due to atrial and ventricular contractions respectively. Hence the PR interval represents the time taken for the impulse to travel from the SA node to the ventricles. The rate of conduction is increased by sympathetic stimulation (via adrenaline) and reduced by parasympathetic stimulation (via acetylcholine). Increased rate of conduction may be seen in people with an additional abnormal conducting pathway (e.g. in Wolff–Parkinson–White syndrome). Supraventricular tachycardia (increased heart rate due to abnormality above the ventricles) results. Measures which reduce the rate of conduction (e.g. stimulation of vagus nerve, adenosine, calcium antagonist, disopyramide, digoxin) may alleviate the condition. Reduced rate of conduction results in heart block. If all the atrial impulses reach the ventricles, the PR interval is prolonged, and the condition is known as first-degree heart block. Second-degree heart block is said to occur if not all atrial impulses reach the ventricles. In third-degree (complete) heart block, the conduction of impulses is completely interrupted.

11.6 A D E

Atrial fibrillation is due to multiple circulating re-entrant excitation in the atria. This results in an irregular and fast atrial rate (up to 500 per minute). Hence the AV node also discharges at an irregular, but slower rate (about 90–150 beats per minutes). P waves cannot usually be detected on the ECG. There are many pathological causes for atrial fibrillation, which include myocardial ischaemia, stenosis of the mitral valve and thyrotoxicosis.

11.7 C E

Cardiac cells are dependent on calcium ions in two ways. Firstly, the pacemaker cells in the SA and AV nodes rely on the slow influx of calcium ions for their automaticity. Secondly, in phase two of the action potential in non-pacemaker cells, a fast influx of sodium ions is followed by a slow influx of calcium ions, which activate contraction of cardiac muscle. Hence calcium channel blockers have potentially two effects. Firstly, they slow the rate of discharge at the SA and AV nodes. Conduction at the AV node is slowed, and the refractory period is prolonged. Thus they are effective in the treatment of supraventricular tachycardia. Secondly, they depress contractility (i.e. they are a negative inotrope).

11.8 B D E

Cardiac glycosides act via two mechanisms. Firstly, they enhance the vagal activity. Hence they reduce conduction through the AV node and are beneficial in supraventricular tachycardia and atrial fibrillation. Secondly, they inhibit the membrane-bound ATPase. ATPase supplies energy for the pump which transports sodium out of and potassium into contracting cells. Hence, inhibition of the enzyme results in an increase in intracellular sodium and a reduction in intracellular potassium. This is accompanied by an increase in extracellular calcium, which accounts for the positive inotropic effect.

11.9 A C

The heart rate is controlled by both sympathetic and parasympathetic nerves to the heart, and the baroreceptor-mediated reflexes. The heart rate is increased during exercise through sympathetic stimulation, and is decreased during sleep through parasympathetic stimulation. Propranolol slows the heart rate through blockage of the β_1-adrengergic receptors, and atropine increases the heart rate by blocking the muscarinic receptors. The heart rate normally varies with the phases of respiration: it increases during inspiration and decreases during expiration. This is due to normal variations in the parasympathetic output to the heart during respiration. In inspiration, impulses from the vagus nerve are decreased.

11.10 A

Ventricular systole follows atrial systole. The mitral and tricuspid valves close at the beginning of ventricular systole. The aortic and pulmonary valves open soon afterwards with the isovolumetric contraction of the ventricles. The P and R waves mark the beginning of the atrial and ventricular systole respectively. During ventricular systole, the left ventricular pressure increases from less than 10 mmHg to about 120 mmHg in the middle of ventricular systole.

11.11 A C

The mitral valve regulates the flow of blood from the left atrium to the left ventricle, and lies posterior to the sternum at the apex of the heart (at the level of the fourth costal cartilage). Whilst the tricuspid valve has three cusps, the mitral valve has two. Since the work done by the left ventricle far exceeds that done by the right ventricle, the associated papillary muscles are much larger than those of the right ventricle. The first heart sound is caused by the vibrations set up by the sudden closure of the mitral valve (and the tricuspid valve to a lesser extent), whilst the second heart sound is associated with the closure of the aortic and pulmonary valves.

11.12 A E

The left atrium forms most of the base, as well as the superior part of the left border of the heart. It receives blood oxygenated during its passage in the lungs from four pulmonary veins. The pulmonary veins enter the left atrium in its posterior wall. Embryologically, a large proportion of the left atrium develops from the primitive pulmonary vein. Hence, a significant proportion of the interior of the left atrium is smooth, apart from the muscular ridges in the auricle.

11.13 A C D E

Cardiac output is the amount of blood pumped out of each ventricle per unit time, whilst the stroke volume is the amount of blood pumped out per beat. Hence cardiac output equals the product of the stroke volume and the heart rate. Traditionally, it may be measured by the Fick method or the indicator dilution method. In the Fick method, oxygen consumption per unit time is measured, and the difference in oxygen concentration in the arterial and venous blood is measured via a cardiac catheter. Cardiac output can be calculated from the equation

Cardiac output = Oxygen consumption per unit time/(Arterial oxygen concentration – Venous oxygen concentration)

In the indicator dilution method, a dye is injected into the vein, and the log of the arterial concentration of the dye is plotted against time. Cardiac output can be calculated from the amount of dye injected and the instantaneous concentration of the indicator in the arterial blood.
In clinical practice, cardiac output can be calculated more easily by estimating the velocity and volume of blood passing through heart valves. These parameters can be measured using echocardiography and Doppler techniques.

11.14 B C D

Cardiac output is equal to the product of heart rate and stroke volume. Hence either an increase in heart rate or an increase in stroke volume would result in an increase in cardiac output. Stimulation of the sympathetic nervous system results in an increase in both the stroke volume and the heart rate. According to Starling's law, the energy of contraction of a cardiac muscle fibre is proportional to its initial length (the preload). For the heart, the length of the muscle fibres is proportional to the end-diastolic volume. Hence the stroke volume increases with the ventricular end-diastolic volume. In the abnormal heart, however, the stroke volume may decrease with increasing ventricular end-diastolic volume above a certain threshold. The arterial pressure is equal to the product of the peripheral resistance and the cardiac output. Standing motionless increases venous pooling of the blood in the legs, and hence reduces the venous return. This reduces the end-diastolic volume and the stroke volume.

11.15 A D E

During exercise, cardiac output may increase up to seven-fold. This is brought about by an increase in both stroke volume and heart rate. The heart rate increases rapidly due to stimulation of the sympathetic nervous system, and the stimulatory effect of the increased carbon dioxide on the medulla. The enhanced activity of the muscle pumps increases the venous return, which contributes to the increase in cardiac output. The arterioles in the muscles dilate due to local mechanisms (fall in local oxygen, and increase in carbon dioxide and other metabolites). This greatly reduces the peripheral resistance. Hence, whilst the systolic pressure may rise slightly during exercise, the diastolic pressure remains constant or falls slightly.

11.16 B C D E

Cardiac failure is said to occur when the heart is unable to pump blood from the ventricles at a rate required for the metabolism of the body. This is often due to reduced capacity of the heart to pump blood (low output failure). However, it may also be caused by increased demands of the body for blood (e.g. in the presence of severe anaemia or pregnancy). Hence cardiac failure may occur in spite of a normal cardiac output, and the condition is known as high output failure. In the early stages of heart failure, the heart may pump sufficient blood by its compensating mechanisms (e.g. by increasing ventricular end-diastolic volume, according to Starling's law). However, in later stages, this may be ineffective, and cardiac output may decrease with an increase in ventricular end-diastolic volume on exercise. If the heart failure exists for some time, the heart may attempt to cope with the demand by ventricular hypertrophy. Ventricular dilatation may result from the extra workload. However, a consequence of the law of Laplace is that the tension in a distensible object to create a given pressure is proportional to its radius. Hence, even more work is needed from the dilated ventricles.

11.17 A B C E

Although the failure of one ventricle may result in the failure of the other, often only one ventricle is failing in the early stages. The commonest causes of left ventricular failure are ischaemic heart disease (e.g. acute myocardial infarct), systemic hypertension and valvular diseases. Ischaemic heart disease affects the ability of the heart to pump blood, whilst systemic hypertension and some valvular disease (e.g. aortic stenosis) provide extra workload on the ventricles. Cardiomyopathy represents cardiac diseases not caused by the above aetiologies or congenital heart diseases. Chronic obstructive airways disease may cause right heart failure.

11.18 D E

Drugs may relieve cardiac failure by reducing the venous return and ventricular filling pressure (preload), reducing the peripheral resistance (afterload), or increasing the contractility of the myocardium (positive inotropic effect). Diuretics increase salt and water loss from the body and reduce venous return. Hence their main mechanisms of action is to reduce preload. Nitrates dilate the smooth muscle of venous capacitance vessels and hence reduce the ventricular filling pressure. Hence, they also act by reducing preload. Hydralazine relaxes the arterial smooth muscle and reduces peripheral resistance. Hence it reduces afterload. ACE prevents the conversion of angiotensin I to the active component angiotensin II, which is a strong arterioconstrictor. This also prevents the formation of aldosterone, which promotes retention of sodium and water. Hence ACE inhibitor has the effect of reducing afterload (by reducing arterioconstriction) and preload (by reducing sodium and water retention). Cardiac glycosides (e.g. digoxin) stimulate cardiac contractility by inhibiting membrane-bound ATPase.

11.19 A B D E

Cardiac failure results in congestion of the pulmonary veins and an increase in pulmonary venous pressure. This results in pulmonary oedema, and patients often complain of breathlessness especially while lying flat, and at night. When the patient lies flat, there is increased venous return. The kidneys often attempt to compensate for cardiac failure by retaining sodium and fluid. As a result, there is widespread systemic venous congestion. The liver is often congested and enlarged. The ventricles may dilate, but this increases the workload of the heart further (see question 11.15).

11.20 B C E

The arch of the aorta is developed from the embryological fourth aortic arch on the left side. On the right side, the embryological fourth aortic arch becomes the proximal part of the right subclavian artery. The embryological sixth aortic arch becomes the ductus arteriosus, which joins the left pulmonary artery with the arch of the aorta. The left recurrent laryngeal nerve, which is the nerve of the sixth pharyngeal arch on the left side, hooks around the arch of the aorta and the ligamentum arteriosum. The coronary arteries are branches of the ascending aorta. The branches of the arch of aorta are the brachiocephalic artery (which divides to right common carotid and right subclavian arteries), left common carotid artery and left subclavian artery.

11.21 A C D E

The pericardium is a double-walled sac which encloses the heart and the roots of the great vessels. It consists of the fibrous and serous pericardium. The fibrous pericardium is inelastic. The serous pericardium consists of the parietal and the visceral layers. The visceral layer is the continuation of the external layer of the epicardium, the external layer of the heart wall. The pericardial cavity is the space between the visceral and parietal layers of the serous pericardium. It contains a small quantity of clear fluid which minimises friction during the cardiac cycle. Inflammation of the pericardium is called pericarditis, and is commonly caused by viral infection. The characteristic symptom is precordial pain. As the surfaces of the pericardium are rough, a friction rub may be heard with a stethoscope. Extensive fluid in the pericardial cavity may be caused by stab wounds to the heart causing the pericardial cavity to be filled with blood. This may seriously restrict the movement of the heart (cardiac tamponade) and cause circulation failure.

11.22 B C E

Compared to arterial walls, the arteriolar walls contain a lower proportion of elastic tissues but a higher proportion of smooth muscle. The smooth muscle is constricted by stimulation of the noradrenergic nerve fibres. Hence the arterioles contribute significantly to the total peripheral resistance, and a small change in the diameter of the vessels results in a large change in the peripheral resistance. The arterioles only contain about 1% of the blood volume. The major capacitor of blood is the venous system.

11.23 A C D

The arterial pressure is the product of cardiac output and peripheral resistance. Peripheral resistance decreases with vasodilatation. Hence the arterial pressure decreases with vasodilatation. Cardiac output is equal to the product of heart rate and stroke volume (the volume of blood pumped by the left ventricle per contraction). Hence an increase in the heart rate or stroke volume increases the arterial blood pressure in the absence of other regulatory mechanisms.

11.24 B D

The arterial pressure in any vessel becomes higher the lower the vessel is vertically. This is due to the effect of gravity. If the sphygmomanometer method is used, the recorded blood pressure would appear lower if the mercury column is raised. If a narrow cuff is used to measure blood pressure in an obese person, the fatty tissue dissipates some of the cuff pressure, and the recording would be abnormally high. For the same reason, the blood pressure recorded would be inappropriately high if the same cuff is used over the legs. The palpation method with the sphygmomanometer usually underestimates the blood pressure, as it is difficult to determine exactly when the first beat is felt.

11.25 C D

There is no universal definition of clinical hypertension, and it should not be diagnosed on a single blood pressure reading, as the high reading may be due to anxiety. Hypertension is more common with increasing age, and there is an inherited component. As blood pressure is equal to the product of cardiac output and peripheral resistance, increase of either cardiac output or peripheral resistance will cause an increase in arterial blood pressure. Clinically, however, sustained hypertension is almost always due to abnormally high peripheral resistance.

11.26 A D E

In over 90% of cases of hypertension, no obvious causes are found (i.e. essential hypertension). The known causes for hypertension include renal disease (e.g. chronic renal failure, acute glomerulonephritis, renal artery stenosis), endocrine diseases (e.g. Cushing's disease, Conn's syndrome with excessive aldosterone secretion), coarctation of the aorta and drug treatment (e.g. corticosteroid therapy). Aortic stenosis is associated with a narrow pulse pressure, but not arterial hypertension.

11.27 A B C D E

Although benign hypertension may be symptomless, patients are at risk of developing atherosclerosis and consequently ischaemic heart disease. Also, they have increased risk for intracerebral haemorrhage, aortic dissection and subarachnoid haemorrhage (from rupture of berry aneurysms). Hence benign hypertension is a serious condition needing prompt treatment.

11.28 B C D

Antihypertensives may act by depleting body sodium and reducing plasma volume (e.g. diuretics); reducing cardiac output by reducing heart rate and/or myocardial contractility (e.g. β-adrenergic blockers); reducing peripheral resistance by dilating arterioles (e.g. calcium blockers, ACE inhibitors); or dilating venous capacitance vessels to reduce venous return (e.g. nitrates, some calcium blockers).

11.29 B C D E

Atherosclerosis affects large and medium-sized arteries. Lesions often begin as fatty streaks. In those who are predisposed to arteriosclerosis, they may progress to fibrolipid plaques. Haemorrhage and thrombi may occur in the plaques. This may lead to total occlusion of the blood supply to important organs such as the coronary arteries.

11.30 A B E

Risk factors for increased atherosclerosis include increased age, hypertension, male sex, high LDL-cholesterol level, obesity and diabetes mellitus. Other less important factors include lack of exercise and low social class. A high level of HDL-cholesterol appears to protect against atherosclerosis.

11.31 –

The oxygen consumed by the heart is directly proportional to the work done by the heart. The work done by the heart is proportional to the product of the heart rate, the stroke volume, and the arterial pressure. By the law of Laplace, the tension in the wall of the heart to sustain a given pressure is proportional to its radius. Hence dilatation of the ventricles results in an increase in work done and oxygen consumed. Sympathetic stimulation results in an increase in stroke volume, heart rate and peripheral resistance. Hence the oxygen consumed is increased.

11.32 A B D

The heart is particularly susceptible to ischaemia, and it is particularly important to match coronary blood flow with the oxygen consumption by the heart. Coronary blood flow depends on three factors: the pressure gradient, chemical factors and neural factors. Probably several chemical factors are involved. Hypoxia, acidosis and an increase in lactic acid and adenosine cause coronary vasodilatation and consequent increased coronary blood flow. As these factors are normally associated with increased metabolic demand on the heart, a balance between supply and demand for oxygenation can be achieved. Neural factors include α-adrenergic receptors (stimulus of which causes coronary vasoconstriction) and β-adrenergic receptors (stimulation of which causes coronary vasodilatation).

11.33 A D E

Both the right and left coronary arteries arise from the ascending aorta just above the aortic valve. Obstruction of the right coronary artery results in inferior myocardial infarction. The right coronary artery gives off the right marginal artery at the inferior border of the heart, which supplies the right ventricle. Obstruction of this branch is unlikely to result in significant myocardial infarct. The most important branch of the right coronary artery is the posterior descending artery, which supplies both ventricles. The left coronary artery has two major branches: the left anterior descending artery, which supplies both ventricles and the interventricular septum, and the circumflex branch, which supplies the left atrium and left ventricle. Obstruction of the left anterior descending artery results in anterior infarction, whilst obstruction of the circumflex artery results in lateral infarction.

11.34 A B C D

Most ischaemic symptoms of the heart are caused by atherosclerosis, either via stenosis of the coronary artery or atherosclerosis with superimposed thrombi. Occasionally, angina symptoms may be experienced by those with no minimal atherosclerosis, and their symptoms may be due to coronary artery spasm. Rarely, severe aortic stenosis may cause ischaemic symptoms by impairing coronary blood flow. Whilst pericarditis may cause precordial pain, the pain is secondary to inflammation and not ischaemia.

11.35 A E

The size of a myocardial infarct is likely to be significant if a major branch of the coronary artery is obstructed, the degree of obstruction is large, and there is a lack of anastomosis between the obstructed artery with the rest of the coronary circulation. Administration of intravenous streptokinase and oral aspirin immediately after a myocardial infarct has been proven to reduce the size of the infarct. Continuous exercise in spite of ischaemic symptoms increases the oxygen demand of the heart, and is liable to increase the size of the infarct.

11.36 A B E

The three established classes of anti-anginal drugs are organic nitrates, β-adrenergic blockers and calcium channel blockers. Organic nitrates act mainly by dilating the capacitance veins (hence reducing the preload) and dilating the main coronary arteries. The β-adrenergic blockers block the β-adrenergic receptors, and hence slow the heart rate, reduce the mechanical contractility of the heart and reduce the peripheral resistance. Calcium channel blockers act by dilating the arterioles (hence reducing the peripheral resistance), dilating the coronary arteries and reducing the contractility of the heart.

11.37 A B C

The histological changes of myocardial infarcts follow a predictable sequence. No changes are usually seen in the first 18 h. Acute inflammatory response occurs between the first and second day. Necrosis occurs between the third and fourth day. Granulation tissue starts to develop after the first week and fibrosis occurs after about two weeks of infarct. Between the first 24–48 h the affected cardiac muscle may appear pale and oedematous and acute inflammatory changes may be seen microscopically. This may be associated with a transient increase in white cell count. The immediate ECG changes are ST elevation due to delayed depolarisation of the infarcted cells. Q waves are due to failure of the infarcted cardiac muscles to contribute to the positivity of the QRS complex, and usually appear at least a few days later.

11.38 C

Although less than 5% of the circulating blood is in the capillaries, the capillary circulation plays an important role in the delivery of oxygen and nutrients to the tissue, as well as the removal of carbon dioxide and other waste products from the tissue. Capillary hydrostatic pressures differ according to the tissues, but capillary pressures at the arteriole and venule end are typically about 30 and 15 mmHg respectively. The osmotic pressure gradient across the capillary wall is roughly constant along the capillary. The rate of filtration along any point along the capillary depends on the balance of hydrostatic and osmotic pressure gradients (Starling forces), and differs according to the tissues. For example, fluid moves out of the capillaries along almost their entire length in the renal glomerulus, but into the capillaries along almost their entire length in the intestines. Over 80% of the filtered fluid in the capillaries is returned to the circulation via reabsorption and the rest via the lymphatics.

11.39 A C

See question 11.38 above. Albumin molecules are too large to diffuse across the capillary wall.

11.40 A E

The pathway for circulation of blood in the adult heart is as follows:

- Deoxygenated blood enters the right atrium via the superior and inferior vena cava
- Deoxygenated blood enters the right ventricle from the right atrium
- Deoxygenated blood is ejected to the lungs by the right ventricle via the pulmonary arteries
- Oxygenated blood is returned from the lungs to the left atrium via the pulmonary veins
- Oxygenated blood enters the left ventricle from the left atrium
- Oxygenated blood is ejected into the aorta by the left ventricle

11.41 B D

Deoxygenated blood from the body returns to the heart via the superior and inferior vena cava. It enters the right atrium and is directed to the right ventricle via the tricuspid valve. It is ejected by the right ventricle through the pulmonary valve into the pulmonary arteries, where it enters the lung capillaries to be reoxygenated. The oxygenated blood leaves the lung via the pulmonary veins and enters the left atrium, where it is directed to the left ventricle through the mitral valve. The oxygenated blood is then ejected by the left ventricle through the aortic valve into the aorta.

11.42 B E

The correct pathways for the flow of oxygenated blood entering the fetal circulation from the placenta are:

- Blood enters through the umbilical veins towards the liver
- Blood flows directly through the ductus venosus into the inferior vena cava, bypassing the liver
- Blood enters the right atrium
- Blood is shunted across the left atrium through the foramen ovale
- Blood enters the left ventricle
- Blood is ejected into the ascending aorta, and supplies the brain and heart

11.43 B

The correct pathways for the flow of deoxygenated blood returned from the fetal head and neck are:

- Blood enters the right atrium via the superior vena cava
- Blood enters the right ventricle via the tricuspid valve
- Blood enters the pulmonary artery, and is shunted across to the descending aorta via the ductus arteriosus
- Blood is returned to the placenta via the umbilical arteries

11.44 B C

See questions 11.42 and 11.43 above for the pathways of the oxygenated and deoxygenated blood. Oxygenated blood mixes with deoxygenated blood at several sites: the inferior vena cava, the right atrium, the left atrium, and at the entrance of the ductus arteriosus into the descending aorta. However, blood in the inferior vena cava and ascending aorta are mostly well oxygenated, whilst blood in the superior vena cava, pulmonary veins and descending aorta are mostly deoxygenated.

11.45 B D

It is important to note the following general points about systolic pressure:

- The ventricles have much higher systolic pressure than the corresponding atria
- The right ventricle and pulmonary arteries have equal systolic pressures
- The left ventricle and the aorta have equal systolic pressures
- The left side of the heart has much higher systolic pressure than the right

The approximate normal systolic pressures are:

- Right atrium – 8 mmHg
- Right ventricle (= pulmonary artery) – 25 mmHg
- Left atrium – 10 mmHg
- Left ventricle (= aorta) – 120 mmHg

11.46 A B E

The usual primary cause of cardiac failure is reduced myocardial contractility. This causes reduced effective arterial blood volume. In order to maintain the blood pressure, both the sympathetic nervous system and the renin–angiotensin system are stimulated. The stimulation of the sympathetic nervous system explains why sweatiness and tachycardia are common in cardiac failure. The activation of the sympathetic nervous system and renin–angiotensin system results in renal vasoconstriction, reduction in glomerular filtration rate, and increased tubular reabsorption of sodium and water. Increased secretion of aldosterone also increases tubular reabsorption of sodium and water. Hence the urinary excretion of sodium and water is reduced, and oedema results.

11.47 B C D

Whilst most peripheral pulses can be used to assess the pulse rate and rhythm, the pulse character (e.g. volume, the rate of rise and decline) is best assessed at an accessible large artery close to the heart. At a small peripheral artery far away from the heart, the pulse may be 'damped'. Clinically, the brachial, carotid and femoral pulses are the best sites for assessing pulse character.

11.48 C D

Central cyanosis causes blue lips and tongue, and is due to a reduction in the oxygen saturation of arterial blood. Central cyanosis may be caused by heart or lung diseases. Blue hands and feet may be due to either central cyanosis or poor circulation to the limbs. If a patient's hands were blue, but the lips and tongue were of normal colour, the cause cannot be central cyanosis, but due to poor circulation to the limbs (peripheral cyanosis). Causes include cold weather, Raynaud's phenomenon or a low cardiac output.

11.49 D

Blood from the internal jugular vein enters the right atrium via the superior vena cava without passing through any valves. This is why the jugular venous pulse gives valuable information about the haemodynamics of the right atrium. The internal jugular vein is more reliable than the external jugular vein in this respect, as the latter may be kinked. The internal jugular vein lies deep to both the sternal and clavicular heads of the sternomastoid muscle. Hence, examination of the jugular venous pulse is easier if the neck muscles are relaxed. Unlike arterial pulses, venous pulses cannot be palpated. They can only be seen.

11.50 D

The jugular venous pressure is the *vertical height* (in centimetres) of the jugular venous pulse from the sternal angle. In a healthy subject, the jugular venous pressure is less than 2 cm. Hence the venous pressure would not be visible in the upright position. If a healthy subject were to lie horizontally, the internal jugular vein would be completely extended, and the jugular venous pulse could not be seen. Hence the pulse is examined with the subject lying at 45° to the horizontal. The subject should be examined with the head turned slightly to the left. Turning the head as far as possible to the left would tense the right sternomastoid muscle and obscure the jugular venous pulse. If the jugular venous pressure is extremely high, the jugular venous pulse may be above the level of the earlobe and therefore could not be seen.

11.51 C D E

The jugular venous pulse mainly reflects the haemodynamics in the right atrium. The correct causes for the phases of the jugular venous pressures are:

- 'a' wave – atrial systole
- 'c' wave – transmission of pressure to atrium from onset of ventricular systole
- 'a–x' descent – atrial relaxation
- 'x–v' ascent – filling of blood from venae cavae
- 'v–y' descent – emptying of blood from right atrium into right ventricle
- 'y–a' ascent – filling of blood from venae cavae until next cycle begins

11.52 B

The correct associations between the heart conditions and their associated jugular venous pulse abnormalities are:

- Atrial fibrillation – absent 'a' waves (due to ineffective atrial contractions)
- Complete heart block – cannon waves (due to occasional contraction of the right atrium against a closed tricuspid valve)
- Superior vena caval obstruction – raised venous pressure with little or no pulsation
- Tricuspid stenosis – slow 'v–y' descent (slow emptying of blood from right atrium into right ventricle)
- Tricuspid incompetence – giant 'v' wave

11.53 B E

The apex beat is defined as the furthest point laterally and inferiorly on the left side of the precordium at which a cardiac impulse is palpable. In healthy subjects, the apex beat lies at the left fifth intercostal space on the mid-clavicular line. A laterally displaced apex beat may be due to left ventricular enlargement, or a right-sided space-occupying lesion (e.g. right-sided pneumothorax).

11.54 C E

Cardiac thrills are palpable vibrations synchronous with certain phases of the cardiac cycle. Like cardiac murmurs, they are caused by turbulent blood flow. In fact, cardiac thrills can be regarded as murmurs which are so loud that they are palpable. Whilst soft systolic murmurs may be innocent, cardiac thrills are always pathological.

11.55 A

The first heart sound occurs at the beginning of the ventricular systole, and is caused by the closure of the mitral and the tricuspid valves. Hence it is louder at the apex of the heart. The first heart sound has a lower pitch and a longer duration than the second because the mitral and tricuspid valves close more gradually than the pulmonary and aortic valves.

11.56 B D E

The second heart sound is caused by the brisk closure of the aortic and pulmonary valves at the end of diastole. Hence it is better heard at the base than the apex of the heart. Since it has a high pitch, it is best heard with the diaphragm of the stethoscope, as the diaphragm filters out low-pitched sounds and helps to identify the high-pitched sounds. Closure of the aortic valve usually precedes the pulmonary valve. As the difference is more pronounced in inspiration than expiration, the second heart sound usually appears single on expiration, but is split during inspiration.

11.57 A C

The types of second heart sound abnormalities can be deduced by the facts that closure of the aortic heart valve usually precedes the pulmonary valve, and that the difference is more pronounced in inspiration than expiration. The correct types of second heart sound abnormalities are:

- Aortic stenosis – soft aortic component
- Pulmonary hypertension – loud pulmonary component
- Right bundle branch block – wide splitting (as the pulmonary component is delayed)
- Left ventricular outflow obstruction – reverse splitting
- Pulmonary stenosis – wide splitting

(Fixed splitting occurs in atrial septal defect as the pressure of left and right atria is equal throughout the cardiac cycle.)

11.58 A C

If one remembers that murmurs radiate in the direction of the blood flow which causes the murmur, then the sites of radiation of murmur can be deduced. The sites of radiation are:

- Aortic stenosis – upper right sternal edge and neck
- Aortic regurgitation – down left sternal edge
- Mitral stenosis – apex of the heart
- Pulmonary regurgitation – left sternal border
- Ventricular septal defect – lower sternal edge

12. The respiratory system
Questions

12.1 The following are present in the respiratory bronchioles:

A Cartilage
B Cilia
C Smooth muscle
D Muscarinic receptors
E β-Adrenergic receptors

12.2 Gas exchange may occur across the walls of:

A The alveoli
B The bronchi
C The respiratory bronchioles
D The acini
E The terminal bronchioles

12.3 Surfactant:

A Is secreted by type I pneumocytes in the alveoli
B Increases the surface tension of the fluid lining the alveoli
C Increases the compliance of the lungs
D Increases the work of breathing
E Is a carbohydrate

12.4 The right main bronchus:

A Is wider than the left main bronchus
B Is longer than the left main bronchus
C Divides into two secondary bronchi
D Is more likely to be entered into by a foreign body than the left main bronchus
E Is circulated by a complete ring of cartilage

12.5 The following statements about lung volumes are true:

- **A** The vital capacity is the amount of air that moves into the lungs on maximal inspiration after maximal expiratory effort
- **B** The residual volume is the volume of air in the lungs at the end of passive expiration
- **C** The tidal volume is the amount of air that moves into the lungs on maximal inspiratory effort after passive expiration
- **D** The expiratory reserve volume is the amount of air left in the lungs after passive expiration
- **E** The inspiratory reserve volume is the amount of air that moves into the lungs on maximal inspiratory effort after normal inspiration

12.6 The following statements about respiratory dead spaces are true:

- **A** The anatomical dead space never exceeds the physiological dead space
- **B** The anatomical dead space may be significantly increased by pulmonary emboli
- **C** The physiological dead space may be significantly increased by pulmonary emboli
- **D** The anatomical dead space may be significantly increased by breathing through a long tube
- **E** The physiological dead space may be significantly increased by breathing through a long tube

12.7 The following statements about lung ventilation and perfusion are true:

- **A** Perfusion at the apices of the lungs is higher than at the bases of upright normal lungs
- **B** Ventilation at the apices of the lungs is higher than at the bases of upright normal lungs
- **C** The ventilation/perfusion ratio at the apices is higher than at the bases of upright normal lungs
- **D** Cyanosis may result if there is widespread ventilation–perfusion mismatch
- **E** A reduced level of carbon dioxide in the blood may result from widespread ventilation–perfusion mismatch

12.8 The following parameters of respiratory function tests are significantly lower than normal in fibrosis of the lungs:

- **A** Peak expiratory flow rate
- **B** Forced expiratory volume in 1 s (FEV_1)
- **C** Vital capacity (VC)
- **D** Forced expiratory ratio (FEV_1/VC)
- **E** Carbon monoxide transfer (T_{CO})

12.9 The following parameters of respiratory function tests are significantly lower than normal in bronchial asthma:

A Peak expiratory flow rate
B FEV_1
C VC
D FEV_1/VC
E T_{CO}

12.10 The following statements about haemoglobin are true:

A It is a globular protein
B It consists of six subunits
C There is one haem moiety per haemoglobin molecule
D The haem moiety contains ferric iron (Fe^{3+})
E In normal human adults, all haemoglobin molecules are of the same type

12.11 The following statements about the reaction of haemoglobin and oxygen are true:

A Haemoglobin increases the oxygen-carrying capacity of the blood by about two-fold
B The globin molecules bind to the oxygen molecules
C Each haemoglobin molecule is capable of binding up to four oxygen molecules
D Binding of the haemoglobin with the first oxygen molecule reduces the affinity for binding to a second oxygen molecule
E Binding to an oxygen molecule increases the likelihood of the haem moieties assuming a tense (T) state

12.12 When the oxygen–haemoglobin dissociation curve is shifted to the right:

A A higher partial pressure of oxygen is required for haemoglobin to bind to a given amount of oxygen
B It becomes easier to oxygenate the blood in the pulmonary capillaries
C The oxygen saturation of haemoglobin is higher for a given partial pressure of oxygen
D It becomes easier for the blood in the capillaries to deliver oxygen to the tissues
E It is almost always clinically undesirable

12.13 The following factors shift the oxygen–haemoglobin dissociation curve to the right:

A Increase in temperature
B Increase in pH
C Increase in (2,3-DPG) 2,3-diphosphoglycerate
D Living at high altitude
E Exercise

12.14 Myoglobin:

- **A** Is mainly found in skeletal muscles
- **B** Can bind up to four oxygen molecules per molecule of myoglobin
- **C** Has a sigmoid oxygen–haemoglobin dissociation curve
- **D** Has an oxygen dissociation curve to the right of the haemoglobin curve
- **E** Can easily deliver oxygen to haemoglobin in the blood

12.15 The following statements about the transport of carbon dioxide in blood are true:

- **A** A higher proportion of oxygen than carbon dioxide is dissolved in the plasma
- **B** Most of the carbon dioxide is transported by forming carbamino compounds with haemoglobin
- **C** Oxygenated blood carries more carbon dioxide than deoxygenated blood
- **D** Carbonic anhydrase facilitates the formation of carbamino-haemoglobin
- **E** The role of the red blood cells in carbon dioxide transport is insignificant

12.16 Compared to the red blood cells in the arterial blood, those in the venous blood:

- **A** Contain more bicarbonate ions
- **B** Contain more chloride ions
- **C** Contain more hydrogen ions
- **D** Contain more oxygen
- **E** Are larger

12.17 The following may occur in the airways of patients with extrinsic asthma:

- **A** The bronchi are hyperreactive to common stimuli
- **B** Excessive histamine is released from mast cells
- **C** Oedema occurs in the mucosa of the bronchioles
- **D** There is excessive mucus secretion from the bronchioles
- **E** An excess of IgM is produced

12.18 The following types of drugs are useful in the treatment or prevention of asthma owing at least partly to the mechanism stated:

- **A** Corticosteroids – reduction in bronchial hyperreactivity
- **B** Sodium cromoglycate – prevents the release of mediators from mast cells
- **C** β_1-Adrenoceptor agonists – dilate narrowed bronchioles
- **D** Methylxanthines (e.g. theophylline) – adenosine agonists
- **E** Antimuscarinic agents (e.g. ipratropium) – reduction in bronchial hyperreactivity

12.19 The following statements about neural control of breathing are true:

A The neural control of respiration always overrides chemical control mechanisms
B The neural system for voluntary control of respiration is located at the pons
C The neural system for automatic control of respiration is located at the medulla oblongata
D The expiratory and inspiratory muscles are generally reciprocally innervated
E Diseases which interfere with the automatic control of respiration always disrupt voluntary control as well

12.20 The following changes will result in a significant increase in respiratory minute volume in a normal subject under normal conditions:

A Decrease in arterial pH from 7.31 to 7.15
B Increase in inspired carbon dioxide level by 20%
C Decrease in inspired carbon dioxide level by 20%
D Increase in inspired oxygen by 20%
E Decrease in inspired oxygen by 20%

12.21 The following factors significantly contribute to the increase of ventilation rate immediately before and during vigorous exercise:

A Psychic stimuli
B Afferent impulses from muscle and joint proprioceptors
C Reduced sensitivity of chemoreceptors to carbon dioxide
D Fluctuations in arterial carbon dioxide level
E Increased production of lactic acid

12.22 Causes of oxygen deficiency at the tissue level include:

A Ventilation–perfusion mismatch
B Anaemia
C Carbon monoxide poisoning
D Stagnation at the tissue
E Cyanide poisoning

12.23 Respiratory failure may result from:

A Severe muscle diseases
B Lung fibrosis
C Ventilation–perfusion mismatch
D Shunt of blood from the venous to the arterial circulation through a defect in the ventricular septum
E Severe kyphoscoliosis (abnormal curvature of the spine)

12.24 Significant clinical improvement can be expected from administering 100% oxygen for hypoxia due to the following conditions:

A Shunting of blood from the venous to the arterial circulation due to congenital abnormalities of the heart
B Severe chronic obstructive airway disease with chronic carbon dioxide retention
C Acute asthmatic attack
D Fibrosis of the lung
E Pneumonia

12.25 The long-term consequences of reduced ventilation may include an increase in:

A Arterial partial pressure of oxygen
B Arterial partial pressure of carbon dioxide
C Plasma pH
D Plasma HCO_3^-
E Renal reabsorption of HCO_3^-

12.26 The following statements about chronic respiratory alkalosis are true:

A Loss of acid by vomiting is a cause
B Hysterical hyperventilation is a cause
C The arterial partial pressure of CO_2 is characteristically raised
D The plasma pH is characteristically raised
E The plasma HCO^- is characteristically raised

12.27 The following statements about cough are true:

A It is usually initiated by irritation of the lining of the trachea or larynx
B It is usually preceded by a deep inspiration
C Expiration is forced against a closed glottis
D It is important in expelling foreign bodies from the respiratory tract
E It always serves a useful purpose

12.28 The following statements about neural control of cough are true:

A It is under substantial voluntary control
B Stimuli to the trachea or larynx are the main afferent inputs of the cough reflex
C The main centre for the autonomic control of the cough reflex is located in the pons
D The cough centre in the brain stem receives inputs from the cerebral cortex
E Increased partial pressure of carbon dioxide in the arterial blood stimulates the cough reflex

12.29 The following measures may be effective in relieving cough:

- **A** Ceasing smoking
- **B** Staying in a dry atmosphere
- **C** Oral administration of a thick syrup with no active pharmacological ingredient
- **D** Oral codeine
- **E** Water inhalation as an aerosol

12.30 Potential sources of pulmonary emboli include thrombi from:

- **A** The leg veins
- **B** The pulmonary veins
- **C** The pelvic veins
- **D** The femoral arteries
- **E** The brachial arteries

12.31 Significant risk factors for pulmonary embolism include:

- **A** Frequent physical exercise
- **B** Pregnancy
- **C** Taking oral contraceptive pills
- **D** High cholesterol level
- **E** Recovery from a major operation

12.32 Possible sequelae of pulmonary emboli include:

- **A** Pulmonary infarct of a lung segment
- **B** Pulmonary hypertension
- **C** Arterial hypertension
- **D** Pulmonary oedema
- **E** Sudden death

12.33 Causes of pulmonary arterial hypertension include:

- **A** Pulmonary emboli
- **B** Chronic obstructive airway disease
- **C** Myocardial infarction
- **D** Mitral stenosis
- **E** Ventricular septal defect

12.34 Causes of pulmonary oedema include:

- **A** Left ventricular failure
- **B** Mitral stenosis
- **C** Low plasma albumin level
- **D** Pulmonary stenosis
- **E** Bronchial carcinoma

12.35 The following muscles are active during forced inspiration:

- **A** The diaphragm
- **B** Internal intercostal muscles
- **C** External intercostal muscles
- **D** Sternocleidomastoid muscles
- **E** Anterior abdominal wall muscles

12.36 The following statements about emphysema are true:

- **A** The disease is usually localised to a few bronchopulmonary segments of the lungs
- **B** It is defined clinically as productive cough for three months in two consecutive years
- **C** The air spaces distal to the terminal bronchioles are permanently enlarged
- **D** The elastin in the walls of the airspaces is thickened
- **E** It occurs much more commonly in people with α1-antitrypsin deficiency

12.37 Risk factors for bronchial carcinoma include:

- **A** Passive cigarette smoke
- **B** Exposure to asbestos
- **C** Excess alcohol intake
- **D** Increased exposure to radon
- **E** Low-fibre diet

12.38 The following statements about an open pneumothorax are true:

- **A** Air is accumulated between the layers of parietal pleura and visceral pleura
- **B** It may result from penetrating wound to the parietal pleura
- **C** The lung on the affected side expands
- **D** The intrapleural pressure on the affected side is lower than the other side
- **E** Air enters the pleural cavity during expiration

12.39 Squamous cell bronchial carcinomas:

- **A** Are usually peripheral
- **B** Arise from squamous metaplasia
- **C** Metastasise early to distant sites
- **D** Usually secrete ectopic ADH
- **E** Are the commonest histological type of bronchial carcinoma

12.40 The vocal folds:

- **A** Are wide open during speech production
- **B** Are longer in females than in males
- **C** Are adducted by the posterior cricoarytenoid muscles
- **D** Are paralysed when the recurrent laryngeal nerves are damaged
- **E** Are controlled by the actions of the extrinsic laryngeal muscles

12.41 The trachea is palpable:

- **A** Above the hyoid bone
- **B** Above the suprasternoid notch
- **C** Throughout its entire course
- **D** In all subjects
- **E** Only on swallowing

12.42 The following lesions cause deviation of the trachea to the opposite side:

- **A** Lymphoma in the mediastinum
- **B** Collapse of the upper lobe of the lung
- **C** Enlarged thyroid gland
- **D** Fibrosis of the upper lobe of the lung
- **E** Asthma

12.43 The following observations in the adult may suggest respiratory diseases:

- **A** The anteroposterior diameter of the chest measures half that the lateral diameter
- **B** A respiratory rate of 15 breaths per minute
- **C** Maximum chest expansion of about 2 cm
- **D** Contraction of sternomastoid and scaleni muscles on normal inspiration
- **E** Pursed lips on expiration

12.44 Causes of dullness to percussion over an area of the lung field include:

- **A** Pulmonary collapse
- **B** Pulmonary effusion
- **C** Pneumothorax
- **D** Pulmonary emphysema
- **E** Pulmonary consolidation

12.45 Bronchial breath sounds:

- **A** Resemble sounds produced at the larynx
- **B** Indicate that the relevant major bronchus is completely obstructed
- **C** May be heard even when the vocal resonance is reduced
- **D** Are usually heard more loudly during inspiration than expiration
- **E** Are continuous between the end of inspiration and the beginning of expiration

12 The respiratory system
Answers

12.1 B C D E

Cartilage protects against collapse of the respiratory passages, and is present in the walls of the trachea and bronchi only. Cilia are present from the trachea down to the respiratory bronchioles, and are important in protecting the lungs from microorganisms. Smooth muscle is present in all the bronchioles. Contraction of the smooth muscle results in bronchospasm and wheezing. The epithelium of both the bronchi and bronchioles is innervated by both muscarinic receptors and β_2-receptors, which mediate bronchoconstriction and bronchodilation respectively. This is important clinically, as muscarinic antagonists (e.g. ipratropium) and β_2-adrenoceptor agonists (e.g. salbutamol) are effective in the treatment of bronchospasm due to asthma.

12.2 A C D

As bronchioles branch, those which are less than 2 mm in diameter are called terminal bronchioles. The terminal bronchioles branch into respiratory bronchioles. The alveoli have flat walls. The respiratory system distal to the terminal bronchioles is comprised of acini, where gas exchange occurs.

12.3 C

Surfactant is secreted by type II pneumocytes in the alveoli, and is essentially a mixture of lipids and proteins, the major component being dipalmitoylphosphatidylcholine. Its main action is to lower the alveolar surface tension, which is an important factor in determining the stretchability (or compliance) of the lung. Stiff lungs have low compliance. Compliance is formally defined as the change in lung volume per unit change in airway pressure. The energy expended on inflating a compliant lung is much less than that of a stiff lung.

12.4 A B D

The right main bronchus is wider, longer and more vertical than the left main bronchus. This is clinically important, as, foreign bodies are more likely to enter the right than the left main bronchus. The right main bronchus divides into three secondary (lobar) bronchi, whereas the left main bronchus divides into two secondary bronchi. Each of these secondary bronchi correspond to a lobe of the lung: the superior lobe, the middle lobe (right lung only) and the inferior lobe.

12.5 E

The amount of air which moves into the lungs with each inspiration is the tidal volume. The amount of air which moves into the lungs with maximal inspiratory effort at the end of a normal inspiration is the inspiratory reserve volume. Similarly, the amount of air which moves out of the lungs with maximal expiration after passive expiration is the expiratory reserve volume. The inspiratory capacity is equal to the sum of the tidal volume and inspiratory reserve volume. Similarly, the expiratory capacity is equal to the sum of the tidal volume and expiratory reserve volume. The vital capacity is the amount of air that moves into the lungs with maximal inspiratory effort after passive expiration. The residual volume is the volume of air left in the lungs on maximal expiration. Hence the total lung capacity is equal to the sum of the vital capacity and the residual volume.

12.6 A C D E

The anatomical dead space is the volume of respiratory system from the mouth and nose to the terminal bronchioles. The gas in this space is not involved in gas exchange, and measures about 150 ml. The physiological dead space is the volume of gas which is not involved in gas exchange. For normal lungs, the two spaces are almost identical. However, if some alveoli are not perfused by capillaries, or if there is excessive air in alveoli necessary to oxygenate the alveolar capillaries, this also contributes to the physiological dead space. Pulmonary emboli may cause ventilation–perfusion mismatch, and hence may increase the physiological dead space, but not anatomical dead space. However, breathing through a long tube increases both the anatomical and the physiological dead space, since the air in the tube is not involved in gas exchange.

12.7 C D E

In the upright normal lungs, both perfusion and ventilation decline linearly from the bases to the apices of the lungs. However, the rate of decline is greater for perfusion, and the ventilation/perfusion ratio is higher in the apices than in the bases of the lungs. Widespread ventilation–perfusion mismatch would result in the failure of the blood in the lung capillaries to be reoxygenated, and cyanosis may occur. Severe ventilation–perfusion mismatch results in carbon dioxide retention.

12.8 B C E

Lung diseases may be categorised into obstructive or restrictive defects, or a mixture of the two types of defects. The vital capacity is the amount of air that moves into the lungs with maximal inspiratory effort after passive expiration. Hence it is usually normal in pure obstructive defects, but is reduced in the presence of restrictive defects such as lung fibrosis, oedema or chest wall deformities. The forced expiratory volume (FEV_1) is the maximum volume of air expelled from the lungs within the first second after maximal inspiration. It depends both on the vital capacity as well as the degree of airway obstruction. Hence it is reduced both in restrictive and obstructive defects. However, the FEV_1/VC ratio depends mainly on the airway obstruction, and is low in obstructive defects but normal or even high in restrictive defects. The transfer factor for carbon monoxide (T_{CO}) is the amount of carbon monoxide absorbed when air containing a known concentration of carbon monoxide is inhaled and the breath is held for 15 s before exhalation. It is a measure of pulmonary gas exchange. Hence it is reduced in restrictive defects but is normal in pure obstructive defects.

12.9 A B D

See Question 12.8 above.

12.10 A

The haemoglobin molecule plays an important role in carrying oxygen in the red blood cells. It is a globular protein made up of four subunits. In normal human adults, most haemoglobin is of the type haemoglobin A, which consists of four polypeptide chains: two α chains and two β chains. However, a small proportion of the haemoglobin is haemoglobin A_2, which consists of two α chains and two δ chains. This is clinically important, as the proportion of haemoglobin A_2 increases in diseases with defective β chain production. There is a haem moiety conjugated to each polypeptide chain. The haem moiety is a porphyrin derivative containing ferrous iron, and is responsible for binding to oxygen molecules. When exposed to various oxidising drugs, the ferrous iron may be converted to ferric iron, forming methaemoglobin. Methaemoglobin is dark-coloured, and may give rise to bluish discoloration of the skin resembling cyanosis.

12.11 C

Haemoglobin increases the oxygen-carrying capacity of the blood by about 70-fold. The haem moiety binds to the oxygen molecules. Since there are four haem moieties per haemoglobin molecule, up to four oxygen molecules may bind to one haemoglobin molecule. The haem moieties may assume either a relaxed (R) or tense (T) state, depending on the distance between the two β chains. Binding to an oxygen molecule increases the likelihood of an R state, which favours further oxygen binding. Hence, binding to an oxygen molecule increases the affinity for binding to a second oxygen molecule. This explains the sigmoid-shaped oxygen–haemoglobin dissociation curve.

12.12 A B

In the oxygen–haemoglobin dissociation curve, the partial pressure of oxygen is represented on the horizontal axis, whilst the percentage oxygen saturation is represented on the vertical axis. If the curve is shifted to the right, the oxygen saturation of haemoglobin is lower for a given partial pressure of oxygen. Conversely, a higher partial pressure of oxygen is required for haemoglobin to bind to a given amount of oxygen. In other words, the haemoglobin molecule holds less tightly to the oxygen molecules. The venous blood haemoglobin oxygen saturation is about 75%, whilst the arterial blood haemoglobin oxygen saturation is about 97%. Since the oxygen dissociation curve for haemoglobin is sigmoid, the oxygen–haemoglobin dissociation curve is steeper at the 75% than the 97% oxygen saturation point. Hence, if the oxygen–haemoglobin dissociation curve is shifted to the right, it is becomes easier to oxygenate the oxygen in the pulmonary capillaries, but more difficult for the blood in the capillaries to deliver oxygen to the tissues. Hence it may be clinically desirable to shift the oxygen–haemoglobin dissociation curve in the tissues to the right.

12.13 A C D E

Shifts of the oxygen–haemoglobin dissociation curve are important mechanisms to ensure oxygen is effectively delivered to the tissues. Increase in temperature, reduction in pH and increase in 2,3-DPG shift the oxygen–haemoglobin dissociation curve to the right, reduce the affinity of haemoglobin for oxygen, and ease the delivery of oxygen to the tissues. Living at high altitude usually triggers an increase in 2,3-DPG. During exercise, a combination of a temperature increase, a reduction in pH and an increase in 2,3-DPG shifts the oxygen–haemoglobin dissociation curve to the right. Furthermore, the steep part of the curve is in operation as partial pressure of oxygen is low. Hence more oxygen is released to the tissues for the given oxygen gradient.

12.14 A

Myoglobin is mainly found in the skeletal muscle. Its function is to extract oxygen from haemoglobin in the blood and deliver it to the exercising skeletal muscles. Each myoglobin molecule can only bind to one oxygen molecule, and thus has a hyperbolic oxygen–haemoglobin dissociation curve. The oxygen dissociation curve of myoglobin is well to the left of the haemoglobin curve, and it is therefore efficient in extracting oxygen from haemoglobin.

12.15 –

Several mechanisms are responsible for carbon dioxide transport, and there are significant roles for both the plasma and the red cells. Almost 90% of the carbon dioxide is transported as bicarbonate ions, about 5% is dissolved, and about 5% is transported as carbamino-haemoglobin. A negligible amount of oxygen is dissolved, but carbon dioxide is about 20 times more soluble than oxygen. Deoxygenated blood carries more carbon dioxide than oxygenated blood (Haldane effect), and this facilitates the uptake of carbon dioxide from the tissues and its delivery to the pulmonary capillaries. Most carbon dioxide is transported as bicarbonate ions. Carbon dioxide enters the red blood cell, and is hydrated to H_2CO_3. This process depends on the enzyme carbonic anhydrase. H_2CO_3 is then dissociated into hydrogen and bicarbonate ions. About 70% of the bicarbonate ions enters the plasma by exchanging with a chloride ion.

12.16 A B C E

See also Question 12.15 above. Carbon dioxide enters the red blood cell, and is converted to H_2CO_3 with the action of carbonic anhydrase. It is then dissociated into hydrogen and bicarbonate ions. Hence venous blood contains more bicarbonate and hydrogen ions. About 70% of the excess bicarbonate ions move out of the red blood cells and are exchanged for chloride ions. Hence, there are more chloride ions in the red blood cells in the venous than the arterial blood. Since the red cell in the venous blood contains extra osmotically active particles (chloride or bicarbonate ions), the cells swell.

12.17 A B C D

Asthma is defined as hypersensitivity of the bronchial tree with intermittent narrowing of the airways. Extrinsic (atopic) asthma may be triggered by common stimuli such as food, house dust mites and pets. Narrowing of the airways is mediated by release of histamine and slow-reacting substance of anaphylaxis (SRS-A) from inflammatory cells such as mast cells via type I hypersensitivity reaction. Excess IgE may be produced. The hypersensitivy reaction may lead to bronchial obstruction, mucus plugging of the bronchi and mucosal oedema of the bronchioles.

12.18 A B

Anti-asthmatic drugs may act by reducing bronchial hyperreactivity, reducing bronchial inflammation, and dilatation of the narrowed bronchi. Corticosteroids act by generally reducing bronchial hyperreactivity, and they may also inhibit the release of mediators from inflammatory cells. Sodium cromoglycate was thought to act mainly by preventing the release of mediators from mast cells, but it may also act on other inflammatory cells or on local axon reflexes. The adrenoceptors in the bronchi are mainly of the β_2 type, and agonists to these receptors act by dilating narrowed bronchioles. Methylxanthines have two modes of action: adenosine receptor antagonists and phosphodiesterase inhibitors. Antimuscarinic agents act as competitive inhibitors of muscarinic receptors, and induce dilatation of narrowed bronchioles.

12.19 C D

Respiration is controlled by both neural and chemical mechanisms. The neural control is usually moderated by chemical control. However, chemical control may override neural control in some situations. An example is that chemical control may initiate inspiration if the breath is voluntarily held for a prolonged period of time. The voluntary and automatic neural control mechanisms are entirely separate. The voluntary system is located in the cerebral cortex and sends impulses to the respiratory motor neurones in the medulla via the corticospinal tract, whilst the automatic neural system is located in the medulla. This may be clinically important. For example, diseases which affect the medulla may result in the loss of automatic control without affecting the voluntary control (Ondine's curse). To coordinate the breathing movements, motor neurones supplying the inspiratory muscles are inhibited whilst those supplying the expiratory muscles are activated, and vice versa.

12.20 A B

The chemoreceptors which mediate the chemical control of respiration are situated at the medulla oblongata near the respiratory centre. The carotid and aortic bodies (situated at the carotid bifurcation and near the arch of the aorta respectively) are sensitive to hypoxia. In general, chemical control tends to restore the arterial blood gases to their normal levels. Hence, a reduction in pH, an increase in carbon dioxide and a reduction in oxygen tend to result in an increase in ventilatory response. However, under normal conditions, the control of carbon dioxide is more sensitive than oxygen. With a normal level of carbon dioxide, the ventilatory response to hypoxia is slight when the partial pressure of oxygen of the inspired air is over 60 mmHg (a reduction of over 40% below normal). One reason for this is that a slight increase in ventilatory response results in a reduction in carbon dioxide and pH. However, when the partial pressure of oxygen of the inspired air is below 60 mmHg, a marked increase in ventilatory response occurs.

This usual respiratory drive by carbon dioxide is of clinical importance, as a high concentration of oxygen may be given to a patient with intact chemical control of respiration for acute hypoxia (e.g. acute asthma) without seriously reducing the respiratory drive.

12.21 A B D E

Several factors contribute to the increased ventilation rate immediately before and during exercise. Immediately before exercise, psychic stimuli and afferent impulses from muscle and joint proprioceptors to the respiratory centre may increase the ventilation rate. During moderate exercise, the arterial oxygen, carbon dioxide and pH do not change much. However, the chemoreceptors may become more sensitive to fluctuations in carbon dioxide levels, which results in an increase in ventilation rate during exercise. In vigorous exercise, pH drops as a result of excessive lactate production. Arterial carbon dioxide may rise and arterial oxygen may drop slightly. All these factors may result in stimulation of the chemoreceptors in the medulla and cause an increase in ventilation rate.

12.22 A B C D E

Oxygen deficiency at the tissue level is known as hypoxia. This may be caused by a low oxygen partial pressure in the arterial blood (hypoxic hypoxia), lack of oxygen-carrying capacity of the blood (anaemic hypoxia), inadequate blood flow to the tissues (ischaemic hypoxia) or inability of the tissue to make use of the available oxygen (histotoxic hypoxia). Causes of hypoxic hypoxia include lung diseases and shunting of blood from the venous to the arterial circulation. Anaemic hypoxia may be caused by either anaemia or carbon monoxide poisoning. Carbon monoxide combines with haemoglobin to form a compound (carbonmonoxyhaemoglobin) which cannot bind to oxygen. Histotoxic hypoxia may be caused by cyanide poisoning, which inhibits enzymes (e.g. cytochrome oxidase) involved in the tissue oxidative processes.

12.23 A B C E

Respiratory failure occurs when hypoxia and carbon dioxide retention occur as a result of ineffective gas exchange between the alveoli and the pulmonary capillaries. This may be caused by ventilation defects, perfusion defects or defects of gas exchange. Causes of ventilation defects include mechanical factors (e.g. obesity, severe abnormal curvature of the spine), muscle weakness (e.g. due to muscular dystrophy or motor neurone disease) or loss of lung volume (e.g. collapse of the lobe of a lung). Ventilation – perfusion mismatch may be caused by multiple pulmonary emboli. Defects of gas exchange may be caused by pulmonary fibrosis or emphysema. Whilst shunting of blood from the venous to the arterial circulation can cause hypoxia, it is not a cause of respiratory failure.

12.24 C D E

100% oxygen therapy increases the alveolar partial pressure of oxygen, and is useful in hypoxia caused by ventilation defects or gas-exchange defects. Hence it is effective for pneumonia and fibrosis of the lung,. It is also partially effective in treating hypoxia due to ventilation – perfusion mismatch. However, increasing the alveolar partial pressure of oxygen will have no effect on the shunting of blood from the venous to the arterial circulation. 100% oxygen is effective and safe in acute asthma, as the chemoreceptors at the medulla are driven by increased carbon dioxide level. However, in a patient with severe chronic obstructive airway disease and chronic carbon dioxide retention, the chemoreceptors at the medulla may not be sensitive to carbon dioxide level. Instead, respiration is driven by hypoxia. Therefore administering 100% oxygen may be dangerous as it may depress the respiratory drive and cause respiratory arrest.

12.25 B D E

Reduced ventilation immediately results in a rise in the arterial partial pressure of carbon dioxide, and a reduction in the arterial partial pressure of oxygen. Since carbon dioxide equilibrates with H_2CO_3, which is in turn in equilibrium with H^+ and HCO_3^-, the pH decreases. This is uncompensated respiratory acidosis. In the long term, the respiratory acidosis is compensated, though only partially, by increased renal secretion of H^+ and reabsorption of HCO_3^-. Hence the plasma HCO_3^- is raised in the compensated respiratory acidotic state.

12.26 B D

Respiratory alkalosis is caused by excessive ventilation as in hysterical hyperventilation. Excessive carbon dioxide is washed out from the lungs, and the arterial partial pressure of carbon dioxide decreases. As a result, the pH increases. In chronic respiratory alkalosis, the kidneys attempt to compensate for the alkalosis by reduced secretion of H^+ and reduced reabsorption of HCO_3^-. Hence the plasma HCO_3^- level decreases.

12.27 A B C D

Cough may be valuable in expelling foreign bodies and secretions from the respiratory tract. However, cough unproductive of sputum sometimes serves no useful clinical purpose. Cough is usually initiated by irritation of the lining of the trachea, larynx or pharynx. During coughing, expiration is forced against a closed glottis, and it is usually preceded by a deep inspiration.

12.28 A B D

Like most other autonomic reflexes, the main centre for the autonomic control of the cough reflex is located in the medulla oblongata. The main afferent inputs are from stimuli to the trachea, larynx or pharynx. However, it also receives neural inputs from the cerebral cortex, and cough is under substantial voluntary control. Changes in the partial pressure of carbon dioxide are monitored by the chemoreceptors which regulate respiratory drive, but do not affect the cough reflex.

12.29 A C D E

In the treatment of cough, the causes of the cough (e.g. infection, tumour) must be diagnosed and appropriately treated. If the cough still persists and is unproductive, it may be treated by measures which reduce the peripheral stimuli for the cough reflex or act on the central nervous system. Measures which would reduce the peripheral stimuli include ceasing smoking, staying in a warm, moist environment, the use of water inhalation as an aerosol, or the oral administration of a demulcent which coats and soothes the pharynx (e.g. simple linctus). Drugs which act centrally are mostly opioids (e.g. codeine, pholcodine).

12.30 A C

Emboli which reach the lung originate from the venous circulation and the right side of the heart. The commonest source of pulmonary emboli is venous thrombosis from the leg veins. The rest usually originate from pelvic veins.

12.31 B C E

Pulmonary emboli frequently originate from venous thrombi in the leg veins. Most venous thrombi are initiated at the venous valves, as they tend to encourage turbulent blood flow. The venous flow of blood from the legs depends on calf muscle contraction. Hence immobilisation is a major risk factor for pulmonary emboli. During a surgical operation, blood pressure may fall, and stasis may occur in the leg veins. Hence, the risk of pulmonary emboli is increased in the immediate post-operative period after a major operation. Other risk factors include malignancy (which may increase blood viscosity), oral contraceptive pills (which increase the risk for both arterial and venous thrombi) and pregnancy. High cholesterol level is a risk factor for atherosclerosis and arterial thrombosis.

12.32 A B E

The sequelae of pulmonary emboli depend on the size of the emboli and where they are lodged. A large pulmonary embolus lodged at the bifurcation of the pulmonary artery (saddle embolus) will significantly deprive both lungs of their blood supply. It is a frequent cause of sudden death. Alternatively, the patient may complain of severe chest pain with intense breathlessness, cyanosis and shock. If an embolus is lodged at a lobar or segmental artery, it may lead to the infarction of a lobe or segment. If there are multiple small pulmonary emboli, this will lead to gradual blockage of the pulmonary arterioles and pulmonary arterial hypertension. Pulmonary oedema may be caused by increased pulmonary venous hydrostatic pressure.

12.33 A B C D E

Pulmonary arterial hypertension may be classified according to the site of the pathology in relation to the pulmonary capillaries: pre-capillary, capillary or post-capillary. 'Pre-capillary' causes include multiple pulmonary emboli and shunt of blood from the left to the right side of the hèart as in ventricular septal defects. 'Capillary' causes are primary lung diseases, and include lung fibrosis and chronic obstructive airway disease. 'Post-capillary' causes are due to high pressure in the pulmonary venous system resulting in back-pressure in the pulmonary arterial system.

Examples are any causes of left ventricular failure and mitral stenosis.

12.34 A B C

The general causes of pulmonary oedema include increased pulmonary venous hydrostatic pressure, reduced plasma oncotic pressure, increased permeability of the alveolar capillary wall and blockage of the lymphatic drainage. The commonest cause of pulmonary oedema is increased pulmonary venous hydrostatic pressure due to left ventricular failure. Other causes of increased pulmonary venous hydrostatic pressure are mitral stenosis and severe aortic stenosis. A low plasma albumin level results in reduced plasma oncotic pressure. Increased permeability of the alveolar capillary wall may be caused by toxic fumes.

12.35 A C D

The diaphragm is the most important inspiratory muscle, and accounts for over three-quarters of the increase in intrathoracic volume during inspiration. The accessory inspiratory muscles (scalene and sternocleidomastoid muscles) lift the thoracic cage to increase the intrathoracic volume in laboured respiration. These muscles are clinically important, as they may be seen to contract actively in the presence of moderately severe respiratory diseases, as in an acute asthmatic attack. Another group of inspiratory muscles are the external intercostal muscles, which run obliquely downwards and forwards from one rib to the rib below. Contraction of these muscles increases the anteroposterior diameter of the chest. The main group of expiratory muscles are the internal intercostal muscles, which run obliquely downwards and backwards from one rib to the rib below. Contractions of these muscles pull the rib cage downwards and decrease the intrathoracic volume. Expiration may also be assisted by contraction of the muscles of the anterior abdominal wall, which both increases the intra-abdominal pressure and pulls the rib cage downwards.

12.36 C E

Chronic bronchitis and emphysema usually coexist. Both are diffuse diseases usually affecting all lobes of the lungs to some extent. Whilst chronic bronchitis is defined clinically as productive cough for three months in two consecutive years, emphysema is defined anatomically as enlargement of the air spaces in the alveoli due to destruction of elastin in their walls. In emphysema, the air spaces distal to the terminal bronchioles are permanently enlarged. Both chronic bronchitis and emphysema usually occur in smokers. The majority of people with deficiency of the enzyme α_1-antitrypsin also develop this disease. α1-Antitrypsin is an acute-phase protein which inhibits the enzyme elastase as well as other protein-denaturing enzymes. This may explain why elastin in the walls of the alveoli is destroyed in these patients.

12.37 A B D

Known risk factors for bronchial carcinoma include cigarette smoking, passive cigarette smoke, occupational exposure to asbestos and chromate, and exposure to excessive radiation. Radon is a radioactive gas. There is no evidence that excessive alcohol or low-fibre diet is associated with bronchial carcinoma.

12.38 A B

The pleural cavities are potential spaces between the layers of parietal pleura and visceral pleura. Normally, the pressure in the pleural cavities is below atmospheric pressure. Air may enter the pleural cavities either if a lung ruptures or a hole is created on the parietal pleura by a penetrating wound. The lung on the affected side collapses due to elastic recoil. The intrapleural pressure on the affected side becomes atmospheric, which is higher than the other side. Thus the mediastinum is shifted towards the normal side. The intrapleural pressure usually decreases normally during inspiration to allow lung expansion and increases during expiration. Hence air enters the pleural cavity during inspiration.

12.39 B E

Just over half of all bronchial carcinomas are of the squamous cell type. About 30% are small cell carcinomas, and just over 10% are adenocarcinoma. Large cell carcinomas are rare. Squamous cell carcinomas arise from squamous metaplasia, and usually arise at the hilum. They tend to metastasise locally to hilar lymph nodes, and distant metastases are rare. Whilst small cell carcinomas are prone to produce ectopic ADH and ACTH, squamous cell carcinomas usually produce ectopic PTH.

12.40 D

The vocal folds control sound production. They consist of elastic tissues derived from the cricothyroid ligaments, and the vocalis muscles. They are wide open during forced inspiration, half-open during normal inspiration, and approximate each other during speech production. The pitch of the voice is controlled by alteration of the length of the vocal folds. They are shorter in women than in men, which accounts for the higher pitch of a woman's voice. Whilst the extrinsic muscles of the larynx control the movement of the larynx as a whole, the length of the vocal folds is indirectly controlled by the intrinsic muscles of the larynx. The posterior and the lateral cricoarytenoid muscles are the main abductors and adductors of the vocal folds respectively. All the intrinsic muscles of the larynx except the cricothyroid are supplied by the recurrent laryngeal nerve. Hence paralysis of the vocal folds may result if it is damaged during surgery, and the patient may present with hoarseness or aphonia.

12.41 B

The trachea is palpable only for the upper 5 cm below the cricoid cartilage and above the suprasternal notch. To find the trachea clinically, the forefinger should be introduced just above the suprasternal notch. It may not be palpable in some subjects, especially the obese.

12.42 A C

Displacement of the trachea may be caused by thyroid, mediastinal and intrathoracic lesions. Mediastinal lesions may include lymphoma or carcinoma. Lesions affecting the upper parts of the lungs are especially likely to cause tracheal deviation. However, in collapse or fibrosis of the upper lobe of the lung, the trachea is deviated to the opposite side.

12.43 D E

The anteroposterior diameter of the chest is usually between 50% and 70% that of the lateral diameter. An increase in the anteroposterior diameter (i.e. barrel chest) may indicate respiratory diseases such as emphysema. The normal respiratory rate in adults is about 12–15 breaths per minute. The maximum chest expansion should be above 5 cm. The intercostal muscles and the diaphragm are usually sufficient for normal respiration. Use of accessory respiratory muscles such as sternomastoids and scaleni may indicate respiratory diseases. Pursed lips during expiration is characteristic of patients with diseases associated with air trapping in the alveoli such as emphysema. This is because the manoeuvre increases the pressure inside the bronchi, and hence delays the collapse of the bronchial wall.

12.44 A B E

Normal lung resonance is due to air in the lung tissues. Dullness to percussion may be due to separation of the chest wall from the underlying lung tissues by pleural fluid (i.e. pleural effusion) or thickened pleural tissue. Alternatively, it may be due to loss of air in the lung tissues (e.g. in consolidation of fibrosis). Pneumothorax or emphysema is associated with hyperresonance.

12.45 A

Normal vesicular breath sounds are caused by the change in the quality of the breath sounds at the larynx on its passage through the normal lung tissues to the stethoscope over the chest wall. Bronchial sounds are heard if the lung tissues become more solid and conduct sound more effectively, and they resemble the sounds produced at the larynx. Hence, the presence of bronchial breathing indicates that the relevant bronchi are patent, and that the consistency of the lung tissues has become more solid (e.g. in consolidation). Bronchial sounds are equally loud and long during inspiration and expiration, and there is a pause between the end of inspiration and the beginning of expiration. Since the presence of bronchial sounds indicates that the underlying lung tissues conduct sounds better than normally, the vocal resonance is always increased.

13. The gastrointestinal system
Questions

13.1 The actions of the following muscles of mastication are correctly matched:

A Masseter – elevation of mandible
B Temporalis (anterior fibres) – depression of mandible
C Temporalis (posterior fibres) – retraction of mandible
D Medial pterygoid – depression and protrusion of mandible
E Lateral pterygoid – elevation and protrusion of mandible

13.2 The functions of saliva include:

A Lubricating food and facilitating swallowing
B The breakdown of proteins into amino acids
C Increasing the acidity of the gastric juice
D The breakdown of nucleic acids into nucleotides
E The breakdown of starch into oligosaccharides

13.3 Salivary secretion is increased under the following conditions:

A The smell of food
B Stimulation of sympathetic fibres at the lower end of the oesophagus
C Stimulation of vagal fibres at the lower end of the oesophagus
D Oral atropine
E The passage of food through the pylorus of the stomach

13.4 The following structures and their secretion are correctly matched:

A Parietal (oxyntic) cells – mucin
B Parietal (oxyntic) cells – intrinsic factor
C Chief (peptic) cells – hydrochloric acid
D G cells in the antrum – gastrin
E Glands in the cardia of the stomach – pepsinogen

13.5 The following gastric secretions and their main functions are correctly matched:

- **A** Mucin – neutralisation of acid
- **B** Intrinsic factor – facilitates breakdown of proteins
- **C** Gastrin – facilitates breakdown of fats
- **D** Pepsinogen – facilitates breakdown of carbohydrates
- **E** Hydrochloric acid – bactericidal actions

13.6 Gastric acid secretion is increased by stimulation of the following receptors:

- **A** Histamine H_1 receptors
- **B** Noradrenaline receptors
- **C** Dopamine receptors
- **D** Gastrin receptors
- **E** Muscarinic receptors

13.7 Gastric acid secretion is increased by the following:

- **A** Stimulation of the vagus nerve
- **B** The presence of food in the stomach
- **C** The presence of fat and acid in the duodenum
- **D** The smell of food
- **E** High blood glucose level

13.8 The following significantly predispose to peptic ulcers:

- **A** *Helicobacter pylori* infection
- **B** Oral treatment with non-steroidal anti-inflammatory drugs
- **C** Excess secretion of gastrin
- **D** Excess alcohol intake
- **E** Excessive peristalsis of the intestines

13.9 The following drugs are correctly paired with their mechanisms of action, and are effective in the treatment of peptic ulcers:

- **A** Magnesium trisilicate – reduction of gastric acid secretion
- **B** Ranitidine – muscarinic receptor antagonist
- **C** Bismuth – enhances mucosal resistance
- **D** Omeprazole – inhibition of the H^+, K^+-ATPase
- **E** Chlorpheniramine – histamine H_2 antagonist

13.10 Complications of duodenal ulcers include:

- **A** Haemorrhage
- **B** Obstruction due to fibrous stricture
- **D** Bacterial infection
- **C** Peritonitis due to perforation
- **E** Malignancy

13.11 Carcinomas of the stomach:

- **A** Are commoner in the United Kingdom than in the Far East
- **B** Have increased in incidence in the last 50 years

C Are predisposed to by chronic gastritis
D Are mostly of the squamous type
E Usually present before they spread beyond the stomach wall

13.12 The following statements about the intestines are true:

A Both circular and longitudinal muscles are present in the walls
B The venous blood is drained into the inferior vena cava
C The outer myenteric plexus mainly mediates the secretion of gastrointestinal hormones
D Both sympathetic and parasympathetic nervous systems supply the intestinal walls
E They receive arterial blood supply from branches of the external iliac arteries

13.13 The area of small intestinal mucosa available for absorption is increased by:

A Villi
B Crypts
C Microvilli
D Peyer's patches
E The length of the intestine

13.14 Malabsorption may result from:

A Pancreatic disease
B Poor dietary intake
C Coeliac disease
D Surgical resection of small bowel
E Diverticulitis affecting the sigmoid colon

13.15 The following gastrointestinal hormones and their actions are appropriately paired:

A Gastrin – reduces gastrointestinal mobility
B Secretin – increase volume and alkalinity of pancreatic juice
C Vasoactive intestinal polypeptide (VIP) – inhibits intestinal secretion
D Substance P – increases intestinal motility
E Cholecystokinin – pancreozymin (CCK-PZ) – increases pancreatic secretion

13.16 The vomiting centre receives significant neural input from the following sources:

A The chemoreceptor trigger zone (CTZ)
B The acoustic system
C The vestibular system
D The peripheral organs such as the heart and biliary tree
E The cerebellum

13.17 The following types of drugs are potentially effective in alleviating vomiting:

- **A** Muscarinic receptor agonists
- **B** Dopamine receptor antagonists
- **C** Histamine H_2 receptor antagonists
- **D** Serotonin receptor agonists
- **E** Nicotinic receptor antagonists

13.18 The following measures may reduce symptoms of gastro-oesophageal reflux:

- **A** Lying down after a meal
- **B** Avoid being overweight
- **C** Antacids
- **D** Antimuscarinic drugs
- **E** Metoclopramide

13.19 A large proportion of the following substances are absorbed in the colon:

- **A** Water
- **B** Amino acids
- **C** Carbohydrates
- **D** Fats
- **E** Sodium

13.20 Disaccharides include:

- **A** Glucose
- **B** Sucrose
- **C** Lactose
- **D** Starch
- **E** Fructose

13.21 Amylase:

- **A** Is secreted by the salivary glands
- **B** Is secreted by the small intestine
- **C** Is secreted by the pancreas
- **D** Functions optimally when the pH is 8
- **E** Breaks down disaccharides into monosaccharides

13.22 The following statements about carbohydrate digestion are correct:

- **A** Starch is broken down into glucose in the stomach
- **B** Sucrose is broken down into glucose and fructose in the lumen of the small intestine
- **C** Lactose is broken down into glucose and galactose at the brush border of the small intestinal mucosa
- **D** Maltose is broken down into fructose and galactose at the brush border of the small intestinal mucosa
- **E** Deficiency in intestinal lactase may result in diarrhoea

13.23 The following enzymes play significant roles in the digestion of lipids:

- **A** Lingual lipase
- **B** Stomach lipase
- **C** Pancreatic lipase
- **D** Jejunal lipase
- **E** Ileal lipase

13.24 The following statements about fat absorption are true:

- **A** Lipid is delivered to the intestinal mucosa in the form of micelles
- **B** Most of the lipids are absorbed in the terminal part of the ileum
- **C** Lipid is transported into intestinal mucosa cells as triglycerides
- **D** Triglycerides leave the intestinal mucosa and enter the portal vein
- **E** About 50% of all ingested lipids are absorbed

13.25 The following enzymes play significant roles in the digestion of proteins:

- **A** Lingual pepsin
- **B** Stomach pepsin
- **C** Stomach trypsin
- **D** Pancreatic chymotrypsin
- **E** Pancreatic carboxypeptidase

13.26 Coeliac disease:

- **A** Occurs in one in every 2 million people in the United Kingdom
- **B** Results from sensitivity to gliaden in gluten
- **C** Has a strong association with HLA-B8
- **D** Is more common in those with a positive family history
- **E** Affects the duodenum more severely than the ileum

13.27 Coeliac disease is associated with:

- **A** Villous atrophy
- **B** Crypt atrophy
- **C** Reduced surface area for absorption
- **D** Normal absorption of amino acids
- **E** Long-term development of malignant lymphoma

13.28 Microorganisms which may cause gastroenteritis include:

- **A** *Salmonella*
- **B** *Campylobacter*
- **C** *Staphylococcus*
- **D** *Escherichia coli*
- **E** Small round structured viruses

13.29 Stimulant laxatives:

A Include lactulose
B Include senna
C May cause abdominal cramps
D Act by increasing the number of osmotically active particles in the stool
E Swell rapidly with water

13.30 Bulk laxatives:

A Include methylcellulose
B Include bran
C Increase the volume of intestinal contents
D Increase the pressure within the intestinal lumen
E Are useful in irritable bowel syndrome

13.31 Crohn's disease characteristically:

A Causes skip lesions
B Spares the terminal ileum
C Causes diffuse mucosal inflammation
D Affects all layers of the bowel
E Causes deep fissures

13.32 The indirect inguinal hernia:

A Is caused by a weakened posterior wall of the inguinal canal
B Can be controlled by finger pressure just above the midpoint of the inguinal ligament
C May extend to the testis
D Is palpable below the pubic tubercle
E Is palpable medial to the pubic tubercle

13. The gastrointestinal system
Answers

13.1 A C

The correct actions of the muscles of mastication are:

- Masseter – elevation of mandible
- Temporalis (anterior fibres) – elevation of mandible
- Temporalis (posterior fibres) – retraction of mandible
- Medial pterygoid – elevation and protrusion of mandible
- Lateral pterygoid – depression and protrusion of mandible

13.2 A E

Saliva performs a number of functions. It contains the digestive enzymes salivary α-amylase (which breaks starch down into oligosaccharides) and lingual lipase (which converts triglycerides into fatty acids). It contains mucins which help to lubricate food and facilitate swallowing. It is slightly alkaline and helps to neutralise the acid refluxed into the oesophagus. It also contains IgA, lysozyme and lactoferrin, which have antibacterial actions. Saliva does not facilitate the digestion of proteins or nucleic acids.

13.3 A C

Reflex secretion of saliva occurs at the sight or smell of food. Pavlov showed that reflex secretion can be conditioned to occur as a result of a stimulus (e.g. the sound of a bell) which immediately precedes the presentation of food. Stimulation of the parasympathetic supply to the salivary glands increases salivary production, and this may be achieved by food stimulating the vagal fibres at the lower end of the oesophagus. Anticholinergic drugs reduce salivary secretion and may cause dry mouth. Stimulus of the sympathetic nerve supply generally causes vasoconstriction of the salivary glands, and may explain the association of stress with dry mouth (e.g. during public speaking).

13.4 B D

Several substances are secreted in the stomach. Mucus (which contains mucin) is secreted by the glands in the cardia and pylorus of the stomach. This is important in protecting the gastric epithelium from damage by gastric acid. Parietal cells in the body of the stomach secrete hydrochloric acid and intrinsic factor.

Hydrochloric acid is useful for its bactericidal activity; it helps to digest proteins and allows pepsin to function optimally. It also stimulates the flow of bile and pancreatic juice. Intrinsic factor is important in the absorption of vitamin B_{12}. The chief (peptic) cells secrete pepsinogens, which are the precursors of pepsins. Pepsins break down proteins and polypeptides into smaller polypeptides. The G cell in the antrum of the stomach produces gastrin. Gastrin stimulates gastric acid and pepsin secretion, as well as the growth of the mucosa of the stomach and the intestines.

13.5 E

See question 13.4 above.

13.6 D E

Gastric acid secretion by the parietal cells is increased by stimulation of the histamine H_2 receptors, the muscarinic M_3 receptors, the gastrin receptors and prostaglandin E_2 receptors. Intracellular calcium acts as the second messenger for gastrin and muscarinic receptors, whereas cAMP acts as the second messenger for the histamine H_2 and prostaglandin E_2 receptors. The hydrogen ions produced in the parietal cells are transported into the gastric lumen by H^+, K^+-ATPase.

13.7 A B D

Gastric acid secretion is regulated by cephalic factors, local factors in the stomach and intestinal factors. Cephalic factors include sight, smell and thought of food, low plasma glucose level, as well as other stimuli which are conditioned with the presence of food. These factors increase gastric acid secretion via vagal stimulation. Food in the stomach increases acid secretion via local reflex in the stomach wall. Intestinal factors, acids, fats and carbohydrates in the duodenum inhibit gastric acid secretion.

13.8 A B C D

The mucosal barrier of the stomach protects the gastric epithelium from damage by the acid. Hence, risk factors for peptic ulcers are those which increase acid secretion or reduce mucosal resistance. *Helicobacter pylori* infection and treatment with non-steroidal anti-inflammatory drugs both reduce mucosal resistance of the stomach to acid. High levels of gastrin and excess alcohol increase acid secretion.

13.9 C D

Drugs for peptic ulcers act either by neutralising excess acid secreted, reducing the secretion of acid, or enhancing the mucosal resistance of the stomach to acid. Antacids such as magnesium trisilicate neutralise excess acid in the stomach. Drugs which reduce acid secretion may act by blocking histamine H_2 receptors (e.g. cimetidine, ranitidine); blocking muscarinic receptors (e.g. pirenzepine); or inhibiting the enzyme H^+,K^+-ATPase, which catalyses the pump for the transport of H^+ out of the parietal cell in exchange for K^+ (e.g. omeprazole). Chlorpheniramine is an H_1 antagonist and cannot be used to treat peptic ulcers.

13.10 A B D

Duodenal ulcers may heal completely. Complications include penetration and erosion of adjacent organs such as the liver; haemorrhage, resulting in altered blood in stools or blood in the vomit; perforation, resulting in severe chemical peritonitis as gastric contents enter the peritoneal cavity; and obstruction due to fibrous stricture. Malignancy occurs rarely following gastric ulcers, but duodenal ulcers are not predisposed to malignancy.

13.11 C

Carcinomas of the stomach are much commoner in the Far East than in the United Kingdom. The incidence has decreased over the past 50 years throughout the world, the reasons for which are not clear. Most carcinomas are adenocarcinomas, and may have progressed from epithelial metaplasia or dysplasia. Chronic atrophic gastritis is an important predisposing factor. As carcinomas of the stomach cause little or no symptoms in the early stages, most carcinomas present when they are clinically advanced with metastases.

13.12 A D

Although there are minor local differences, the structure of the walls of the gastrointestinal tract is broadly similar There are usually two longitudinal muscle layers with one layer of circular muscle layer in between. There are two major networks of nerve fibres: an outer myenteric plexus and an inner submucous plexus. In general, the inner submucous layer regulates the secretion of exocrine and endocrine secretion by cells, whilst the outer myenteric plexus regulates the control of peristaltic activity. These plexuses also receive extrinsic innervation from both sympathetic and parasympathetic nervous systems. The blood supply to the intestines is usually derived directly from branches of the abdominal aorta. The venous blood in drained via the portal vein to the liver. This is important clinically as orally administered drugs may undergo metabolism before reaching the systemic circulation.

13.13 A C E

The main functions of the small intestine are the digestion of food and absorption of nutrients. A large area of small intestinal mucosa is necessary for optimum absorption. This is achieved in several ways. Firstly, the small intestine is long (over 2.5 m). Secondly, the mucous membrane is thrown into fingerlike projections called villi. Thirdly, the edges of the cells (enterocytes) which make up the villi are themselves divided into smaller microvilli. As a result, the total area for absorption approaches 200 m^2. The enterocytes originate in the crypts, but migrate up the villi and ultimately shed into the intestinal lumen. Peyer's patches are dense aggregates of lymphoid tissue.

13.14 A C D

Malabsorption describes the failure of the intestines to absorb the nutrients available in the ingested food. Digestion and absorption of food mainly occur in the small intestines, and digestion is dependent on the appropriate pancreatic enzymes. Hence, malabsorption may be due to deficiency of digestive enzymes (e.g. pancreatic disease or specific biochemical disorders) or small intestine diseases. The small intestine diseases may be due to a decrease in the length of the small bowel (e.g. following surgical resection), or due to a reduction in absorption surface (e.g. coeliac disease or giardiasis). Disorders affecting only the large bowel are unlikely to result in significant malabsorption.

13.15 B D E

Gastrointestinal hormones are polypeptides secreted in the gastrointestinal mucosa. Many gastrointestinal hormones have been identified, and their integrated actions are important in the regulation of gastrointestinal motility and secretion. The sight and smell of food, and the presence of food in the stomach, initiate gastrin secretion, which stimulate both acid secretion and increased motility. On the other hand, acid in the upper intestine stimulates the secretion of secretin, which increases the alkalinity and volume of pancreatic enzyme. This acts as negative feedback to neutralise the acid. VIP stimulates intestinal secretion, whilst substance P and somatostatin inhibit intestinal secretion. CCK-PZ is stimulated by food and acid in the duodenum, and its action is to increase pancreatic secretion and contract the gallbladder. Again, this serves to neutralise the acid. A number of polypeptides are involved in the coordination of a peristaltic movement. Acetylcholine and substance P are responsible for the contraction behind a stimulus, whereas NO and VIP are responsible for the relaxation in front.

13.16 A C D

Vomiting is controlled by the vomiting centre in the medulla oblongata. It coordinates the act of vomiting on receiving inputs from various sources. These include the chemoreceptor trigger zone (which is sensitive to the action of drugs and other chemicals), the periphery (e.g. the heart, biliary tree), cortical centres and the vestibular system (which initiates vomiting in motion sickness).

13.17 B

The vomiting centre in the medulla contains cholinergic (muscarinic) and histamine H_1 receptors. Hence antimuscarinics and histamine H_1 receptor antagonists are potential anti-emetics.

Some drugs (e.g. cyclizine) have both antimuscarinic and antihistamine H_1 receptor activity. The chemoreceptor trigger zone (CTZ) contains dopamine D_2 receptors. Hence antagonists to these receptors are potentially good anti-emetics. Examples are metoclopramide and domperidone. However, these drugs also act peripherally on the gut by reducing the tone of the oesophageal sphincter, relaxing the pyloric antrum and increasing peristalsis. Serotonin 5-HT_3 receptor antagonists (e.g. ondansetron) are also effective anti-emetics. They probably both act centrally on the CTZ and peripherally.

13.18 B C E

Normally, contraction of the lower oesophageal sphincter prevents reflux of gastric contents into the oesophagus. If the sphincter becomes incompetent, reflux of acid into the lower oesophagus occurs, and this causes symptoms of heartburn and oesophagitis. Lying down after a meal or bending would encourage reflux. Elevating the head of the bed may minimise reflux. Antacids, histamine H_2 antagonists or proton pump inhibitor (e.g. omperazole) reduce acid secretion and hence the symptoms. Metoclopramide increases the tone of the lower oesophageal sphincter and increases gastric emptying, and may alleviate symptoms. Antimuscarinics tend to relax the lower oesophageal sphincter and exacerbate the symptoms.

13.19 A E

The main functions of the colon are to absorb water and sodium. Amino acids, carbohydrates and fats are mostly absorbed in the small intestine.

13.20 B C

Starch is a glucose polymer and is a polysaccharide. Disaccharides include maltose (glucose–glucose), lactose (galactose–glucose) and sucrose (fructose–glucose). Glucose, galactose and fructose are monosaccharides.

13.21 A C

Amylase is an enzyme secreted by both the salivary gland and the pancreas. Its main action is to break down starch into the disaccharide maltose. This digestive action occurs both in the mouth and the small intestine. However, it does not occur in the stomach, as the enzyme functions optimally at a pH of between 6 and 7.

13.22 C E

Starch is broken down into disaccharides in the lumen by amylase. In general, oligosaccharides are broken down into monosaccharides in the brush border of the small intestinal epithelial cells. Different oligosaccharides are broken down by different enzymes. For example, maltose is broken down by maltase and sucrase, sucrose is broken down by sucrase, and lactose is broken down by lactase. Many negroes and orientals have a genetic lactase deficiency. Hence they are unable to digest lactose (which is present in milk). The osmotic pressure generated by these disaccharides may draw water into the bowel lumen and cause diarrhoea.

13.23 A C

The digestion of fats starts in the mouth by lingual lipase secreted by glands on the dorsal surface of the tongue, and accounts for about a quarter of fat digestion. Most fat digestion occurs in the duodenum by pancreatic lipases. There are at least two pancreatic lipases.

13.24 A

Lipids are emulsified in the small intestinal lumen by the detergent action of bile, and are delivered to the intestinal mucosa in aggregates called micelles. Lipids diffuse out of the micelles near the brush border of the small intestine, and most of the lipids are absorbed in the duodenum and jejunum. Fatty acids and monoglyceride enter the mucosal cell, in which triglycercide is synthesised. It is exocytosed into the extracellular space, from where it enters the lymphatic system. Over 90% of all ingested lipids are absorbed.

13.25 B D E

Protein digestion starts in the stomach, where stomach pepsins break down proteins into polypeptides. Pepsin no longer functions when it reaches the duodenum, as it requires an acidic pH to function optimally. In the intestines, the polypeptides are further broken down at the interior peptide bonds by endopeptidases such as trypsin, chymotrypsins and elastase. The pancreas also produces carboxypeptidases which act at the carboxy ends of the polypeptides.

13.26 B C D E

Coeliac disease occurs in one in every 2000 people in the United Kingdom, and is more prevalent in Ireland. It results from sensitivity to gliadin in gluten. However, genetic factors are also important. It is more likely to occur in those with a positive family history, and there is a strong association with HLA-B8. It affects the proximal small intestine most, probably due to a higher exposure to gliadin. Hence coeliac disease is often confirmed by histological examination of a jejunal biopsy.

13.27 A C E

Normally, cells are continually shed from the tips of the villi, and replaced by migration of cells from the crypts. In coeliac disease, the villous cells are lost at an increased rate, which often results in total villous atrophy. Hence malabsorption occurs for oligosaccharides, fatty acids and amino acids. The crypts attempt to compensate for this by hypertrophy and increased mitosis. Coeliac disease predisposes to the development of malignant lymphoma of the small bowel.

13.28 A B C D E

Gastroenteritis can be caused by different microorganisms. Viruses are the commonest cause. Small round structured viruses commonly occur in winter, and may cause outbreaks of gastroenteritis in schools or nursing homes. Rotaviruses often occur in children. Bacterial infections may be associated with poor food hygiene, and are usually transmitted by infected meat. *Campylobacter* is the commonest bacterial gastroenteritis and is usually transmitted by infected poultry. A particular type of *Escherichia coli* may be associated with renal failure. *Staphylococcus aureus* can rarely caused fatal gastroenteritis.

13.29 B C

Stimulant laxatives include glycerol, senna and danthrons. They act by increasing the intestinal motility, and may directly stimulate the sensory endings in the lumen of the colon. Hence they may cause abdominal cramps, and should never by used when mechanical obstruction is a possibility. Osmotic diuretics such as lactulose increase the number of osmotically active particles in the stool. Bulk laxatives such as methlycellulose and ispahula husk swell rapidly with water.

13.30 A B C E

Bulk laxatives occur naturally as dietary fibres in vegetables and fruits. They also include bran, methycellulose and ispahula husk. They act by increasing the volume of intestinal contents so that large soft bulky stool can be formed. It is important that the fluid intake is adequate for this to occur. As a result, the pressure within the intestinal lumen is reduced. Besides simple constipation, bulk laxatives are also useful in diverticulosis (partly caused by increased intestinal pressure) and irritable bowel syndrome.

13.31 A D E

About two-thirds of all Crohn's disease affects the small intestine only, and the terminal ileum is characteristically affected. Unlike ulcerative colitis, Crohn's disease is characterised by 'skip lesions' – segments of diseased bowel separated by segments of apparently normal bowel. Hence mucosal inflammation is usually patchy. Whilst ulcerative colitis generally affects the superficial layer of the bowel, Crohn's disease characteristically affect all layers of the bowel. It often causes deep fissures.

13.32 B C E

Both inguinal and femoral hernias occur near the groin. The femoral canal lies below the inguinal ligament. All inguinal hernias appear through the external inguinal ring, which lies above and medial to the pubic tubercle. Hence inguinal hernia is palpable medially and above the pubic tubercle. An indirect inguinal hernia occurs due to persistence of the processus vaginalis. Hence it may extend to the testis. After reduction, it is controllable by pressure over the internal inguinal ring, which lies just above the mid-inguinal point. By contrast, direct inguinal hernia is caused by weakness of the posterior wall of the inguinal canal. Hence it is not controllable by pressure over the internal inguinal ring.

14. The liver and biliary system
Questions

14.1 The liver:

- **A** Is attached to the abdominal wall via the falciform ligament
- **B** Is attached to the diaphragm via the falciform ligament
- **C** Is easier to palpate in a clinical examination during expiration than inspiration
- **D** Is covered with peritoneum for over 75% of its surface
- **E** Lies more interiorly in the supine than in the erect position

14.2 Extensive communications between the left and the right lobes of the liver exist between their:

- **A** Arterial blood supply
- **B** Venous drainage
- **C** Biliary drainage
- **D** Portal venous supply
- **E** Nerve supply

14.3 The portal venous system:

- **A** Provides a little less than 50% of the blood supply to the liver
- **B** Carries blood from the gastrointestinal tract to the liver
- **C** Carries blood from the spleen to the liver
- **D** Has a mean pressure of about 70 mmHg
- **E** Contains valves

14.4 Sites of communication between the portal and the systemic venous systems include the:

- **A** Gastro-oesophageal region
- **B** Ileal region
- **C** Caecal region
- **D** Anorectal region
- **E** Periumbilical region

14.5 Clinical portal hypertension may directly cause:

- **A** Haemorrhoids
- **B** An enlarged spleen
- **C** Oesophageal varices
- **D** Dilating tortuous veins radiating from the umbilicus
- **E** Elevated blood pressure

14.6 Functions of the liver include:

- **A** Synthesis of albumin
- **B** Synthesis of amino acids
- **C** Secretion of bile
- **D** Production of corticosteroids
- **E** Storage of glycogen

14.7 The following statements about a liver lobule are true:

- **A** Blood flow is outward from the central vein
- **B** Bile flows inwards towards the central vein
- **C** The tissues nearest the central vein are most vulnerable to anoxic injury
- **D** Each hepatocyte is adjacent to several bile canaliculi
- **E** Branches of the hepatic artery run in the centre of the lobule close to the central vein

14.8 The following substances are produced by the healthy liver:

- **A** Aspartate aminotransferase (AST)
- **B** Alkaline phosphatase
- **C** γ-glutamyltransferase (γ-GT)
- **D** β-Human chorionic gonadotrophin (β-hCG)
- **E** α-Fetoprotein (AFP)

14.9 The following biochemical abnormalities are caused by primary liver failure:

- **A** Reduced albumin
- **B** Prolonged prothrombin time
- **C** Increased AST
- **D** Reduced γ-GT
- **E** Greatly elevated alkaline phosphatase

14.10 Causes for acute liver cell injury include:

- **A** Hepatitis A infection
- **B** Hepatitis C infection
- **C** α1-Antitrypsin deficiency
- **D** Primary biliary cirrhosis
- **E** Paracetamol

14.11 Liver diseases which may be caused by alcohol include:

- **A** Acute hepatitis
- **B** Chronic hepatitis
- **C** Fatty change
- **D** Micronodular cirrhosis
- **E** Liver cysts

14.12 Probable mechanisms for alcohol to cause liver disease include:

- **A** Accumulation of glycogen in liver cells
- **B** Accumulation of fats in liver cells

C Toxicity of alcohol to liver cells
D Deposition of elastin in liver cells
E Stimulation of collagen synthesis in liver cells

14.13 Cirrhosis of the liver:
A Often affects only one of the four lobes
B May recover completely with time
C Is usually caused by necrosis of individual liver cells (apoptosis)
D Is characterised by fibrosis
E Is characterised by nodular regeneration

14.14 Causes of cirrhosis include:
A Wilson's disease
B Hepatitis B infection
C Hepatitis A infection
D Haemochromatosis
E Primary biliary cirrhosis

14.15 Cirrhosis of the liver may lead to:
A Liver failure
B Liver cell carcinoma
C Gallstones
D Cardiac failure
E Portal hypertension

14.16 Liver cell carcinoma:
A Is commoner in Europe than South East Asia
B Is more commonly preceded by micronodular than macronodular cirrhosis
C Characteristically produces AFP
D Is often multifocal
E Is predisposed to by aflatotoxins

14.17 Significant constituents of bile include:
A Bilirubin
B Cholic acid
C Alkaline phosphatase
D Acid phosphatase
E Cholesterol

14.18 Substances whose absorption or excretion is severely reduced in the presence of obstruction in the bile ducts include:
A Carbohydrates
B Fats
C Proteins
D Bilirubin
E Vitamin K

14.19 The following statements about bile salts are true:

- **A** They are mainly synthesised by the bile ducts
- **B** They are discharged into the distal part of the stomach
- **C** A little less than 30% are reabsorbed in the small intestine
- **D** About 50% are reabsorbed in the large intestine
- **E** The reabsorbed bile salts are transported back to the liver via the portal vein

14.20 Unconjugated bilirubin:

- **A** Is formed by the breakdown of haemoglobin in the blood
- **B** Is mostly bound to albumin in the circulation
- **C** Is conjugated to glucuronic acid in the blood
- **D** Cannot be absorbed in the intestine
- **E** Can be excreted in the urine

14.21 Conjugated hyperbilirubinaemia may result from:

- **A** Increased breakdown of red blood cells
- **B** Reduced concentration of albumin
- **C** Reduced entry of bilirubin into liver cells
- **D** Intrahepatic bile duct obstruction
- **E** Extrahepatic bile duct obstruction

14.22 Extrahepatic bile duct obstruction is associated with:

- **A** Increased urinary urobilinogen concentration
- **B** Pale stools
- **C** Pruritis
- **D** A markedly raised serum alkaline phosphatase level
- **E** A low haemoglobin level

14.23 Significant functions of the gallbladder include:

- **A** Secretion of cholesterol
- **B** Formation of bile pigments
- **C** Storage of bile between periods of digestion
- **D** Concentration of bile
- **E** Secretion of digestive enzymes

14.24 Cholecystokinin (CCK):

- **A** Is secreted by the gallbladder
- **B** Produces contraction of the gallbladder
- **C** Increases the secretion of digestive enzyme from the pancreas
- **D** Stimulates the secretion of secretin from the small intestine
- **E** Is secreted in response to an increasing concentration of free bilirubin in the blood

14. The liver and biliary system Answers

14.1 A B D

The liver is the largest abdominal organ, and accounts for about 2% of the body weight in adults. The superior and anterior surfaces in contact with the diaphragm and the anterior abdominal wall respectively, and the falciform ligament attaches the liver to both these structures. As the diaphragm moves downwards with inspiration, the liver moves with it. Hence it is easier to palpate the liver during inspiration in a clinical examination. The liver also occupies a more inferior position in the erect than in the supine position due to gravity. As the liver develops between two layers of ventral mesentry embryologically, the surface of the liver is covered almost completely with peritoneum. The only exception is the bare area on its posterior surface.

14.2 –

The left and the right lobes of the liver are separated by the gallbladder fossa and the fossa for the inferior vena cava, and they function independently of each other. They receive their own arterial and portal venous blood supplies, and have their own venous and biliary drainage. The caudate lobe and most of the quadrate lobe of the liver function as the left lobe of the liver. The liver is innervated by the sympathetic and parasympathetic nervous systems via the hepatic plexus. However, there is no extensive communication between the nerve supplies to the right and the left lobes.

14.3 B C

The portal venous system carries blood from the gut, the spleen, the gallbladder and the pancreas to the liver. It provides about 70% of the blood supply to the liver, the other 30% being provided by the hepatic artery. Whilst the hepatic arterial pressure is about 90 mmHg, the portal venous pressure is only about 10 mmHg. The low portal venous pressure allows blood to flow from the mesenteric veins to the liver. In the presence of obstruction in the liver (e.g. due to cirrhosis), the portal venous pressure rises. As there are no valves in the portal veins, the blood flow can be reversed and portal venous blood can be returned to the inferior vena cava via the systemic-portal collateral circulation.

14.4 A D E

There are four main areas of portal – systemic anastomosis: in the gastrointestinal region, in the anorectal region, in the para-umbilical region and in the retroperitoneal region mainly between the splenic and the left renal veins. This is important clinically, as in the presence of portal hypertension dilated tortuous veins develop in these regions to cause haemorrhoids, oesophageal varices, caput medusae (veins radiating from the umbilicus) and enlarged spleen.

14.5 A B C D

See question 14.4 above. Ascites may also develop in portal hypertension. An increase in portal venous pressure (portal hypertension) does not affect the arterial blood pressure.

14.6 A C E

The liver performs many essential functions. The main functions are the formation and secretion of bile; inactivation of toxins and hormones; synthesis of important proteins (e.g. albumin, acute-phase proteins, some of the clotting factors, hormone-binding proteins); and the metabolism of carbohydrate, fats and proteins. The liver is the main storage site for glycogen. It breaks down amino acids to form urea (deamination).

14.7 C D

The liver is organised into lobules. In the centre is the central vein, which drains blood from branches of the portal vein and hepatic artery at the periphery. Hence blood flows inwards through the sinusoids towards the central vein. The central veins of the lobules then form the hepatic veins, which drain into the inferior vena cava. The blood in the sinusoids closest to the central vein is least oxygenated, and hence the tissues around the central vein are most prone to anoxic injury (e.g. in cardiac failure). Each liver cell is adjacent to several bile canaliculi, and the bile drains towards branches of the bile ducts in the portal space at the periphery of the lobule. Branches of the hepatic artery, portal vein and bile ducts run close together in the portal space.

Another way to describe the organisation of the liver is that it is divided into acini, with the portal space at the centre and the central veins in the periphery.

14.8 A C

AST, alanine aminotransferase (ALT) and γ-GT are produced by the healthy liver, and they are useful in diagnosing diseases of the liver cells. In the past, γ-GT was used clinically as a marker of excessive alcohol intake, although a raised level is not specific to liver injury by alcohol. Alkaline phosphatase is produced in the biliary system, and an elevated level indicates biliary obstruction. AFP is produced by primary liver cell tumour.

14.9 A B C

See question 14.8 above. As the liver is the prime producer of both albumin and the vitamin K-dependent clotting factors, a low albumin and a prolonged prothrombin time may occur in liver failure. A greatly elevated level of alkaline phosphatase occurs in biliary obstruction.

14.10 A B E

Causes of acute liver cell injury include viral infections (e.g. hepatitis viruses, alcohol, drugs (e.g. paracetamol) and toxins. Primary biliary cirrhosis and α_1-antitrypsin deficiency usually cause chronic injury and cirrhosis.

14.11 A B C D

Alcohol causes a spectrum of liver diseases. Fatty change is a benign abnormality, and is characterised by fat globules within the cytoplasm of the liver cells. It may proceed to acute hepatitis with acute inflammation. Mallory's hyaline (intracytoplasmic aggregates of filaments in liver cells) is a characteristic histological feature. Alcohol may also cause chronic hepatitis and cirrhosis. Alcohol is the commonest cause of micronodular cirrhosis (i.e. with nodules less than 3 mm diameter).

14.12 B C E

The probable mechanisms for alcohol liver disease are diversion of cellular energy from fat metabolism (hence causing an accumulation of fats in liver cells), direct toxicity of alcohol to liver cells, and stimulation of collagen synthesis (hence causing fibrosis).

14.13 D E

Liver cells can usually regenerate in response to injury. However, if there are repeated injuries which affect the architecture of the liver, repair may not restore the architecture. In cirrhosis, there is diffuse irreversible disturbance of the liver architecture. Fibrosis and nodular regeneration are characteristic. In nodular regeneration, the organisation of the lobules is lost. Cirrhosis is more likely following bridging necrosis, with areas of necrosis in the lobules extending from the central area to the portal spaces.

14.14 A B D E

Hepatitis B, hepatitis C and alcohol are the common causes of cirrhosis. Other causes include haemochromatosis (associated with excess iron deposition), Wilson's disease (a genetic disease associated with abnormal copper deposition), primary biliary cirrhosis (an autoimmune disease) and α_1-antitripysin deficiency.

14.15 A B E

Cirrhosis of the liver may cause liver failure if a critical proportion of functioning liver cells are lost. Cirrhosis may cause portal hypertension by an increase in the vascular resistance at the sinusoids. Cirrhosis due to any aetiology predisposes to liver cell carcinoma.

14.16 C D E

All cases of cirrhosis predispose to liver cell carcinoma, but the risk is especially high for macronodular cirrhosis (i.e. nodules more than 3 mm in diameter). As nodules in cirrhosis are multifocal, liver cell carcinoma which occurs in cirrhotic livers also tends to be multifocal. Hepatitis B infection is an important predisposing factor on its own, and may partly explain the higher prevalence in some parts of the world such as South East Asia. Aflatotoxin (a toxin produced by the fungus *Aspergillus flavus*) may also cause liver cell carcinoma. Liver cell carcinoma characteristically produces AFP, which is clinically used as a diagnostic marker.

14.17 A B C E

Water constitutes over 95% of bile in the bile ducts. Bile salts, bile pigments, cholesterol and lecithin are important constituents. Bile salts are either sodium or potassium salts of bile acids, of which cholic acid and chenodeoxycholic acid are the most important. Bile pigments are mainly bilirubin and biliverdin, and account for the brown colour of the bile. The relative proportions of bile salt, cholesterol and lecithin determine the solubility of cholesterol, and are important in the formation of gallstones. Alkaline phosphatase is also present, and accounts for the greatly elevated level of the enzyme in obstructive jaundice compared with jaundice due to liver disease. Acid phosphatase is mainly secreted by the prostate gland.

14.18 B D E

The function of bile salts is to prepare for the digestion and absorption of fats. Bile salts reduce surface tension, and are important for the emulsification of fat before it is digested and absorbed in the small intestine. Also, bile salts have both a hydrophilic and a hydrophobic end. Hence bile salts tend to form cylindrical discs (micelles) and tend to keep fats in solution. In the absence of bile salts, the absorption of fat and fat-soluble vitamins (e.g. vitamins A, D, E and K) is severely reduced. Bile pigments consist mostly of biliverdin and bilirubin, and the biliary system is essential for their excretion.

14.19 E

Bile salts are synthesised in the liver. The bile enters the gallbladder, where the bile salts are concentrated by the reabsorption of water, and the bile passes through the cystic and the common bile ducts. The common bile duct joins the pancreatic duct and enters the second part of the duodenum. About 95% of the bile salts are reabsorbed in the small intestine, and re-enter the liver via the portal vein. This enterohepatic circulation is important. For example, fat malabsorption may result from the presence of severe small intestinal disease due to reduced absorption of bile salts, and the inability of the liver to keep up with its synthesis.

14.20 A B E

Most of the bilirubin is formed by the breakdown of haemoglobin. The unconjugated bilirubin is mostly bound to albumin, and only a small proportion is free. Free bilirubin enters the liver cells and becomes conjugated to glucuronic acid. The reaction is catalysed by the enzyme glucuronyl transferase. The conjugated bilirubin is then secreted into the bile. Unlike unconjugated bilirubin, conjugated bilirubin cannot be absorbed in the intestine. Hence it is excreted by the gut, and accounts for the characteristic colour of the stool.

14.21 D E

Bilirubin is conjugated in the liver cells. Hence increased breakdown of red blood cells (i.e. haemolysis) and reduced entry of bilirubin into liver cell, or defective conjugation (e.g. due to glucoronyl transferase deficiency), result in unconjugated hyperbilirubinaemia. However, intrahepatic or extrahepatic bile duct obstruction results in conjugated hyperbilirubinaemia.

14.22 B C D

Extrahepatic bile duct obstruction results in conjugated hyperbilirubinaemia. Characteristic symptoms include jaundice, dark urine (due to conjugated bilirubin in the urine), pale stools (due to lack of bile pigments reaching the large intestine) and pruritus (due to increased bile salts in the blood). Increased urinary urobilinogen is due to unconjugated hyperbilirubinaemia.

14.23 C D

The gallbladder is not essential, as most subjects with their gallbladders removed surgically enjoy good health. The main functions of the gallbladder are to concentrate the bile and store the bile between periods of digestion.

14.24 B C D

In the past, it was thought that one hormone (cholecystokinin) stimulates the contraction of the gallbladder and another (pancreozymin) stimulates the production of enzyme-rich pancreatic secretion. They have been found to be the same hormone, and is now called cholecystokinin – pancreozymin (CCK-PZ). The hormone exists in several forms, and is secreted in both the small and large intestines. Its secretion is stimulated by the contact of digestive products with the intestinal mucosa, and especially the presence of fatty acids in the duodenum. Hence digestion is facilitated by the release of bile from the gallbladder and digestive enzymes from the pancreas. Furthermore, CCK-PZ stimulates the secretion of secretin from the small intestine. This increases the secretion of bicarbonate into the pancreatic juice.

15. The endocrine system
Questions

15.1 Physiological functions regulated by the hypothalamus include:

- **A** Temperature
- **B** Vomiting
- **C** 'Fight, fright and flight' defensive response
- **D** Blood pressure control
- **E** Sleep – wake cycle

15.2 Leptin:

- **A** Is a protein
- **B** Acts on the hypothalamus
- **C** Is found at a higher concentration in men than women
- **D** Is found at a higher concentration in obese than non-obese subjects
- **E** Increases food intake

15.3 The level of thirst is significantly increased by a reduction of:

- **A** Plasma osmolality
- **B** Plasma angiotensin II level
- **C** Plasma renin level
- **D** Extracellular volume
- **E** Intracellular volume

15.4 Physiological mechanisms for increasing the body temperature include:

- **A** Erection of hairs in the skin
- **B** Sweating
- **C** Shivering
- **D** Cutaneous vasoconstriction
- **E** Increased secretion of adrenaline

15.5 Hormones secreted by the hypothalamus into the portal hypophyseal vessel include:

A Vasopressin (ADH)
B Thyrotrophin-releasing hormone (TRH)
C Prolactin-prohibiting hormone
D Adrenocorticotrophic hormone (ACTH)
E Oxytocin

15.6 Vasopressin:

A Is a nonapeptide (consists of nine amino acids)
B Is secreted in the anterior pituitary gland
C Is secreted directly by nerve cells
D Has a half-life of about 24 h
E Causes sodium retention

15.7 Factors which decrease the secretion of vasopressin include:

A Consumption of alcohol
B Haemorrhage
C Oral consumption of water
D Raised plasma osmolality
E Erect posture

15.8 In nephrogenic diabetes insipidus:

A The plasma vasopressin level is low
B The subject often drinks a large quantity of water (polydipsia)
C Urine output is low
D The urine osmolality is high
E Synthetic vasopressin may alleviate the symptoms

15.9 The following statements about inappropriate ADH secretion are true:

A Bronchial carcinoma is a recognised cause
B It often occurs following an operation
C The plasma sodium concentration is often abnormally high
D The extracellular volume increases
E Demeclocycline is a recognised treatment

15.10 Direct actions of oxytocin include:

A An increase in the volume of milk produced by the breast
B Facilitation of the ejection of milk from the ducts of the breast
C Contraction of the perineal muscle during labour
D Contraction of the smooth muscle of the uterus
E Contraction of the smooth muscle of the bladder

15.11 The following statements about the pituitary gland are true:

A It lies inferior to the optic chiasma
B It lies in the ethmoidal bones
C It is supplied by branches of the internal carotid artery

- **D** The posterior pituitary develops from an evagination from the roof of the pharynx embryologically
- **E** The anterior pituitary develops from an evagination of the floor of the third ventricle embryologically

15.12 The following statements about thyroid hormones are true:

- **A** The thyroid gland produces more triiodothyronine (T_3) than thyroxine (T_4)
- **B** T_3 is more active than T_4
- **C** Reverse T_3 (RT_3) is more active than T_3
- **D** About 20% of T_4 in the plasma is bound to protein
- **E** T_4 can be converted into T_3 in the liver

15.13 Thyroid hormones:

- **A** Bind to receptors in the cytoplasm
- **B** Inhibit membrane-bound Na^+,K^+-ATPase activity
- **C** Alter the rate of protein synthesis by binding to the ribosomes
- **D** Increase the rate of mobilisation of fatty acids
- **E** Decrease the overall rate of oxygen consumption

15.14 Physiological effects of thyroid hormones include an increased rate of:

- **A** Carbohydrate absorption
- **B** Protein synthesis
- **C** Muscle breakdown
- **D** Glucagon synthesis
- **E** Fatty tissue synthesis

15.15 The following statements about the relationship between thyroid hormones and catecholamines are true:

- **A** Thyroid hormones increase the concentration of plasma catecholamines
- **B** Thyroid hormones are competitive inhibitors of plasma catecholamines
- **C** Thyroid hormones increase the number of β-adrenergic receptors
- **D** Thyroid hormones increase the affinity of catecholamines to β-adrenergic receptors
- **E** The effect of thyroid hormones may be partially reduced by propranolol

15.16 The following statements about the control of thyroid hormone secretion are true:

A Increased free T_4 increases the rate of TRH secretion
B Increased free T_4 decreases the rate of thyroid-stimulating hormone (TSH) secretion
C Increased free T_3 decreases the rate of TSH synthesis
D Increased catecholamines decrease the rate of TSH synthesis
E Increased thyroxine-binding globulin (TBG) increases the rate of TSH secretion

15.17 Recognised clinical features of hyperthyroidism include:

A Tremor
B Weight gain
C Hypothermia
D Sweating
E Increased heart rate

15.18 Recognised biochemical abnormalities of hypothyroidism due to thyroid disease include:

A A raised free T_4 level
B A raised plasma TSH level
C A poor TSH response to a test dose of TRH
D A raised plasma thyroxine-binding globulin
E A low total plasma T_3 level

15.19 Carbimazole:

A Is an antagonist of T_4 at the thyroid hormone receptor
B Increases thyroid hormone synthesis
C Exerts its maximal clinical effect within 24 h of administration
D Usually results in reduction in the size of the goitre
E May cause acute reduction in neutrophil count

15.20 Grave's disease:

A Is the commonest cause of hyperthyroidism
B Is usually associated with diffuse goitre
C Is associated with autoantibodies to thyroglobulin
D May be associated with exophthalmos
E Occurs more frequently in men than women

15.21 Long-acting thyroid stimulator (LATS):

A Is an autoantibody to thyroid epithelial cells
B Is an IgM
C Is associated with accumulation of mucopolysaccharides in the dermis of the shins (pretibial myxoedema)
D Inhibits the formation of thyroid hormones
E Is characteristically associated with Hashimoto's disease

15.22 The following statements about thyroid carcinomas are true:

A They are commoner than benign thyroid tumours
B Papillary carcinoma is commoner than other types of thyroid carcinomas
C Anaplastic carcinoma has a worse prognosis than follicular carcinoma
D Follicular carcinoma often metastasises to bone
E Medullary carcinoma often secretes calcitonin

15.23 The following statements about the thyroid gland are true:

A It is surrounded by a sheath derived from the pretracheal fascia
B The isthmus lies anterior to the second to fourth rings of the trachea
C It is developed from the endoderm embryologically
D Embryological incomplete descent may result in lingual thyroid
E The recurrent laryngeal nerves lie posteromedial to the lobes

15.24 The following statements about calcium metabolism are true:

A Just less than half of the body calcium is in the skeleton
B Just over half of the calcium excretion takes place in the kidneys
C The amount of calcium bound to protein varies with the plasma protein concentration
D Calcium can be actively transported from the gut lumen into the capillaries
E There is usually no exchange of calcium between bones and extracellular fluid in healthy individuals

15.25 Total body calcium is generally higher in:

A Teenagers than childhood
B Those aged 50 than those aged 30
C The elderly than those aged 50
D Women than men of the same age
E Post-menopausal women than pre-menopausal women

15.26 Effects of vitamin D include increased:

A Active transport of calcium from the intestinal lumen to the capillaries
B Calcium reabsorption from the kidneys
C Calcium secretion in the kidneys
D Stimulation of osteoclasts in bone
E Stimulation of osteoblasts in bone

15.27 The following statements about the various forms of vitamin D are true:

A The normal diet contains cholecalciferol (vitamin D_3)
B The synthesis of cholecalciferol (vitamin D_3) from 7-dehydrocholecholesterol requires sunlight
C The conversion of 25-hydroxycholecalciferol to 1, 25-dihydroxycholecalciferol takes place in the kidneys
D The conversion of 25-hydroxycholecalciferol to 24, 25-dihydroxycholecalciferol takes place in the liver
E 24,25-Dihydroxycholecalciferol is more active than 1, 25-dihydroxycholecalciferol

15.28 The following are important mechanisms for the regulation of the plasma level of the active form of vitamin D:

A High plasma calcium stimulates the formation of 25-hydroxycholecalciferol
B High plasma calcium stimulates the formation of 1, 25-dihydroxycholecalciferol
C High plasma phosphate stimulates the formation of 1, 25-dihydroxycholecalciferol
D High parathyroid hormone stimulates the formation of 1, 25-dihydroxycholecalciferol
E High parathyroid hormone stimulates the formation of 24, 25-dihydroxycholecalciferol

15.29 The following statements about the parathyroid glands are true:

A There are normally six parathyroid glands
B The superior parathyroid glands normally lie on the anterior surface of the thyroid gland
C The superior parathyroid glands normally lie outside the fascial sheath of the thyroid gland
D The inferior parathyroid glands are occasionally found within thymic tissue in the superior mediastinum
E They secrete calcitonin

15.30 Parathyroid hormone:

A Is a tripeptide
B Is secreted by the superior, but not the inferior, parathyroid glands
C Increases bone formation
D Increases plasma phosphate
E Indirectly increases calcium absorption from the intestine

15.31 Abnormal findings in pseudohypoparathyroidism include low:

A Plasma calcium
B Plasma phosphate
C Plasma parathyroid hormone
D Urinary phosphate excretion
E Plasma protein

15.32 Calcitonin:

- **A** Increases plasma calcium
- **B** Inhibits bone resorption
- **C** Increases urinary calcium excretion
- **D** Increases absorption of calcium from the gut
- **E** Is a recognised treatment for Paget's disease

15.33 Clinical features of hypercalcaemia include:

- **A** Tetany
- **B** Convulsions
- **C** Muscle weakness
- **D** Polyuria
- **E** Tiredness

15.34 Recognised causes of hypercalcaemia include:

- **A** Bone metastases
- **B** Ectopic PTH secretion from squamous bronchial carcinoma
- **C** Chronic renal failure
- **D** Vitamin D deficiency
- **E** Sarcoidosis

15.35 Secondary hyperparathyroidism:

- **A** Is usually caused by a parathyroid adenoma
- **B** Is associated with a high plasma calcium level
- **C** May be due to renal failure
- **D** May progress to tertiary hyperparathyroidism
- **E** Is best treated by parathyroidectomy

15.36 Recognised temporary treatment for hypercalcaemia due to primary hyperparathroidism include:

- **A** Adrenocortical steroid
- **B** Intravenous saline and frusemide
- **C** Thiazide diuretics
- **D** Dialysis
- **E** Calcitonin

15.37 Bisphosphonates may be used to treat:

- **A** Osteoporosis
- **B** Osteomalacia
- **C** Hypercalcaemia
- **D** Osteoarthritis
- **E** Paget's disease

15.38 Hormones normally secreted by the islets of Langerhans in the pancreas include:

A Insulin
B Gastrin
C Glucagon
D Somatostatin
E Cholecystokinin – pancreozymin

15.39 The following statements about insulin are true:

A It consists of four amino acid chains
B Disulphide bridges link separate amino acid chains
C There are major differences in the structure between pig and human insulin
D Humans receiving beef insulin often develop antibodies against it
E Human insulin may be manufactured by recombinant DNA technique

15.40 Physiological effects of insulin include decreased:

A Transport of glucose into cells
B Transport of amino acids into cells
C Plasma potassium level
D Protein synthesis
E Glycogen synthesis

15.41 Insulin receptors:

A Are not found outside the pancreas
B Each consist of two α-and two β-glycoprotein subunits
C Are usually in the nuclei
D Decrease in number with increasing plasma insulin level
E Increase in number in obesity

15.42 The results of a standard glucose tolerance test depend significantly on:

A The rate of intestinal absorption of glucose
B The rate of entry of glucose into cells
C The uptake of glucose by the brain
D The rate of glycogen synthesis by the liver
E The rate of glucose uptake by red blood cells

15.43 Recognised effects of a high plasma glucose level include:

A Presence of glucose in the urine
B Dehydration
C Thirst
D Polyuria
E Reduction in HbA_{1c} level

15.44 Metabolic changes associated with diabetes mellitus include:

A Intracellular hyperglycaemia
B Glycogen depletion

C Increased formation of ketone bodies
D Greatly positive nitrogen balance
E Excess acetyl CoA formation

15.45 In diabetic ketoacidosis:

A There is an accumulation of ketone bodies in the plasma
B There is an accumulation of total body sodium
C The total body potassium is depleted
D The plasma potassium is usually low
E The respiratory rate may be abnormally fast

15.46 Sulphonylureas:

A Increase insulin synthesis in the islet cells
B Are indicated for patients with total deficiency of insulin
C May cause hyperglycaemia in normal subjects
D Frequently cause weight loss
E Usually become more effective after regular usage for a few years

15.47 Biguanides:

A Include glibenclamide
B Are mainly used to treat insulin-dependent diabetes mellitus
C Reduce the production of glucose in the liver
D May cause lactic acidosis
E Are not suitable for obese patients

15.48 Compared to type II diabetes, type I diabetes (i.e. juvenile-onset, insulin-dependent diabetes)

A Is more likely to present with ketoacidosis
B Is associated with higher insulin secretion
C Has a higher monozygotic twin concordance
D Is more likely to be autoimmune in aetiology
E Is more likely to be triggered by viral infection

15.49 The following diseases are commoner in patients with diabetes mellitus:

A Myocardial infarction
B Cerebrovascular disease
C Peripheral vascular disease
D Retinopathy
E Nephropathy

15.50 Glucagon:

A Increases the breakdown of glycogen
B Increases the plasma glucose level
C Is broken down in the liver
D May act via cAMP as a second messenger
E Stimulates the secretion of insulin

15.51 The following increase the secretion of glucagon:

A High plasma glucose
B High plasma insulin
C Exercise
D Sympathetic nervous stimulation
E High plasma amino acids

15.52 Symptoms of hypoglycaemia may include:

A Palpitations
B Sweating
C Confusion
D Convulsions
E Drowsiness

15.53 The following hormones increase as a compensatory response to hypoglycaemia:

A Growth hormone
B Adrenaline
C Aldosterone
D Cortisol
E Glucagon

15.54 Physiological effects of growth hormone include:

A Linear elongation of long bones after the epiphyses have fused
B An increase in the breakdown of proteins
C A reduction of the breakdown of glycogen in the liver
D Reduction in insulin secretion
E An increase in the plasma free fatty acid

15.55 Somatomedins:

A Are growth factors
B Are secreted by the liver
C Are secreted in response to growth hormone
D Can stimulate both skeletal and cartilage growth
E Are increased in untreated diabetes mellitus

15.56 The following hormones and the sites of secretion are correctly matched:

A Mineralocorticoid – zona fasciculata of adrenal cortex
B Sex hormones – zona glomerulosa of adrenal cortex
C Dopamine – adrenal medulla
D Adrenaline – adrenal medulla
E Glucocorticoids – zona reticularis of adrenal cortex

15.57 Compared to adrenaline, noradrenaline produces a significantly higher:

A Peripheral resistance in the circulation
B Heart rate

C Diastolic blood pressure
D Pulse pressure
E Level of fear and anxiety

15.58 The following statements about the synthesis of glucocorticosteroids are true:

A Cholesterol acts as the precursor
B Mitochondrial enzymes are essential
C Intracellular cyclic AMP acts as a second messenger
D It is initiated by ACTH binding to a nuclear receptor
E Some of the metabolic pathways are common to those for mineralocorticoid synthesis

15.59 Recognised pharmacological uses of systemic adrenal steroids include:

A Collagen disorders (e.g. systemic lupus erythematosus)
B Anaphylactic shock
C Rejection of transplanted kidneys
D Severe asthmatic attack
E Idiopathic thrombocytopenia purpura

15.60 Recognised side effects of long-term administration of steroids include:

A Postural hypotension
B Osteomalacia
C Depression
D Peptic ulceration
E Increased susceptibility to infection

15.61 Conditions which are associated with a low plasma ACTH but a high plasma cortisol level include:

A Addison's disease
B Psychologically stressful situations
C Panhypopituitarism
D Primary adrenal tumour
E Ectopic ACTH-secreting bronchial carcinoma

15. The endocrine system
Answers

15.1 A C E

The hypothalamus plays an extremely important role for both endocrine control and the regulation of many autonomic functions. It exerts its endocrine control mainly via its neural connections with the posterior pituitary gland and its hormonal connections with the anterior pituitary gland. The hypothalamus also regulates several important physiological body functions. They include control of temperature, appetite, thirst, sexual behaviour and the defensive reactions. There is good evidence that the suprachiasmatic nuclei of the hypothalamus receive input from the eyes via the retinohypothalamic fibres, and control many circadian rhythms including body temperature rhythms and sleep–wake cycles. Vomiting, cough and blood pressure control are mediated by centres in the medulla oblongata.

15.2 A B D

Leptin is a protein containing 167 amino acids, and has only been recently isolated. It acts on the hypothalamus to decrease food intake and increase energy consumption. Leptin level can be measured by radioimmunoassay. Leptin levels appear to correlate directly with the proportion of body fat. Hence obese subjects have a higher concentration than non-obese subjects, and women have a higher concentration than men. It appears that leptin is important in controlling the body's store of fat by providing feedback to the hypothalamus on the total body fat store.

15.3 D

The level of thirst is usually controlled by two factors: plasma osmolality and the extracellular volume. An increase in plasma osmolality (e.g. in dehydration due to water loss, infusion of hypertonic solution) stimulates the osmoreceptors in the anterior hypothalamus, which results in an increased level of thirst. A reduction in extracellular volume (e.g. in haemorrhage) stimulates the baroreceptors, which causes an increase in the plasma level of renin and angiotensin II. This leads to an increased level of thirst.

15.4 A C D E

Body temperature may be increased either by producing more heat or reducing heat loss. Mechanisms for producing more heat include voluntary muscle contraction and shivering. Secretion of adrenaline or noradrenaline will increase heat production in the short term, and thyroid hormone may increase heat production in the longer term. Mechanisms for minimising heat loss include constriction of the blood vessels in the skin and erection of hairs in the skin.

15.5 B C

The hypothalamus controls the release of anterior pituitary hormones by secreting releasing and inhibiting hormones into the portal hypophyseal vessel, but the secretion of posterior pituitary hormones is controlled by direct neural connection between the supraoptic and paraventricular nuclei of the hypothalamus and the posterior pituitary gland. Hormones secreted by the posterior pituitary gland include vasopressin (antidiuretic hormone) and oxytocin. Most of the anterior pituitary hormones are mainly controlled by releasing hormones, apart from prolactin, which is mainly controlled by prolactin-inhibiting hormone. The releasing hormones secreted by the hypothalamus into the portal hypophyseal vessel include corticotrophin-releasing hormone (CRH), TRH, luteinising hormone-releasing hormone (LHRH) and growth hormone-releasing hormone (GRH). There are only two types of inhibiting hormones: prolactin-inhibiting hormone (PIH) and growth hormone–inhibiting hormone (GHIH). ACTH is secreted by the anterior pituitary gland and its release is controlled by CRH.

15.6 A C

Vasopressin is secreted in the posterior pituitary gland by nerve cells and released directly into the circulation. Like oxytocin, it consists of nine amino acids (i.e. a nonapeptide). It has a short half-life (less than half an hour), and hence the plasma osmolality can be sensitively controlled. Its main effect is to decrease the urinary excretion of water.

15.7 A C

Factors controlling the secretion of vasopressin are similar to those controlling thirst: plasma osmolality and extracellular volume. Hence an increase of the osmotic pressure in the plasma results in stimulus of the osmoreceptors and release of vasopressin. Reduced extracellular volume is detected by the baroreceptors, which mediates the release of vasopressin. The occurs partly due to the release of angiotensin II. Standing slightly reduces the stimulation of the baroreceptors, and hence increases the secretion of vasopressin slightly. Alcohol reduces the secretion of vasopressin. This explains why diuresis occurs after alcohol consumption.

15.8 B

In diabetes insipidus, urinary excretion of water is increased due to reduced reabsorption in the collecting ducts. Hence the urinary volume increases, the urinary osmolality decreases and the plasma osmolality increases. This stimulates thirst, and the subject often drinks a large quantity of water (polydipsia). In most cases, the cause is reduced or absent secretion of vasopressin. In nephrogenic diabetes insipidus, the plasma concentration of vasopressin is normal, but the kidneys fail to respond to the hormone due to a congenital defect of their receptors. Hence treatment with synthetic vasopressin does not usually alleviate the symptoms.

15.9 A B D E

The syndrome of inappropriate ADH secretion is said to occur if the secretion of vasopressin is high in spite of a low osmolality. This may occur because factors other than osmolality facilitate the secretion of vasopressin. An example is in the post-operative operative period when pain and reduced extracellular volume maintain a high level of vasopressin secretion. It may also occur as a result of autonomous secretion of vasopressin by bronchial carcinoma. There are also other causes such as head injury and cerebral tumour. The high level of vasopressin reduces the urinary excretion of water. Hence the extracellular volume and plasma sodium increase due to dilution effect. Demeclocycline (a tetracycline) has been found to reduce the response of the kidneys to vasopressin, and is often useful in treating the condition.

15.10 B D

The main sites of action for oxytocin are the breast and the uterus. Prolactin increases the volume of milk produced by the breast, whilst oxytocin facilitates the ejection of milk available in the breast. Oxytocin causes contraction of the uterine muscle, and the uterine muscle becomes more sensitive to oxytocin during pregnancy. Hence synthetic oxytocin is often used to accelerate labour, and also in the treatment of postpartum haemorrhage in conjunction with ergometrine.

15.11 A C

The pituitary gland is connected to the inferior surface of the brain via the infundibulum, and is well protected in the sella turcica of the sphenoid bone. It lies inferior to the optic chiasma. Hence a large pituitary tumour may involve the optic chiasma and give rise to characteristic visual field defects (bitemporal hemianopia). As a structure of the brain, it is supplied by branches of the internal carotid artery. Embryologically, the anterior and intermediate lobes of the pituitary gland develop from an evagination from the roof of the pharynx (Raphke's pouch), whilst the posterior lobe develops from an evagination of the floor of the third ventricle. Hence only the posterior pituitary belongs to the brain embryologically. This explains why posterior pituitary hormones are secreted directly from neurones with cell nuclei in the hypothalamus, whilst the anterior pituitary hormones are secreted in response to tropic hormones from the hypothalamus in the portal hypophyseal circulation.

15.12 B E

The main hormones secreted by the thyroid gland are T_4, T_3 and RT_3. T_4 constitutes over 90% of the hormones secreted, whilst T_3 accounts for less than 4% and RT_3 accounts for less than 2%. However, T_3 is more active than T_4, whilst RT_3 is inactive. Most of the plasma T_3 is produced by peripheral conversion from T_4 in tissues such as the liver and the kidneys. About 99.8% of plasma T_4 is bound to proteins. Hence the total plasma thyroid hormone may not reflect the true thyroid status of the subject. Measurement of free thyroid hormones or an indirect measure of their free concentration is important.

15.13 D

Thyroid hormones act by entering the cell and binding to receptors in the nucleus; the resulting hormone–receptor complex then binds to the DNA. This affects the rate of protein synthesis. In general, thyroid hormones increase the overall metabolic rate and rate of oxygen consumption. This is partly achieved by an increases in Na^+,K^+-ATPase activity. The rate of absorption of carbohydrates and mobilisation of fatty acids are increased.

15.14 A C

In general, thyroid hormones increase the rate of catabolism and decrease the rate of anabolism. Hence carbohydrates are absorbed and utilised at a high rate. The rate of fatty acid and protein breakdown is increased, but their rate of synthesis is reduced.

15.15 C D E

The actions of thyroid hormones and catecholamines are very similar and are closely interrelated. They both increase the metabolic rate. This is because thyroid hormones (T_3 and T_4) increase both the numbers of β-adrenergic receptors and the affinity of catecholamines to the receptors. Hence the tissue becomes more sensitive to catecholamines. This is important clinically. Thyroid hormones cause increased heart rate, sweating and tremor mainly through this effect, and this effect can be reduced by β-adrenergic antagonists. Hence it is essential to administer propranolol or other β-adrenergic antagonists in the immediate treatment of severe hyperthyroidism to protect against cardiotoxicity.

15.16 B C

The secretion of thyroid hormones is mostly regulated by the negative feedback control exerted by free T_3 and T_4 on both the hypothalamus and the pituitary gland. The main control mechanism is that an increase in either free T_3 or T_4 inhibits the secretion of TRH from the hypothalamus, which results in a reduction in both the synthesis and secretion of TSH from the pituitary gland. However, an increase in free T_3 or T_4 also blocks the usual increase in TSH in response to TRH. Catecholamines and TBG play no part in the regulation of thyroid hormone secretion.

15.17 A D E

Many of the clinical features of hyperthyroidism can be deduced from the known effects of thyroid hormones. Increased sensitivity of the β-adrenergic receptors to catecholamines gives rise to increased heart rate, tremor, mental agitation and sweating. Weight loss and heat intolerance result from increased metabolic rate. Diarrhoea, palpitations, muscle weakness and increased tendon reflex are other features of hyperthyroidism.

15.18 B E

Hypothyroidism is most commonly due to primary disease of the thyroid, especially Hashimoto's disease (an autoimmune disorder). However, hypothyroidism may also be secondary to pituitary or hypothalamic failure. The biochemical abnormalities differ depending on the site of the disease. In primary hypothyroidism, all total and free thyroid hormones are low. This causes an increase in the secretion of TRH from the hypothalamus and TSH from the pituitary gland via its feedback loop. The TSH response to TRH is exaggerated. The concentration of plasma-binding proteins is not affected.

15.19 B E

Carbimazole belongs to a class of drugs known as thionamides. Its antithyroid action is due to a reduction in the synthesis of thyroid hormone both by inhibiting the incorporation of iodine and the conversion of T_3 and T_4 to iodotyrosines. The drug produces no significant clinical effects until the existing stores are exhausted, which may take up to three months. A decrease in T_4 results in increased synthesis and secretion of TSH from the pituitary gland, which may cause thyroid gland enlargement. Carbimazole and other thionamides rarely cause an acute aplastic anaemia or reduced granulocyte count, which may be fatal. Therefore it is essential to check the white cell count should a patient on carbimazole develop symptoms suggestive of an infection such as sore throat.

15.20 A B D

Grave's disease is the commonest cause of hyperthyroidism. It is a thyroid-specific autoimmune disease, and is usually associated with the production of long-acting thyroid stimulator (LATS). Autoantibodies to thyroglobulin are associated with Hashimoto's disease. Like most autoimmune disorders, it occurs more commonly in women than men. It causes a diffuse enlargement and increased vascularity of the thyroid gland. Clinically, the increased vascularity may be detected by a bruit over the gland. LATS mimics TSH by stimulating thyroid to secrete thyroid hormones. It also causes exophthalmos (accumulation of fat in orbital tissues), pretibial myxoedema and clubbing of the fingers (accumulation of mucopolysaccharides in the dermis).

15.21 A C

LATS is an autoantibody to thyroid epithelial cells and is characteristically associated with Grave's disease. It is an IgG, and hence may cross the placenta and give rise to symptoms of hyperthyroidism in the infant. It stimulates the thyroid gland to increase the formation of thyroid hormones. It is also associated with infiltration of the orbital tissues by fat (which results in exophthalmos) and accumulation of mucopolysaccharides in the dermis (which results in pretibial myxoedema and clubbing).

15.22 B C D E

Most thyroid tumours are benign, and thyroid carcinomas are quite rare. Amongst the thyroid carcinomas, about 60% are papillary carcinomas. They usually occur in young adults, and have the best prognosis. Follicular carcinoma constitutes about a quarter of all thyroid carcinomas. They occur in young adults and middle-aged people. They often spread via the bloodstream to the bones or lungs. However,they respond well to radioactive iodine. Anaplastic carcinomas constitutes only about 10–15% of all thyroid carcinomas. They usually occur in the elderly, and have the worst prognosis. Medullary carcinomas are derived from the C-cells and commonly secrete calcitonin. They are often associated with other endocrine neoplasia such as phaeochromocytoma.

15.23 A B C D E

The thyroid gland consists of two lobes connected by a narrow isthmus. It is surround by a sheath derived from the pretracheal fascia, which also adheres to the larynx. This explains why the thyroid gland moves with the larynx on swallowing. This phenomenon is valuable in deciding whether a neck swelling originates from the thyroid clinically. The thyroid gland develops from an endodermal outgrowth from the floor of the pharynx. The site of origin is on the tongue, the foramen caecum. Normally, the thyroid descends to its normal adult position. Incomplete descent may result in thyroid tissue being found at any point between the base of the tongue and the trachea. The isthmus lies anterior to the second and fourth rings of the trachea; the lobes of the thyroid gland lie lateral to the trachea. Hence clinical enlargement of the thyroid gland may compress the thyroid gland and cause airway obstruction. The recurrent laryngeal nerves lie posteromedial to the lobes in the groove between the trachea and the oesophagus, and may be liable to damage in a thyroidectomy operation.

15.24 C D

About 99% of the total body calcium is in the skeleton. Normally, about 90% of all calcium excreted appears in the faeces, and only 10% appears in the urine. This loss of calcium is replaced by net absorption of calcium from the diet. Calcium can be reabsorbed by either active transport or passive diffusion. There is usually a continuous exchange of calcium between the bones and extracellular fluid, although there might be little or no net transfer of calcium between two body compartments in healthy individuals. About half of the total plasma calcium is bound to proteins. This proportion increases with increasing plasma protein concentration and decreasing plasma pH.

15.25 A

Total body calcium is an index of bone mass. In osteoporosis, there is a net excess of bone resorption over bone formation, and people with osteoporosis are liable to develop fractures, especially of the femur. Normally, the bone mass increases in childhood during growth until early adulthood. Thereafter, the bone mass gradually declines. Men generally have higher bone mass than women. In women, the loss of bone mass accelerates after the menopause. Hence fracture of the femur is commoner in the elderly and in women especially after the menopause.

15.26 A B D E

Vitamin D increases the plasma calcium by its effect on the intestines, the kidneys and bone. It increases the absorption of calcium by stimulating the active transport of calcium from the intestinal lumen. The urinary excretion of calcium is reduced by increasing calcium reabsorption in the kidneys. It stimulates the maturation of both osteoblasts (which mobilise calcium from bone) and osteoclasts (which form bone utilising plasma calcium). However, the net effect is mobilisation of calcium from bone.

15.27 A B C

There are two sources of vitamin D_3: dietary and conversion from 7-dehydrocholecholesterol. Sunlight is required for the latter. Vitamin D_3 is converted to 25-hydroxycholecalciferol in the liver. It is then converted in the proximal tubules of the kidneys either to the active form, 1,25-dihydroxycholecalciferol, or to the relatively inactive form, 24,25-dihydroxycholecalciferol. The quantity of

24,25-dihydroxycholecalciferol is tightly controlled by the plasma calcium and phosphate level.

15.28 D

The most active form of vitamin D is 1,25-dihydroxycholecalciferol. It is tightly regulated, and is synthesised by conversion in the renal tubules from 25-hydroxycholecalciferol. The level of 25-hydroxycholecalciferol itself is not tightly regulated. When the synthesis of the 1,25-dihydroxycholecalciferol is increased, the synthesis of the inactive 24,25-dihydroxycholecalciferol is decreased, and vice versa. When the plasma calcium is high, the secretion of parathyroid hormone is decreased. This decreases the synthesis of 1,25-dihydroxycholecalciferol in the kidneys. A high plasma level of phosphate directly inhibits the synthesis of 1,25-dihydroxycholecalciferol in the kidneys.

15.29 D

There are normally two superior and two inferior parathyroid glands. They normally lie posterior to and within the fascial sheath of the thyroid gland. Hence the parathyroid glands can be accidentally removed in thyroidectomy. The superior glands are usually in their normal position. However, the inferior glands are sometimes found more caudal to their normal position, and are occasionally found amongst the thymic tissue in the superior mediastinum. This is because the inferior parathyroid glands and the thymus are closely related in their development, as they are both derived from the third pharyngeal pouch. During thyroidectomy, it is important for the surgeons to locate the parathyroid glands. The parathyroid glands only secrete parathyroid hormones. Calcitonin is secreted by the C-cells of the thyroid gland.

15.30 E

Parathyroid hormone (PTH) is a peptide with 84 amino acids. It is secreted by all four parathyroid glands. It increases plasma calcium and decreases plasma phosphate levels via its direct actions on bones and kidneys, and its indirect action on the intestines. It has an overall effect of mobilising calcium from the bones. PTH decreases the reabsorption of phosphates and increases the reabsorption of calcium from the kidneys. Hence the urinary excretion of phosphate is increased but the urinary excretion of calcium is decreased. PTH does not act directly on the intestine, but it increases the synthesis of 1,25-dihydroxycholecalciferol. This causes an increase in calcium absorption from the intestine.

15.31 A D

In hypoparathyroidism, the level of PTH is low. This leads to a low plasma calcium level, reduced urinary phosphate excretion and a high plasma phosphate level. In pseudohypoparathyroidism, the PTH receptors in the tissues fail to respond to the hormone. Hence, although the parathyroid hormone level is normal or increased, all other biochemical features are similar to hypoparathyroidism. Plasma protein level is not affected.

15.32 B C E

Calcitonin is secreted by the C-cells (parafollicular cells) of the thyroid gland. It acts mainly on the bones and the kidneys to lower the plasma calcium and phosphate levels. It inhibits the osteoclasts and hence inhibits bone resorption. As the disorganised new bone formation in Paget's disease is due to an increased osteoclastic activity, calcitonin is useful in the treatment of Paget's disease. Calcitonin also increases the urinary excretion of calcium, but it has no direct action on the intestine.

15.33 C D E

Calcium is essential for neuromuscular transmission. A low plasma calcium level has an excitatory effect on muscle and nerve cells. Hence hypocalcaemia may give rise to a 'pins and needles sensation', tetany or convulsions. Hypercalcaemia is associated with tiredness, muscle weakness, thirst or polyuria, and constipation.

15.34 A B E

Hypercalcaemia may be caused by primary or secondary bone diseases, excessive PTH secretion, excessive vitamin D or increased sensitivity of receptors to vitamin D. Bone metastases and multiple myeloma are important causes of hypercalcaemia. Excessive PTH may be due to primary or tertiary hyperparathyroidism or ectopic PTH secretion from malignancies. Increased sensitivity of tissues to vitamin D occurs in sarcoidosis.

15.35 C D

Primary hyperparathyroidism is usually caused by parathyroid hyperplasia or a parathyroid adenoma. The plasma calcium level is high, and the plasma PTH level is inappropriately high for the level of plasma calcium. Parathyroidectomy may be required. Secondary hyperparathyroidism is due to a physiological response to a low plasma calcium level caused by a disease outside the parathyroid gland. The parathyroid gland attempts to compensate for the low calcium level by producing more PTH. Renal failure is a common cause. Treatment of the underlying disease is essential. The parathyroid gland in chronic secondary hyperparathyroidsm may become autonomous. This is tertiary hyperparathyroidism, when the plasma calcium level is high.

15.36 B D E

Medical treatment for hypercalcaemia is only a temporary measure to allow more time for the underlying cause to be treated. The first line of treatment is to rehydrate with intravenous saline in order to increase the urinary excretion of calcium. This can be augmented with a loop diuretic such as frusemide. However, thiazide diuretics must not be used as it increases renal reabsorption of calcium. Calcitonin reduces plasma calcium by inhibiting bone resorption and increasing urinary calcium excretion. Bisphosponates may also be used, although they are more useful in hypercalcaemia due to malignancy. Adrenocortical steroid acts by reducing intestinal absorption of calcium, and is useful in hypercalcaemia due to vitamin D intoxication or sarcoidosis with associated hypersensitivity to vitamin D. However, adrenocortical steroid is not useful in hyperparathyroidism. Dialysis may be required for severe cases or in the presence of renal failure.

15.37 A C E

Bisphosphonates reduce the reabsorption of bone by adsorbing onto bone crystals and by inhibiting osteoclast activity. Hence they have been used to treat Paget's disease (which is characterised by increased bone resorption and formation), osteoporosis (with abnormal reduction in the bone mass) and hypercalcaemia due to neoplasia. Osteomalacia is caused by vitamin D deficiency, and the treatment is vitamin D.

15.38 A C D

The islets of Langerhans of the pancreas secrete at least four hormones. Insulin and glucagon are important for regulating the metabolism of carbohydrates, fats and proteins. Somatostatin is important for regulating islet cell secretion. The fourth hormone, pancreatic polypeptide, is primarily concerned with gastrointestinal function. Gastin is secreted by G-cells in the stomach. Cholecystokinin–pancreozymin is secreted in the upper small intestine, and mediates the contraction of the gallbladder and enzymatic secretion of the pancreas.

15.39 B D E

Insulin consists of two amino acid chains linked by disulphide bridges. There are only minor variations in amino acid sequences amongst species. For example, pig insulin only differs from human insulin by one amino acid, and beef insulin by three amino acids. Hence pig and beef insulin are active when given to diabetic humans. However, humans almost invariably develop antibodies to beef insulin after a few months of treatment, although the antigenicity of pig insulin is lower. This reduces the effectiveness of the treatment. Fortunately, this problem can now be avoided as human insulin can be manufactured by recombinant DNA technique.

15.40 C

The overall net effect of insulin is to increase storage of carbohydrates, protein and fat. Hence the transport of glucose and amino acids into cells is increased. The transport of potassium into cells is also increased, and insulin and glucose together are sometimes used to treat hyperkalaemia. Protein synthesis is increased, and protein degradation is reduced. The synthesis of both glycogen and fat is increased.

15.41 B D

Insulin receptors are found in a large variety of cells, and are found on the cell membranes. Each receptor consists of two α-and two β-glycoprotein subunits, but these are synthesised by a single mRNA. When insulin binds to its receptors, they aggregate and are endocytosed into the cytoplasm, where they exert their effects of increasing transport of glucose, amino acids into cells, as well as their effects on other mediators. The insulin–receptor complexes are eventually destroyed in lysosomes. The number and affinity of insulin receptors are closely regulated. Hence the number of receptors decreases with increasing plasma insulin level, and the affinity of receptors increases with decreasing plasma insulin level. The number of receptors decreases in obesity. This is partly explained by a higher plasma insulin level.

15.42 B D

Glucose tolerance refers to the rate of decline of the plasma glucose level to normal after an oral glucose meal. In the glucose tolerance test, a standard glucose load is given orally, and the rate of decline of the plasma glucose level is monitored. The result depends mainly on the rate of entry of glucose into the cells (peripheral utilisation) and the rate of glycogen synthesis by the liver. The rate of glucose absorption is not an important factor. The rates of glucose uptake by the brain and red blood cells do not usually vary much with plasma glucose level.

15.43 A B C D

Some of the clinical features of diabetes result directly from the high plasma glucose level. When the renal threshold for glucose is exceeded, glucose may appear in the urine, and may be detected with a dipstick. High plasma glucose increases the plasma osmolality. This leads to the stimulation of thirst as well as osmotic diuresis. If the plasma level is elevated over a period of time, small amounts of haemoglobin A may be glycosylated to form HbA_{1c}. This is used clinically to monitor diabetic patients in clinical practice, as elevated levels of HbA_{1c} may indicate poor control of diabetes over the previous six weeks.

15.44 B C E

Deficiency of insulin in diabetes mellitus leads to decreased entry of glucose into cells. Hence there is intracellular glucose deficiency. Glycogen synthesis is reduced, and glycogen breakdown increases. Breakdown of adipose tissue and fats leads to an accumulation of acetyl CoA. Entry to the citric acid cycle is decreased due to a deficiency of enzyme converting acetyl CoA to malonyl CoA. Hence, the excess acetyl CoA is converted to ketone bodies, which also appear in the urine. The ketone bodies can be detected in diabetic patients clinically. Deficiency of insulin also leads to decreased entry of amino acids into cells. These amino acids may be used to synthesis glucose in the liver. Hence there is a net breakdown of protein, and there is an overall negative nitrogen balance.

15.45 A C E

In diabetic ketoacidosis, the accumulation of ketone bodies causes excessive hydrogen ions to be released in the plasma. The low plasma pH stimulates the respiratory centre, and results in abnormally deep and fast breathing. Urinary loss of sodium and potassium is excessive partly due to the polyuria associated with increased plasma osmolality. Hence the total body sodium and potassium are depleted. However, the plasma potassium is usually normal. This is partly because the extracellular volume is diminished, and partly because the low insulin level and high plasma H^+ favour potassium to stay in the extracellular fluid rather than in cells.

15.46 –

Sulphonylureas include drugs such as tolbutamide and chlorpropamide. They lower the blood glucose mainly by releasing stored insulin from the islet cells. However, they do not increase insulin synthesis. Hence they should not be used in patients with total deficiency of insulin (e.g. type I diabetes). Sulphonylureas also seem to increase the sensitivity of tissues to insulin. They cause hypoglycaemia in the same way in normal subjects. Sulphonylureas frequently cause weight gain. As diabetes is usually associated with progressive loss of β-cell function, the effectiveness of sulphonylureas usually decreases with time.

15.47 C D

Metformin is the commonest biguanide used in clinical practice. It reduces plasma glucose by decreasing the production of glucose in the liver and enhancing peripheral utilisation of glucose. It does not increase the formation of insulin, and hence is unsuitable for insulin-dependent diabetes mellitus. As it has an anorexic effect and may reduce weight in obese patients, its main use is for obese patients with non-insulin-dependent diabetes mellitus. It may be used in combination with sulphonylureas. It usually does not cause hypoglycaemia on its own. However, it may occasionally cause lactic acidosis, especially if there are other underlying diseases such as septicaemia, liver or renal failure.

15.48 A D E

Type I diabetes is due to impaired β-cell function and inadequate insulin secretion. Subjects often present in childhood with diabetic ketoacidosis, and usually require long-term insulin treatment. There are several hypotheses regarding its aetiology. Subjects often have circulating antibodies to different islet cells, and the disease is thought to be autoimmune. Subjects with certain HLA types (e.g. HLA-DR4) are more likely to develop the disease. The autoimmune disease is thought to be triggered by certain viruses such as Coxsackie B viruses. The monozygotic twin concordance rate is 40%. By contrast, type II diabetes secretes a normal amount of insulin, but there is a reduction in the number of insulin receptors. The disease usually develops in middle age, and ketoacidosis is uncommon. Genetic factors play an extremely important part, as the monozygotic concordance is almost 100%. There is no evidence that it is an autoimmune disease.

15.49 A B C D E

Diabetes mellitus affects both large and small blood vessels. Hence patients with diabetes often develop atherosclerosis at an earlier age, and hence are more at risk of myocardial infarction, cerebrovascular disease and peripheral vascular diseases. It also affects small blood vessels of the kidneys and the retina. Hence subjects may develop nephropathy and retinopathy.

15.50 A B C D E

Glucagon is a polypeptide with 29 amino acids. In the liver, glucagon mediates its effect by increasing cAMP. Glucagon increases the breakdown of glycogen in the liver, which also increases the plasma glucose level. It also increases the conversion of amino acids in the liver to glucose, and increases ketone body formation and the breakdown of fats. Physiologically, it is important that the available glucose is taken up and used by the cells. This is achieved as glucagon is a potent stimulator of insulin secretion, and insulin increases the uptake of glucose by the cells. Glucagon is broken down in the liver. Hence, in patients with liver diseases, the amount of glucagon reaching the circulation may be increased.

15.51 C D E

The secretion of glucagon is mainly stimulated by a reduced plasma glucose level. This provides a feedback mechanism to control the plasma glucose level. Although a high plasma insulin level would result in a reduced plasma glucose level, insulin increases the secretion of GABA from A-cells, which in turn inhibits glucagon secretion. Stimulation of the β-adrenergic receptors results in increased secretion of glucagon. This is important in the 'fight, fright, flight' response of the sympathetic nervous system. Exercise increases the secretion of glucagon at least partly via stimulating the sympathetic nervous system. A high level of plasma amino acids increases the secretion of glucagon, as glucagon is necessary for the conversion of amino acids into glucose.

15.52 A B C D E

When the plasma glucose decreases, the first symptoms to appear are due to increased sympathetic discharge. Hence sweating, palpitations and nervousness occur. As glucose is the only source of fuel for the neural tissues, neurological symptoms appear if the plasma glucose decreases further. Lethargy, coma, convulsions and permanent brain damage may occur depending on the level of hypoglycaemia.

15.53 A B D E

Whilst insulin is the only hormone which lowers the plasma glucose level, there are at least four hormones which increase the plasma glucose level: glucagon, adrenaline, growth hormone and cortisol. All four hormones increase the breakdown of glycogen in the liver. Growth hormone and cortisol increase peripheral utilisation of glucose.

15.54 E

The physiological effects of growth hormone include the growth of long bones before the epiphyses have fused, and metabolic effects on carbohydrates, fat and protein metabolism. Linear growth of the long bones is no longer possible after the epiphyses have fused. Hence excessive growth hormone may cause bone and soft tissue deformities as in acromegaly. Growth hormone increases the breakdown of glycogen in the liver, and hence increases the plasma glucose level. Although growth hormone enhances the response of the tissues to insulin, it has no effect on the plasma insulin level. Growth hormone breaks down fat and increases the plasma fatty acid level, which can be used by tissues as an alternative source of energy.

15.55 A B C D

Somatomedins are polypeptide growth factors which are secreted by the liver and other tissue in response to growth hormone. One of the factors (IGF-1) can stimulate both skeletal and cartilage growth. It is not clear exactly what role somatomedins play in mediating the actions of growth hormone. Somatomedins are decreased in untreated diabetes mellitus, which partly accounts for the increased breakdown of protein.

15.56 C D E

The adrenal medulla secretes catecholamines (adrenaline, noradrenaline and dopamine). The adrenal cortex consists of an outer layer (zona glomerulosa), a middle layer (zona fasciculata) and an inner layer (zona reticularis). The zona glomerulosa secretes mineralocorticoid. Sex hormones are secreted by both the zona fasciculata and zona reticularis. Glucocorticoids are secreted by all three layers.

15.57 A D

Both adrenaline and noradrenaline are produced by the adrenal medulla and the sympathetic nervous system. Whilst the physiological effects of adrenaline and noradrenaline are very similar, there are some minor differences. Both adrenaline and noradrenaline act on the β_1 receptors to increase the force and rate of cardiac contractions. However, noradrenaline produces vasoconstriction in most organs (via α_1 receptors) whilst adrenaline dilates the blood vessels in skeletal muscles and the liver (via β_2 receptors). Hence, whilst the peripheral resistance increases with noradrenaline, it may decrease with adrenaline. Whilst noradrenaline produces an increase of both systolic and diastolic blood pressure, adrenaline tends to produce an increase in systolic blood pressure but decreases the diastolic pressure, hence widening the pulse pressure. Adrenaline tends to produce a higher level of fear and anxiety. It has been found that the ratio of noradrenaline to adrenaline is increased in certain situations (e.g. hypoxia). The significance of this is still not properly understood.

15.58 A B C E

In the synthesis of glucocorticoids, ACTH acts on receptors on the plasma membrane of a cortisol-secreting cells in the zona fasciculata or zona reticularis of the adrenal cortex. This leads to activation of membrane adenyl cyclase, and an increase in intracellular cAMP. The cAMP activates protein kinase, which converts cholesterol esters to cholesterol. Cholesterol is the precursor of all steroids. The cholesterol is transported into mitochondria by a carrier protein. The enzymes responsible for the synthesis of various glucocorticoids and mineralocorticoids are the mitochondrial cytochrome P450s. The products are shuttled between the mitochondria and the smooth endoplasmic reticulum, before the final products are released outside the cell. Mineralocorticoids (e.g. aldosterone) are synthesised by enzymatic conversion of corticosterone.

15.59 A B C D E

Systemic adrenal steroids are used in a wide variety of conditions for their anti-inflammatory and immunosuppressive actions. These include collagen disorders and other autoimmune disorders such as idiopathic thrombocytopenia purpura, anaphylactic shock, organ rejection, severe asthma attack, severe dermatitis, active chronic hepatitis, sarcoidosis and rheumatic fever. Adrenal steroids are occasionally used to replace physiological deficiencies as in Addison's disease.

15.60 C D E

Long-term administration of steroids may induce features of Cushing's syndrome. These include characteristic deposition of fat in the body and face (moon face), striae, hypertension, acne and hirsuitism, and osteoporosis of bone with associated fractures. Other recognised side effects include peptic ulceration, mental symptoms (e.g. depression or psychosis), and increased susceptibility to infection.

15.61 D

Cortisol is normally secreted in the adrenal cortex in response to ACTH. Hence psychologically stressful situations and ectopic ACTH-secreting tumours are associated with raised ACTH and cortisol levels. On the other hand, panhypopituitarism is associated with reduced ACTH and cortisol levels. In Addison's disease, the secretion of cortisol by the adrenal cortex is reduced. This stimulates ACTH secretion. Hence the cortisol level is low but the ACTH level is high. In primary adrenal tumour, the cortisol level may be high. Plasma ACTH level is low due to feedback inhibition from the raised plasma cortisol level.

16. The reproductive system
Questions

16.1 **People with the following sex chromosomal constitutions usually have testes:**

A XX
B XXY
C XO
D XYY
E XXX

16.2 **People with the following sex chromosomal constitutions have significantly abnormal gonadal function:**

A XO
B XX
C XY
D XXY
E XYY

16.3 **The following statements about the genetic control of the embryological development of the gonads are true:**

A A sex-determining region on the X chromosomes (SRX) directs the primordial germ cells to develop into ovaries
B A sex-determining region on the Y chromosome (SRY) directs the primordial germ cells to develop into testes
C The structural genes for developing the gonads are located in the sex chromosomes
D XXY individuals may have both testes and ovaries
E Testosterone is essential for the development of testes

16.4 **The following structures develop from the embryological Wolffian (mesonephric) system:**

A Testes
B The penis
C Ovaries
D Epididymis
E Oviducts

16.5 Structures developed from the Mullerian (paramesonephric) ducts are usually absent in the following individuals:

A Normal people with XY sex chromosomes
B Normal people with XX sex chromosomes
C Complete testicular feminisation syndrome with XY sex chromosomes
D Adrenogenital syndrome (XX individuals with excessive secretion of androgens)
E Turner's syndrome with sex chromosomes XO

16.6 Individuals with complete testicular feminisation syndrome and reared unambiguously as girls from birth usually have female:

A Genetic sex
B External genitalia
C Internal genitalia
D Gender identity
E Gender role

16.7 Prior to any medical treatment, a male to female transsexual almost always has male:

A Genetic sex
B External genitalia
C Internal genitalia
D Gender identity
E Sexual preference

16.8 Compared to puberty in girls, boys have:

A An earlier growth spurt
B A higher growth velocity
C More conspicuous voice changes
D A higher increase in the proportion of body fat
E A higher increase in skeletal mass

16.9 According to the hypothalamic maturation hypothesis for the initiation of puberty:

A The key mechanism is a change in the pituitary sensitivity to gonadotrophin-releasing hormone (GnRH)
B The key mechanism is the secretion of GnRH in a pulsatile manner
C Hypothalamic maturation is not possible in people without functioning gonads
D Gonads of young children cannot be made to respond to hypothalamic signals
E The gonadostat hypothesis is impossible

16.10 The following statements about puberty in developed countries are true:

- **A** There has been a secular trend towards earlier puberty for girls
- **B** There has been a secular trend towards later puberty in boys
- **C** Girls with a body weight below 45 kg are unlikely to have menstruation
- **D** Reduction in exposure to sunlight is associated with earlier puberty
- **E** A low protein diet is associated with earlier puberty

16.11 Causes of delayed puberty in girls include:

- **A** Anorexia nervosa
- **B** Constitutional delay
- **C** Anterior hypothalamic tumour
- **D** Turner's syndrome
- **E** Oestrogen-secreting ovarian tumour

16.12 The intratubular component of the seminiferous tubules of the testis:

- **A** Is associated with the synthesis of spermatozoa
- **B** Is associated with the synthesis of androgens
- **C** Is associated with the synthesis of inhibin
- **D** Is lined by Leydig cells
- **E** Exchanges freely with the extratubular component

16.13 The following statements about the regulation of androgen and spermatozoa synthesis are true:

- **A** Luteinising hormone (LH) is essential for the secretion of testosterone
- **B** Follicule-stimulating hormone (FSH) is essential for the secretion of testosterone
- **C** Oestrogen is essential for effective spermatogenesis
- **D** FSH is essential for effective spermatogenesis
- **E** Testosterone is essential for effective spermatogenesis

16.14 The following statements about ovarian germ cells in a human female are correct:

- **A** The total number reaches a maximum at about 25 years of age
- **B** The total number increases rapidly during puberty
- **C** About 10% result in a functioning corpus luteum
- **D** Selection for pre-antral follicular development is regulated by the pituitary gland
- **E** The ovarian germ cells of a 10-year-old girl can undergo mitosis

16.15 The release of GnRH:

A Stimulates the secretion of FSH
B Stimulates the secretion of LH
C Is usually at a constant rate
D Is from the hypothalamus
E Is usually increased by a high progesterone concentration

16.16 The LH surge in the menstrual cycle:

A Is an example of a positive feedback system
B Is associated with reduced sensitivity of the anterior pituitary to GnRH
C Is associated with increased secretion of GnRH
D Is necessary for ovulation to occur
E Is induced by a progesterone surge

16.17 In females, inhibin:

A Is secreted by the corpus luteum
B Acts to reduce the plasma FSH level
C Acts to reduce the plasma LH level
D Is important in the positive feedback regulation of gonadotrophins
E Acts in a similar way to activin

16.18 The following hormones are generally significantly higher in the luteal than in the early follicular phase in the menstrual cycle:

A Oestrogen
B Progesterone
C FSH
D LH
E Inhibin

16.19 During the late luteal phase of the menstrual cycle:

A The number of progesterone receptors in the uterus increases
B The basal body temperature is higher than in the follicular phase
C The cervix produces thick mucus
D Sperm penetration into cervical mucus is enhanced
E Stromal proliferation occurs in the uterus

16.20 Most combined oral contraceptives ('the pill') consist of:

A Androgen
B Oestrogen
C Progestagen
D Corticosteroids
E Prostaglandins

16.21 Mechanisms of action of combined oral contraceptives include:

A Production of anti-sperm antibodies
B Prevention of fertilisation
C Facilitation of implanted zygote to abort
D Spermicidal activity
E Inhibition of ovulation

16.22 Advantages of combined oral contraceptives over progestagen-only contraceptive ('mini-pills') include reduced likelihood of:

A Contraceptive failure
B Deep-vein thrombosis
C Inhibition of lactation during pregnancy
D Irregular bleeding
E Contraceptive failure if the administration of a pill is inadvertently delayed

16.23 Inhibition of ovulation is a significant mechanism of action for the following contraceptives:

A Progestagen-only pills
B Intramuscular progesterone
C Intrauterine contraceptive device
D Subcutaneous progestagen implant (e.g. Norplant)
E Female surgical sterilisation procedure

16.24 Significant predisposing factors for endometrial carcinoma include:

A Oestrogen replacement therapy after menopause
B Late menarche
C Obesity
D Premature menopause
E Multiple sexual partners

16.25 Primary ovarian tumours:

A May be familial
B Are often associated with an increased plasma CA125 level
C Cause more deaths than endometrial carcinoma
D Are almost always malignant
E May produce oestrogen

16.26 Significant predisposing factors for carcinoma of the cervix include:

A Cigarette smoking
B Frequent sexual intercourse
C Multiple sexual partners
D Human papillomavirus infection
E Late menopause

16.27 The following statements about the female breast are correct:

A Accessory nipples are usually found in the midline
B The lobes secrete milk independent of one another
C The epithelial cells do not produce secretions
D The myoepithelial cells contain contractile proteins
E Each lobe is drained by one lactiferous duct

16.28 The female breasts:

A Require progesterone for their development
B Require oestrogens for their development
C Enlarge rapidly during puberty
D Enlarge rapidly during pregnancy
E Undergo cyclical changes in the absence of pregnancy

16.29 The following substances increase the secretion of prolactin:

A Dopamine
B Bromocriptine
C Phenothiazines (e.g. chlorpromazine)
D Vasoactive intestinal polypeptide (VIP)
E Digoxin

16.30 The following are associated with unusually high plasma prolactin levels in women:

A Breast-feeding
B Pregnancy
C Recent university entry
D Hyperthyroidism
E Pituitary tumour

16.31 An abnormally high plasma level of prolactin in women may cause:

A Impaired fertility
B Loss of menstruation
C Headache
D Loss of libido
E Abnormal milk secretion

16.32 Significant factors for maintaining milk production during breast-feeding include:

A A high oestrogen level
B A high progesterone level
C Suckling
D A high prolactin level
E A high corticosteroid level

16.33 Pharmacological actions of cyproterone acetate in men include:

A Competitive inhibition of peripheral testosterone receptors
B A reduction in sperm counts
C A reduction in sex drive
D Impotence
E Breast enlargement

16.34 Recognised indications for cyproterone acetate include:

A Male contraception
B Male hypersexuality
C Prostatic carcinoma
D Severe acne in women
E Failure to ovulate in women

16.35 After spermatogenesis, the sperms must pass through the following structures before ejaculation:

A Epididymis
B Vas deferens
C Prostatic duct
D Seminal vesicle
E Penile urethra

16.36 Events which normally occur during penile erection include:

A Inhibition of the parasympathetic nervous supply
B Inhibition of the sympathetic nervous supply
C An increase in the arterial smooth muscle tone
D An increase of blood flow into the corpora cavernosa
E An increase in the venous outflow from the corpora cavernosa

16.37 The following neurotransmitters play significant roles in initiating and sustaining penile erection:

A GABA
B Acetylcholine
C Gastrin
D Nitric oxide
E Vasoactive intestinal polypeptide (VIP)

16.38 Recognised local drug treatment for impotence include:

A α-Adrenergic antagonists (e.g. papaverine)
B β-Adrenergic antagonists (e.g. propranolol)
C Corticosteroids (e.g. prednisolone)
D Prostaglandin E_1 (e.g. alprostadil)
E Calcium antagonists (e.g. nifedipine)

16.39 Oral sildenafil (Viagra):

A Is effective in improving spermatogenesis
B Is effective in treating impotence
C Is an inhibitor of cGMP-specific phosphodiesterase
D Increase nitric oxide level in the corpora cavernosum
E Is particularly useful if there is a recent history of myocardial infarct

16.40 The following statements about fertilisation are correct:

A It takes place in the endometrium of the uterus
B Sperm capacitation occurs after the acrosome reaction
C The acrosome reaction occurs after fusion with the oocyte
D Down's syndrome may result if an oocyte is fertilised by two sperms
E The oocyte contains a haploid set of chromosomes before fertilisation

16.41 The following events between fertilisation and implantation and their outcomes are appropriately matched:

A Division of the conceptus into two distinct groups of cells – monozygotic twins
B Two oocytes are separately fertilised by two sperms in the same ovulatory cycle – dizygotic twins
C One oocyte is fertilised by two sperms in the same ovulatory cycle – monozygotic twins
D Two oocytes are fertilised by two sperms in different ovulatory cycles – polyploidy
E Two separately fertilised conceptuses sticking together to form a single conceptus – triploidy

16.42 Human chorionic gonadotrophin (hCG):

A Is secreted by the ovaries
B Binds to LH receptors
C Increases during the luteal phase of the menstrual cycle in the absence of pregnancy
D Consists of two α chains and two β chains
E May be used as a marker of pregnancy

16.43 The following hormones are secreted by the placenta during pregnancy:

A Oestrogen
B Progesterone
C Prolactin
D hCG
E Human placental lactogen

16.44 Amniotic fluid:

- **A** Has a total volume of about 2 litres at 20 weeks pregnancy
- **B** Has a protein content higher than that of normal serum
- **C** Is removed by the fetus from the amniotic cavity by swallowing
- **D** Is partly produced by the fetus micturating into the amniotic cavity
- **E** Contains fetal epithelial cells

16.45 The following abnormalities of amniotic fluid and their possible fetal causes are correctly matched:

- **A** Low amniotic fluid volume (in late pregnancy) – oesophageal atresia
- **B** Excessive amniotic fluid (in late pregnancy) – renal agenesis
- **C** Low α-fetoprotein (AFP) level (in early pregnancy) – spina bifida
- **D** High bilibrubin level (in late pregnancy) – rhesus incompatibility
- **E** Low sphingomyelin : lecithin ratio – immature fetal lungs

16.46 The following diseases may be diagnosed antenatally by amniocentesis or chorionic villous biopsy:

- **A** Duchenne muscular dystrophy
- **B** Cystic fibrosis
- **C** Down's syndrome
- **D** Haemophilia
- **E** Turner's syndrome

16.47 Significant mechanisms protecting the fetus against rejection by the mother's immune system include:

- **A** General immunosuppression by fetal corticosteroids
- **B** Inert properties of the chorionic trophoblast
- **C** Induced tolerance of the mother's immune system
- **D** Barriers to maternal–fetal transmission of antibodies or immune cells
- **E** Binding of fetal antigens to hostile maternal antibodies or immune cells

16.48 Endocrine changes just before parturition include an increase of:

- **A** Oestrogen to progesterone ratio
- **B** Prostaglandin locally in the uterus
- **C** Inhibin
- **D** Oxytocin
- **E** Relaxin

16.49 The following statements about uterine muscle contraction at parturition are true:

A The muscle cells act as a syncytium
B Prostaglandin increase contractility by direct action on prostaglandin receptors
C Oxytocin increases contractility by lowering the excitation threshold
D Contraction is initiated by the release of intracellular calcium
E Pacemakers are usually located near the cervix

16.50 The following measures are effective in initiating labour:

A Prostaglandin vaginal pessary
B Intravenous salbutamol
C Intravenous syntocinon (analogue of oxytocin)
D Artificial rupture of membrane
E Intravenous corticosteroids

16. The reproductive system Answers

16.1 **B D**

The key determinant to whether a person develops testes is the presence of the 'sex-determining region' on the Y chromosome. A person with a Y chromosome has the potential to develop testes, whilst the female gonads (the ovaries) develop in the absence of a Y chromosome. The Y chromosome contains a regulatory gene which controls the expression of other structural genes for developing the testes. The sex chromosomal constitution for normal males and normal females is XY and XX respectively. Turner's syndrome has XO constitution, and 'super females' have XXX constitution. They develop ovaries, although the ovaries of Turner's syndrome often under-develop and fail prematurely. XYY and XXY are the sex chromosomal constitution for 'super males' and Kleinefelter's syndrome respectively. They both develop testes. However, in Klinefelter's syndrome, the germ cells die when they enter meiosis, and the person may become infertile.

16.2 **A D**

See question 16.1 above. A Y chromosome is necessary for the initial formation of testes, and ovaries develop in the absence of a Y chromosome. However, the subsequent abnormal testicular development in Klinefelter's syndrome demonstrates that normal testicular development cannot take place with more than one X chromosome. Similarly, the abnormal ovarian development in Turner's syndrome demonstrates that the presence of more than one X chromosome is necessary for the subsequent normal ovarian development.

16.3 **B**

See also question 16.1. Whilst the formation of testes is dependent on the sex-determining region on the Y chromosome (SRY), the formation of ovaries is by default. The sex-determining region on the Y chromosome is located at the end of the short arm of the Y chromosome, and regulates the activities of many structural genes on various other chromosomes which are required to make the tests. Whilst the testes make testosterone, the development of testes is not dependent on testosterone.

16.4 D

The embryological gonads and external genitalia are capable of differentiating into either male or female structures. However, the embryological internal genitalia of males and females have different origins: the male internal genitalia develop from the embryological Wolffian (mesonephric) ducts to form the epididymis, vas deferens and seminal vesicles, whilst the female internal genitalia develop from the embryological Mullerian (paramesonephric) ducts to form the oviducts, the uterus and the cervix.

16.5 A C

The development of the Wolffian (male) and Mullerian (female) ducts is controlled by different hormones, and is not necessarily related to the genetic sex. The Wolffian ducts persist only in the presence of testosterone secreted by the testes, otherwise they will disappear. On the other hand, the Mullerian ducts will disappear only in the presence of Mullerian inhibiting hormone (MIH) secreted by the testes, otherwise they will persist. Hence, the structures developed from the Wolffian ducts (epididymis, vas deferens, seminal vesicles) are only found in males, and those from the Mullerian ducts (oviducts, uterus, cervix) are only found in females. In testicular feminisation syndrome, the genetic sex is male, and the secretion of androgens is normal. The peripheral tissues are insensitive to androgens, and hence the Wolffian ducts disappear. However, MIH is secreted and causes the Mullerian system to disappear as well. Hence individuals with testicular feminisation syndrome have no internal genitalia structures. Individuals with adrenogenital syndrome have female genetic sex and secrete androgens. However, they do not secrete MIH. Hence they develop the structures derived from both Mullerian and Wolffian ducts. People with Turner's syndrome secrete neither androgens nor MIH, and they develop normal Mullerian duct structures.

16.6 B D E

Individuals with complete testicular feminisation syndrome have XY sex chromosomes and therefore have male genetic sex. The tissues are insensitive to androgens, and hence they have female external genitalia. They have neither female nor male internal genitalia (see question 16.5 above). Gender identity is the self-awareness and personal experience of one's identity as male or female. This depends mainly on the sex assignment at birth and subsequent rearing. Hence individuals with complete testicular feminisation syndromes and reared as girls usually have a female gender identity. Gender role is defined by the way the individuals relate to others about their gender identity.

16.7 A B C

A male to female transsexual is an XY individual with testes and male external genitalia, and yet feels psychologically that he is a female. Hence their genetic sex is male, they have male internal and external genitalia, but they have female gender identity. Prior to medical treatment, their sexual preference may be either male or female.

16.8 B C E

Although many physiological and behavioural changes during puberty are similar in boys and girls, there are a few differences. Puberty in boys is initiated by androgens, but oestrogen is essential for puberty in girls. Whilst the onset of menarche (first menstrual bleeding) in girls is quite definitive, the first ejaculation in boys is less so. The growth spurt in boys is later than in girls, although the average peak height velocity is higher in boys than girls. This partly explains why, although girls are usually taller than boys between the ages of 11 and 14, men are taller than women. The changes in body shape are considerable during puberty. There is a much higher increase in the proportion of body fat in girls than boys, but boys achieve a higher increase in skeletal mass.

16.9 B

There are two main hypotheses for the mechanism for the initiation of puberty: the gonadostat hypothesis and the hypothalamic maturation hypothesis. According to the gonadostat hypothesis, maturation of the feedback system of the hypothalmo-pituitary–gonadal axis is important. Hence changes in the responsiveness of the hypothalamus to oestrogen or testosterone levels and the pituitary of GnRH are important. According to the hypothalamic maturation hypothesis, the maturation of the hypothalamus is the key element, and is independent of the pituitary–gonadal axis. The hypothalamus releases GnRH in a pulsatile manner. According to this hypothesis, hypothalamic maturation may occur in individuals without functioning gonads (e.g. Turner's syndrome), and gonads of young children can be made to respond to pulsatile release of GnRH. Experimental and clinical evidence supports the hypothalamic maturation hypothesis. However, the two hypotheses are not mutually exclusive.

16.10 A C

There has been a secular trend towards earlier puberty in the developed countries amongst both boys and girls. There are many hypothesis for this observation. Firstly, longer days created by artificial light are associated with earlier puberty in some animals. However, this is unlikely to be important in humans. Secondly, improved nutrition may be important. Body weight has been shown to correlate closely with the onset of puberty. Girls under about 47 kg and boys under about 55 kg are unlikely to undergo puberty. However, the precise mechanism for triggering pulsatile secretion of GnRH in the hypothalamus is still unknown.

16.11 A B C D

Delayed puberty in girls is said to occur if menstruation has not occurred by 16 years of age. The commonest cause is constitutional delayed puberty with no organic pathology, and there is often a family history. It appears that the hypothalamic maturation is programmed to be delayed. Pathological causes include pathology in the hypothalamus, pituitary and the ovaries. Girls with anorexia nervosa may fail to reach the critical body weight necessary to trigger hypothalamic maturation. Tumours in the anterior hypothalamus cause delayed puberty, whilst tumours in the posterior hypothalamus cause precocious puberty. Prolactin-secreting pituitary tumours or craniopharyngioma (tumour of Rathke's pouch) are associated with delayed puberty, whilst gonadotrophin-secreting pituitary tumours are associated with precocious puberty. Premature ovarian failure (e.g. Turner's syndrome) is associated with delayed puberty due to lack of oestrogen. On the other hand, oestrogen-secreting ovarian tumour causes precocious puberty.

16.12 A

Two intratubular and extratubular components of the seminiferous tubules of the testis are completely separate. Spermatozoa are synthesised in the intratubular compartment in association with Sertoli cells, whilst hormones (androgens, inhibin, oestrogens) are secreted in the Leydig cells within the extratubular compartment. The two compartments are separated by junctional barriers between adjacent Sertoli cells, and form the blood–testis barrier. As the body's immune system will produce antibodies against spermatozoal antigens which may lead to subfertility, this barrier is important in preventing spermatozoa from leaking into the lymphatic or venous system.

16.13 A D E

The secretion of testosterone by Leydig cells is stimulated by LH secreted by the anterior pituitary gland, and is facilitated by both inhibin and prolactin. Effective spermatogenesis depends on the actions of both testosterone and FSH.

16.14 –

Unlike spermatogenesis, mitosis of ovarian germ cells cease at the time of birth, and meiosis is initiated. Hence a human female has all the egg cells she will ever have (about 7 million) within her ovaries at birth. Thereafter, the total number declines until menopause. About 15–20 follicles are recruited for early antral follicle development in each cycle, and only one becomes the dominant follicle. Hence the proportion of ovarian germ cells which results in a functioning corpus luteum is very small (less than 1%). The mechanisms for selection of cells for pre-antral follicular development are not subject to regulation by factors outside the ovaries, although the exact mechanism is still unclear.

16.15 A B D

GnRH is secreted by the hypothalamus. It is secreted in pulses, and stimulates the secretion of both FSH and LH. Hence the gonadotrophins are also secreted in a pulsatile manner. Both the secretion of GnRH and the response of the pituitary gland to GnRH are important mechanisms for the control of the menstrual cycle in the female. In general, oestrogen usually reduces the pulse amplitude of GnRH secretion at relatively low secretion, and progesterone reduces the pulse frequency of GnRH secretion. This usually acts as a negative feedback system. However, in the luteal phase, a very high level of oestrogen may increase GnRH (and hence LHRH) secretion by a positive feedback system.

16.16 A C D

The LH surge marks the end of the follicular phase of the menstrual cycle, and is essential for the luteal phase and ovulation to take place. The LH surge is an example of a positive feedback system, and is triggered by an oestrogen surge at the end of the follicular phase. This positive feedback system is brought about by a combination of increased pulse amplitude of the GnRH secretion, and increased sensitivity of the anterior pituitary to the released GnRH.

16.17 A B

In the female, inhibin is secreted by the granulosa cells in the late follicular phase and by the corpus luteum. Hence, the plasma level of inhibin starts to increase in late follicular phase, and is highest in the early luteal phase. It acts to reduce plasma FSH level by reducing the anterior pituitary response to GnRH. It has no effect on LH level. It is thought to be important in the negative feedback regulation of gonadotrophins. Activin is another cytokine with an opposite mode of action to inhibin. It generally increases FSH level, but its physiological role is still unclear.

16.18 A B E

In the luteal phase, the corpus luteum secretes large quantities of progesterone, as well as oestrogen and inhibin. Inhibin acts to reduce the FSH level. Oestrogen and progesterone act to suppress the gonadotrophin levels. The presence of progesterone also prevents positive feedback regulation leading to LH surge.

16.19 A B C E

In the early luteal phase of the menstrual cycle, oestrogen induces the synthesis of progesterone receptors in the uterus. This, together with the increasing concentration of progesterone, stimulates secretions from the endometrium (lining of the uterus), stromal proliferation, as well as enlargement of the uterine muscle cells (myometrium). These changes prepare for the implantation of the embryo should fertilisation occur. In the cervix, progesterone changes the nature and amount of glycoproteins produced in the cervical epithelium, and produces a small volume of thick mucus which can only be stretched a short distance before snapping (a low spinnbarkeit). This mucus is relatively impenetrable to sperms. The body temperature also increases slightly under the influence of progesterone. This increase in body temperature and changes in cervical mucus allow women to detect ovulation and work out the 'safe period' using the 'natural' contraceptive method.

16.20 B C

Most combined oral contraceptives consist of an oestrogen and a progestagen. Most combined oral contraceptives contain low-dose oestrogen (20–35 μg), and contraceptives containing 50 μg oestrogen are now seldomly used.

16.21 B E

Combined oral contraceptives act mainly by inhibiting ovulation. This is achieved by oestrogen acting on the hypothalamus to prevent release of GnRH. However, progesterone in the combined oral contraceptives also makes cervical mucus more viscous and hence spermatozoa are less likely to reach the egg cell. Whilst combined oral contraceptives might inhibit the implantation of the zygote into the endometrium, they do not cause an implanted zygote to abort.

16.22 A D E

Combined oral contraceptives have a lower failure rate, and are less susceptible to contraceptive failure due to inadvertent delay or omission of a pill. Whereas an alternative contraceptive method must be used if a mini-pill is delayed for more than 3 h, the combined oral contraceptives are still effective even if an oral pill is delayed for up to 12 h. Furthermore, as the combined oral contraceptives are taken 21 days out of 28, women on combined oral contraceptives experience regular withdrawal bleeding, whereas women on progestagen-only pill may experience either absent, irregular or excessive vaginal bleeding. However, as the oral combined contraceptives contain oestrogen, there is a small increased risk of arterial or venous thromboembolism. As oestrogen inhibits lactation, it is not suitable whilst breast-feeding.

16.23 A B D

Although the key mechanism of action for the progestagen-only contraception method may be to render the cervical mucus inhospitable to sperms, it also inhibits ovulation. This applies whether the progestagens are taken orally, intramuscularly or subcutaneously. Intrauterine contraceptive devices act mainly by preventing implantation of the zygote in the endometrium. In female sterilisation, the oviducts (Fallopian tubes) are blocked by surgical clips. This prevents fertilisation from taking place.

16.24 A C

Endometrial carcinomas are mostly adenocarcinomas. The main risk factor is oestrogen stimulation unopposed by progesterone. Hence hormone replacement therapy with oestrogen (without progesterone) and polycystic ovarian syndrome are significant risk factors. They also occur more commonly in obese women, probably reflecting their higher oestrogen level. Multiple sexual partners are a significant risk factor for cervical but not endometrial carcinoma.

16.25 A B C E

There are many types of primary ovarian tumours, and they may arise from epithelial cells, germs cells or the sex cord stroma. They may be benign or malignant. Some ovarian carcinomas are familial, and a few ovarian cancer genes have recently been identified. As ovarian carcinomas often present late, they cause more deaths than any other gynaecological cancers. The protein CA125 has been found to be raised in cases of ovarian cancer, and it is now widely used as a tumour marker both to aid diagnosis and to monitor therapy.

16.26 A B C D

Squamous carcinoma is the commonest cervical carcinoma. It is likely to be caused by a sexually transmitted agent, such as human papillomaviruses and perhaps herpes simplex virus type 2. In general, increased sexual exposure (e.g. early age of sexual intercourse, frequent sexual intercourse and multiple sexual partners) is a predisposing factor. Cigarette smoking is an independent risk factor. Squamous cervical carcinoma is not hormone-dependent.

16.27 B D E

The female breasts consist of about 15–20 lobes. The lobes are separated from each other by fat and connective tissue. Milk is secreted by acini in each lobule. The acini are lined by epithelial cells which secrete milk. The myoepithelial cells surround the epithelial cells. They contain contractile proteins which contract in response to oxytocin and help to expel any milk synthesised into the ducts. The intralobular ducts drain into extralobular ducts, and they finally drain into the lactiferous ducts and sinuses. Each lobe is drained by one lactiferous duct. Accessory nipples are developmental abnormalities, and they are almost always found along the embryological 'milk line' between the axilla and the groin.

16.28 A B C D E

The hormonal regulation for breast development is complex and still not fully understood. However, it is clear that oestrogen and progesterone are essential. Other hormones which may be important include prolactin, growth hormone, glucocorticoids and insulin. The female breasts grow rapidly during puberty and in pregnancy. This involves both ductular and glandular proliferation, as well as deposition of adipose and connective tissue. The female breasts vary slightly in size and consistency due to variations in oestrogen and progesterone levels throughout the menstrual cycle. After menopause, the ductules and glandular structure involute. In the elderly, the breasts consist of mainly adipose tissue.

16.29 C D E

In diseases associated with a disconnection in the vascular links between the hypothalamus and the anterior pituitary gland, the secretion of prolactin is greatly increased whilst that of other hormones is reduced. Hence the secretion of prolactin from the anterior pituitary is mostly controlled via inhibitory factors from the hypothalamus. Dopamine is the main prolactin inhibitory factor, but GABA (γ-aminobutyric acid) and GnRH may also inhibit the release of prolactin. Bromocriptine is a dopamine agonist, and therefore inhibits the secretion of prolactin. Phenothiazines are dopamine antagonists and hence they increase prolactin secretion. It has been found recently that prolactin-releasing factors also exist. The main prolactin-releasing factor is VIP, but thyrotrophin-releasing hormone (TRH) and oestrogens also stimulate prolactin secretion. Digoxin increases prolactin secretion and may cause breast enlargement in men.

16.30 A B C E

Plasma prolactin levels are usually higher during sleep and decrease when awake. They are also abnormally high in the presence of psychological stress. As the main function of prolactin is to initiate and maintain milk secretion, the plasma level is physiologically high during pregnancy and breast-feeding. An elevated TRH level (e.g. in primary hypothyroidism) may increase prolactin secretion. Greatly elevated levels of prolactin may be due to a prolactin-secreting pituitary microadenoma.

16.31 A B D E

Hyperprolactinaemia is commoner in women than in men. In men a high prolactin level may cause impaired fertility and loss of libido. In women it may cause loss of libido, loss of menstruation, impaired fertility and abnormal milk secretion. Headache may be a symptom of a pituitary tumour, but not hyperprolactinaemia itself.

16.32 C D

Whilst oestrogen and progesterone are important in promoting ductal and lobular growth of the breasts during pregnancy, they inhibit milk secretion. Suckling is important in inducing prolactin release during breast-feeding and hence maintains milk production. Conditioned reflex (e.g. to a baby's cry) may increase the secretion of oxytocin and induce the expulsion of milk into the ducts. However, it does not increase milk production on its own.

16.33 A B C D

Cyproterone acetate is a competitive inhibitor of testosterone receptors in the peripheral tissues. Hence cyproterone acetate would reduce spermatogenesis, sex drive and the ability to sustain erection in men. It does not have an oestrogenic effect, and does not cause breast enlargement.

16.34 B C D

As cyproterone acetate is anti-androgenic, it may be used for management of male hypersexuality. However, it is particularly important to obtain informed consent. Cyproterone acetate is used in prostatic carcinoma as the disease is often androgen-dependent. The anti-androgenic effect of cyproterone may also be useful in treating severe acne or polycystic ovarian syndrome in women. Cyproterone acetate has no effect on ovulation.

16.35 A B E

After spermatogenesis, the spermatozoa are carried through vasa efferentia, and via the epididymis into the vas deferens and the posterior urethra. Semen is formed by a mixture of the spermatozoa with secretions from the prostate and the seminal vesicles.

16.36 B D

Erection is caused by increased blood flow to the corpora cavernosa. This causes venous compression and reduced venous outflow, and hence erection occurs. The initial increase in blood flow is initiated by a reduction in the arterial smooth muscle tone, which is controlled by the opposing effects of sympathetic and parasympathetic nervous supplies. Stimulation of the parasympathetic nervous system stimulates the α-adrenergic receptors, and causes a reduction in the arterial smooth muscle tone and hence penile erection, whilst stimulation of the sympathetic nervous system causes an increase in the arterial smooth muscle tone and hence penile flaccidity.

16.37 B D E

Stimulation of the sympathetic nervous system causes penile flaccidity. Stimulation of the parasympathetic nervous system causes penile erection, and the neurotransmitters implicated are acetylcholine, VIP and nitric oxide. The levels of these neurotransmitters are raised during erection.

16.38 A D

α-Adrenergic antagonists (e.g. papaverine) injected into the corpora cavernosa may be effective in treating impotence as it blocks the sympathetic tone which tends to increase the tone of the arterial smooth muscle. β-Adrenergic antagonists have no effect.

Prostaglandin E_1 (e.g. alprostadil) is a vasodilator and may increase arterial inflow if injected into the corpora cavernosa. Corticosteroids and calcium antagonists have no effect on penile erection.

16.39 B C D

Sildenafil (Viagra) was licensed for the treatment of male impotence in Britain in 1998. It is a potent inhibitor of cGMP phosphodiesterase type 5, the specific isoenzyme found in corpora cavernosa. Hence sildenafil increases cGMP, which in turns increase nitric oxide and decreases the tone of arterial smooth muscle. Its possible cardiovascular side effects have been well publicised, and the drug should not be given to anyone with a history of myocardial infarct within the last six months.

16.40 –

Fertilisation takes place in the Fallopian tube (oviduct). Before the sperm can fuse with the oocyte, it must undergo the acrosome reaction. Before the acrosomal reaction can occur, it must be prepared by the process of sperm capacitation, during which the surface components of the spermatozoa undergo changes. In this acrosome reaction, the acrosomal membrane of the sperm fuses with the overlying plasma membrane, and the contents of the acrosomal vesicle are discharged. This is associated with a large increase in intracellular calcium and cAMP, and the exposed plasma membrane in the equatorial and post-acrosomal membrane is now capable of fusion with the occyte. If the oocyte is fertilised by two sperms, the zygote contains three sets of chromosomes and triploidy results. The resulting triploidy is termed androgenetic triploidy. Before fusion of the gametes, the oocyte is in its second meiotic division, and still contains two sets of chromosomes. It must complete the second meiotic division and get rid of one set of chromosomes via the second polar body. Otherwise, gynogenetic triploidy occurs.

16.41 A B

Normally, the zona keeps the cells of the conceptus together after fertilisation but before implantation. Monozygotic twins result from the division of the conceptus shortly after fertilisation into two distinct groups of cells. The twins are genetically identical. Dizygotic twins result if two oocytes are separately fertilised in the same ovulatory cycle. Their genetic similarities are the same as those between other siblings. Androgenetic triploidy results if one oocyte is fertilised by two sperms in the same ovulatory cycle. Two oocytes fertilised in different ovulatory cycles result in normal siblings. Two separately fertilised conceptuses sticking together to form a single conceptus result in a chimaeric conceptus. The resulting fetus has two genetically different sets of cells.

16.42 B D E

hCG is structurally similar to LH, and consists of two α chains and two β chains. It signals the presence of the conceptus to the mother so that the uterus can be maintained in the luteal phase. It is initially secreted by the cytotrophoblast, and later by the syncytiotrophoblast of the implanting blastocyte from a few days after implantation. Urinary test for the β unit of hCG is widely used for the diagnosis of pregnancy.

16.43 A B D E

The placenta produces several hormones during pregnancy. hCG is important from two to seven weeks of pregnancy. Oestrogen and progesterone are important in maintaining the uterus in the luteal phase thereafter. Human placental lactogen and a placental variant of human growth hormone is produced after the first trimester, but their functions are not entirely clear. In the past, the maternal serum level of some of these hormones has been used as indicators of placental function, and 16α-hydroxylated steroids have been used as indicators of fetal well-being. However, these biochemical markers are now seldom used as ultrasound and Doppler findings have been found to be more reliable.

16.44 C D E

The volume of amniotic fluid produced in pregnancy increases until about 34 weeks. The average amniotic fluid volume at 20 weeks is about 500 ml. Apart from a much lower protein content, the composition of the amniotic fluid is broadly similar to that of normal serum. Before about 20 weeks into pregnancy, the amniotic fluid exchanges freely with the extracellular fluid of the fetus via its lungs, gut and skin. In later stages of pregnancy, micturition of the fetus contributes significantly to amniotic fluid volume. Hence renal agenesis of the fetus (Potter's syndrome) is associated with a low volume of amniotic fluid (oligohydramnios). The fetus swallowing contributes significantly to the removal of amniotic fluid in late pregnancy. Hence an excess of amniotic fluid (polyhydramnios) occurs in mechanical gastrointestinal obstruction (e.g. oesophageal atresia). Skin epithelial cells of the fetus can be found in the amniotic fluid. Hence chromosomal and genetic diseases may be diagnosed by sampling the amniotic fluid (amniocentesis) in early pregnancy.

16.45 D E

As the amniotic fluid exchanges freely with the extracellular fluid of the fetus, abnormalities in the fetus may cause abnormalities in the amniotic fluid. Abnormally low or abnormally high amniotic fluid volume may be due to renal agenesis or oesophageal atresia respectively (see question 16.44 above). A high AFP level in the amniotic fluid may indicate open neural tube defect in the fetus. The maternal serum AFP level may also be raised, although the result is not as reliable as the amniotic fluid level. Maternal AFP level and ultrasound are used as initial screening tests. A high unconjugated bilirubin level in the amniotic fluid in late pregnancy is likely to be due to haemolytic diseases in the fetus. This is usually due to rhesus incompatibility, although the disease is now rare due to the use of anti-D in rhesus-negative mothers after delivery. Amniotic bilirubin level may be used to monitor the disease antenatally. The fetal lung secretes surfactant during late pregnancy, and a lack of surfactant may cause idiopathic respiratory distress syndrome in the newborn baby. A component of the surfactant may be detected in the amniotic fluid in late pregnancy. This is valuable in predicting whether the fetus would develop idiopathic respiratory distress syndrome if delivered prematurely. If the sphingomyelin: lecithin ratio is low (<2), intramuscular corticosteroid or ACTH may be given to the mother at least 48 h before delivery in order to stimulate the fetus lung to produce sufficient surfactant.

16.46 A B C D E

Fetal cells are obtained from both amniocentesis and chorionic villous biopsy. Hence the karyotype of the fetus can be examined for chromosomal abnormalities such as Down's syndrome and Turner's syndrome. Genetic diseases may be diagnosed using recombinant DNA techniques if the relevant gene probes are available. These are now available for cystic fibrosis, haemophilia, Duchenne muscular dystrophy and most haemoglobinopathies.

16.47 B D E

Fetal antigens are different from the maternal antigens. Hence the mother's immune system would reject the fetus if there are no protecting mechanisms. It has been shown that the mother is neither generally immunosuppressed nor tolerant to the fetal antigens during pregnancy. Hence a rhesus-negative mother would react against rhesus-positive antigen on the fetal red cell membrane. The major protecting mechanisms are that the chorionic trophoblast is inert and acts as an immunological filter; some maternal immune cells may not cross the placenta (although IgG does cross the human placenta); and that free fetal antigens may bind to and hence 'mop up' a small quantity of maternal antibodies or immune cells. The last mechanism fails in rhesus incompatibility because the antigen is only present in a small proportion of cells in the body (red blood cells).

16.48 A B D E

To prepare for parturition, the cervix needs to be softened ('ripened'), and the uterus needs to be capable of contracting strongly and in a coordinated manner to expel the fetus. Prostaglandin both softens the cervix and increases the contractility of the uterus, and it is released locally from the cervix and uterus. Oxytocin also increases the contractility of the uterus. The release of both prostaglandin and oxytocin is facilitated by an increase in the oestrogen to progesterone ratio. Relaxin is also released in late pregnancy. It also softens the cervix. It might also soften the ligaments joining individual pelvic bones, and hence facilitate delivery.

16.49 A C D

The uterine muscle cells hypertrophy during pregnancy. They also act as a syncytium so that action potentials can spread via gap junctions. This allows effective and coordinated contraction of the uterus during parturition. The pacemakers are usually at the upper end of the uterus, so that contraction results in expulsion of the fetus. Uterine contraction is initiated by an increase of intracellular calcium. This is regulated by both prostaglandin and oxytocin. Prostaglandin increases the release of calcium from intracellular stores, whilst oxytocin lowers the excitation threshold of the muscle cells.

16.50 A C D

See question 16.49. Clinically, induction of labour may be achieved by artificial rupture of membranes, prostaglandin pessary and intravenous syntocinon. Artificial rupture of membranes causes an sudden release of prostaglandin from the cervix and uterus. Intravenous salbutamol (β-adrengergic agonist) tends to inhibit uterine contraction and prolong labour.

17. The renal and urinary system
Questions

17.1 The urinary concentration is normally significantly higher than the plasma concentration for the following substances:

A Glucose
B Urea
C Sodium ions
D Creatinine
E Albumin

17.2 The following substances are produced by the kidneys:

A Renin
B Aldosterone
C Erythropoietin
D 1,25-Dihydroxycholecalciferol
E Angiotensin II

17.3 The following statements about the kidneys are true:

A The left kidney lies slightly more inferior than the right kidney
B They normally move downwards on inspiration
C They lie in the peritoneal cavity
D They mainly receive parasympathetic innervation
E They are surrounded by fatty tissue

17.4 In contrast to cortical nephrons, juxtamedullary nephrons:

A Are more abundant
B Have longer loops of Henle
C Have glomeruli on the outer portions of the renal cortex
D Do not have vasa recta
E Produce more concentrated urine

17.5 The following structures of juxtamedullary nephrons can be found in the renal medulla:

A Renal glomeruli
B Distal convoluted tubules
C Thin descending limb of the loops of Henle
D Vasa recta
E Collecting ducts

17.6 The ureters:

A Open into the anterior surface of the bladder
B Have fibrous walls
C Are partially innervated via the testicular plexus in the male
D Are separated from the bladder by bicuspid ureteric sphincters
E Run anterior to the parietal peritoneum

17.7 The following structures originate from the ureteric bud in their embryological development:

A The renal pelvis
B Glomeruli
C Loops of Henle
D Collecting ducts
E The ureters

17.8 A horseshoe kidney:

A Results from the degeneration of the ureteric bud
B Results from a defect in the function of the proximal convoluted tubule
C Occurs as a result of abnormal descent of the metanephric mesoderm in its development
D Occurs in less than one out of a million people
E Is associated with fusion of the upper poles of both kidneys

17.9 An inert substance X is not produced, stored or metabolised by the kidneys. It is freely filtered by the kidneys. It is actively secreted but not reabsorbed by the renal tubules. It does not affect renal blood flow. The urine flow is 10 ml/min, the urinary concentration of X is 20 mg/ml, and its plasma concentration is 0.2 mg/ml.

A Substance X is ideal for measuring glomerular filtration rate (GFR)
B Substance X is ideal for measuring effective renal plasma flow
C The effective renal plasma flow is 1 litre/min
D The GFR is less than 1 litre/min
E The clearance of X is greater than the GFR

17.10 Which of the following increase renal blood flow?

A Noradrenaline
B Dopamine
C Exercise
D Renin
E Changing from supine to erect position

17.11 The GFR:

- **A** Is higher in women than in men
- **B** Is higher in neonates than in adults after correction for surface area
- **C** Is higher in the elderly than in younger adults.
- **D** Is normally about 1.8 litres per day (1.25 ml/min) in adults
- **E** May be estimated by creatinine clearance in clinical practice

17.12 The following substances are correctly matched to the mechanism of reabsorption in the proximal renal tubules:

- **A** Mannitol – passive diffusion
- **B** Water – secondary active transport via carrier proteins
- **C** Glucose – primary active transport
- **D** Sodium ions – secondary active transport via carrier proteins
- **E** Lactic acid – passive diffusion

17.13 Fluid at the following sites of the nephron is significantly hypertonic:

- **A** The glomerulus
- **B** Thin descending loop of Henle
- **C** The top of the thick ascending loop of Henle
- **D** Distal tubule
- **E** Medullary portion of the collecting duct

17.14 In the absence of vasopressin (antidiuretic hormone):

- **A** The collecting ducts are highly permeable to water
- **B** Reabsorption of sodium ions in the proximal renal tubules is reduced
- **C** The osmolality of the urine is abnormally low
- **D** The osmolality of the plasma is abnormally low
- **E** The urine volume is abnormally low

17.15 A reduction in the transport of sodium and chloride ions from the thick segment of the ascending loop of Henle:

- **A** May result in increased urinary potassium excretion
- **B** May result in diuresis
- **C** May increase the osmolality in the medullary interstitium
- **D** May be caused by frusemide
- **E** May be caused by thiazides

17.16 Spironolactone:

- **A** Is an aldosterone antagonist
- **B** Decreases the sodium reabsorption in the distal tubule
- **C** May cause hypokalaemia
- **D** Is a more powerful diuretic than frusemide
- **E** Antagonises the diuretic effect of frusemide

17.17 Osmotic diuresis occurs in:

A Mannitol infusion
B Diabetes insipidus
C Diabetes mellitus
D Compulsive water drinking
E Inappropriate ADH secretion

17.18 Recognised indications for frusemide include:

A Congestive heart failure
B Hypokalaemia (low potassium level)
C Hypercalcaemia (high calcium level)
D Hypertension
E Hyponatraemia (low sodium level)

17.19 Sodium excretion from the kidneys increases with:

A Shock
B Massive gastrointestinal haemorrhage
C A high-salt dietary intake
D An abnormally high plasma level of aldosterone
E Hypotension

17.20 The following changes occur in dehydration:

A Renal blood flow decreases
B GFR increases
C The medullary interstitial fluid becomes more hypertonic
D The urine becomes less concentrated
E Less vasopressin is secreted

17.21 The following statements about the transport of hydrogen ions from renal tubular cells into the tubular lumen are true:

A It occurs mainly in the loop of Henle
B Passive diffusion is an important mechanism
C Primary active transport is an important mechanism
D It is coupled with the entry of a sodium ion from the tubular lumen into the tubular cell
E It fails to occur if the pH of the urine is less than 3

17.22 Acetazolamide:

A Is an inhibitor of carbonic anhydrase
B Increases the production of aqueous humour
C Is an effective and commonly used diuretic
D Usually increases the plasma pH
E May be useful in preventing mountain sickness and facilitating acclimatisation at high altitude

17.23 The following buffer systems in the renal tubular lumen are important for effective excretion of hydrogen ions:

A Bicarbonate
B Sulphate
C Phosphate
D Ammonia
E Chloride

17.24 Alkalisation of urine:

A May be achieved by oral ammonium chloride
B Discourages the growth of *Escherichia coli* in urine
C Is useful in the treatment of amphetamine poisoning
D Is useful in the treatment of aspirin poisoning
E Is useful in the treatment of phenobarbitone poisoning

17.25 Recognised pharmacological effects of thiazide diuretics include:

A Increased plasma potassium
B Decreased plasma sodium
C Increased plasma magnesium
D Glucose intolerance
E Increased plasma uric acid

17.26 The following abnormalities frequently occur in renal failure:

A Anaemia
B Metabolic alkalosis
C High plasma urea
D Low plasma creatinine
E High plasma calcium

17.27 The presence of significant quantities of the following substances in urine is characteristic of glomerular damage:

A Urea
B Blood
C Protein
D Amino acids
E Glucose

17.28 Recognised causes of glomerular diseases include:

A Anti-glomerular basement membrane antibodies
B Diabetes mellitus
C Connective tissue disease
D Drugs
E Post-streptococcal infection

17.29 Recognised pathological features of obstructive nephropathy due to ureteric calculi include:

A Dilated renal pelvis
B Constricted renal calyces
C Atrophic renal tissues
D Hydronephrosis
E Dilated bladder

17.30 Pyelonephritis occurs more frequently:

A During pregnancy than at other times for women
B In the presence of vesico-ureteric reflux
C In the presence of urinary tract infection
D In the presence of septicaemia
E Following urethral catheterisation

17.31 Factors which favour the formation of stones in the urinary tract include:

A *Proteus* urinary tract infection
B Hypocalcaemia
C Excess excretion of calcium in urine
D High plasma uric acid level
E High blood cholesterol level

17.32 The following statements about renal cell carcinoma (hypernephroma) are true:

A It is the commonest malignant tumour in men
B It occurs less frequently than transitional cell tumour of the kidney
C Patients frequently present after metastasis has occurred
D It may be associated with polycythaemia (high red cell number)
E It is associated with exposure to aniline dye

17.33 The empty bladder:

A Lies entirely in the pelvis in adults
B Lies entirely in the pelvis in young children
C Can be palpated through the abdominal wall in adults
D Is approximately cuboid in shape
E Is joined at the middle portion of its anterior surface by the two ureters

17.34 The following groups of muscles usually contract during voluntary micturition:

A Perineal muscles
B External urethral sphincter
C Detrusor muscle
D Internal urethral sphincter
E Abdominal wall muscles

17.35 The following statements about neural control of the bladder are true:

- **A** Micturition may occur as a spinal reflex action
- **B** Micturition may be controlled via the higher cortical centre
- **C** The parasympathetic nervous supply to the bladder is active during micturition
- **D** Sympathetic stimulation is associated with contraction of the detrusor muscles
- **E** Sympathetic stimulation is associated with contraction of the external urethral sphincter

17.36 The following groups of drugs are recognised treatment for incontinence of urine due to instability of the detrusor muscle:

- **A** Noradrenaline
- **B** Tricyclic antidepressants
- **C** Antimuscarinic agents
- **D** Cholinergic agents
- **E** Inhibitors of serotonin reuptake

17.37 Causes of muscular hypertrophy of the bladder include:

- **A** Renal cell carcinoma
- **B** Benign prostatic hypertrophy
- **C** Carcinoma of the prostate
- **D** Urethral stricture
- **E** Ureteric calculi

17.38 The following statements about bladder tumours are true:

- **A** Sarcomas are commoner than epithelial tumours
- **B** Squamous cell carcinoma is the commonest epithelial tumour
- **C** They are commonly of the papillary type
- **D** Hydronephrosis in one kidney is a recognised complication
- **E** They are more commonly solitary than multiple

17.39 Significant predisposing factors for transitional cell bladder tumours include:

- **A** Aniline dyes
- **B** Schistosomiasis infection
- **C** Diabetes mellitus
- **D** Smoking
- **E** Excessive alcohol intake

17.40 Acquired bladder diverticula:

- **A** Predispose to calculi formation
- **B** Predispose to urinary tract infection
- **C** Are usually solitary
- **D** Occur more frequently in women than in men
- **E** Are frequently associated with bladder muscle hypertrophy

17.41 The prostate gland:

A Lies lateral to the rectum
B Lies superior to the neck of the bladder
C Can be palpated in a rectal examination
D Surrounds the prostatic urethra
E Produces an acidic secretion

17.42 Benign enlargement of the prostate gland:

A Has a higher incidence in older men
B Is associated with hypertrophy of glandular tissue
C Is caused by a reduction in oestrogen level
D Is associated with multiple circumscribed solid nodules
E May cause trabeculation of the bladder

17.43 Symptoms of benign prostatic enlargement may be partially relieved by:

A Loop diuretics
B α_1-Adrenoceptor antagonist
C β-Adrenoceptor antagonists
D 5 α-Reductase inhibitors
E Synthetic oestrogen

17.44 Clinical prostatic carcinoma:

A Arises most commonly in the lateral lobes
B Is mostly of the squamous cell type
C Is often associated with an abnormal low serum acid phosphatase level
D Is often associated with a raised serum prostatic specific antigen level
E Seldom metastasise to bone

17. The renal and urinary system
Answers

17.1 B D

The kidneys filter a fluid (glomerular filtrate) which resembles plasma in composition. In the renal tubules, over 99% of water and about 99% of solutes are reabsorbed. The proportion of urea and creatinine reabsorbed is only about 53% and 8% respectively, and hence their concentrations in urine are higher than their plasma concentrations. Over 99% of sodium is reabsorbed, and its urinary concentration is normally less than its plasma concentration. Normally, almost 100% of the glucose is reabsorbed, and it is absent in the urine. The presence of glucose in urine may be caused by excessive blood glucose (e.g. in diabetes) or reduced reabsorption of glucose by the kidneys (e.g. renal glycosuria). Although albumin is a relatively small molecule (about 7 nm in diameter), it is negatively charged, and is repelled by the negative charges on the glomerular walls. Hence the urinary concentration of albumin in urine is normally very low.

17.2 A C D

Substances produced by the kidneys include renin, erythropoietin and vitamin D (1,25-dihydroxycholecalciferol). Erythropoietin stimulates red cell production, and is useful clinically for the treatment of anaemia in renal failure. 1,25-Dihydroxycholecalciferol is an active metabolite of vitamin D, and is converted from the less active metabolite 25-hydroxycholecalciferol in the proximal tubules of the kidneys. Renin is produced in the kidneys. Renin converts angiotensionogen into angiotensin I, which is in turn converted by angiotensin-converting enzyme into angiotensin II in the lungs. Aldosterone is produced by the adrenal cortex.

17.3 B E

The kidneys lie behind the peritoneum on the posterior abdominal wall under the costal margin. They are surrounded by fatty tissues (perirenal fat, renal fascia and pararenal fat) which support the kidneys and hold them in position. The right kidney lies lower than the left kidney due to the large size of the right lobe of the liver. Both kidneys move downward during inspiration when the diaphragm contracts. This movement may be detected clinically if the kidneys are abnormally large. The kidneys receive mainly sympathetic innervation via the renal sympathetic plexus. This innervation is important in the control of renin secretion and renal blood flow.

17.4 B C E

There are two types of nephrons. In humans, 85% of nephrons are of the juxtamedullary type and 15% are of the cortical type. The cortical nephrons have their glomeruli in the outer portions of the renal cortex, they have shorter loops of Henle, and consequently are less able to produce concentrated urine. By contrast, the juxtamedullary type have their glomeruli on the outer portions of the renal cortex, have longer loops of Henle, and can produce more concentrated urine. There are also more mitochondria as much energy is required to concentrate the urine in the loops of Henle. Vasa recta are vessels that form hairpin loops alongside the loops of Henle which the efferent arterioles of the juxtamedullary glomeruli drain into. Vasa recta are absent in cortical nephrons.

17.5 C D E

The glomerulus and proximal convoluted tubule can be found in the renal cortex. The loops of Henle lie in the outer and inner medulla. The ascending loops of Henle emerge in the cortex from the medulla and form the distal convoluted tubules. The distal tubules coalesce to form the collecting ducts, which then pass through both the renal cortex and medulla to empty into the pelvis of the kidney. Vasa recta are alongside the loops of Henle and are therefore in the renal medulla.

17.6 C

The ureters drain urine from the pelvis of the kidneys to the posterior surface of the urinary bladder. They are retroperitoneal and run immediately behind the parietal peritoneum. Urine is propelled by peristaltic contraction of the smooth muscle walls. Hence patients with ureteric stones may complain of colicky pain. The ureters pass obliquely through the bladder wall, which tends to keep the ureters closed except during peristaltic waves. This usually prevents reflux of urine up the ureters in adults and older children. However, there are no anatomical ureteric sphincters. Renal scarring may result in children under 5 years of age in the presence of both urinary tract infection and reflux of urine into the ureters. The ureters are innervated by renal, testicular (or ovarian in women) and hypogastric plexuses. The innervation from the testicular plexus explains why patients with ureteric colic may complain of referred testicular pain.

17.7 A D E

The kidneys develop from two different sources of embryological tissues: the metanephric mesoderm and the ureteric bud. The ureteric bud gives rise to the ureter, the renal pelvis, the major and minor calyces and the collecting ducts. The metanephric mesoderm gives rise to the glomeruli, the proximal convoluted tubule, the loop of Henle and the distal convoluted tubule. Hence early splitting of the ureteric bud may result in duplication of the ureter and renal pelvis.

17.8 –

The embryological kidneys usually ascend in the cranial direction during their development. If the two kidneys are very close together during their ascent, the lower poles may fuse, and their ascent may be prevented by the root of the inferior mesenteric artery. This results in the formation of a horseshoe kidney. It is a relatively common congenital abnormality and can be found in about one in every 600 people.

17.9 B C D E

Substances for measuring effective renal plasma flow should have the following characteristics: freely filtered by the kidneys; not affecting the renal blood flow; and not stored, produced or metabolised by the kidneys. Substances actively secreted by the renal tubules would be more suitable, as the venous concentration can be ignored, being much smaller than the arterial concentration. The effective renal plasma flow can then be estimated by the clearance of the substance

$$\text{Clearance} = \frac{\text{Urinary concentration} \times \text{Urine flow}}{\text{Plasma concentration}}$$

Hence,

$$\text{Clearance of X (ml/min)} = \frac{20 \times 10}{0.2} = 1000 \text{ ml/min} = 1 \text{ litre/min}$$

Substances for measuring GFR must also be freely filtered by the kidneys, produce no effect on the renal blood flow, and not stored, produced or metabolised by the kidneys. However, there must be no net reabsorption or secretion by renal tubules. The GFR can be calculated by their clearance as above.

For substances with no net tubular secretion or reabsorption, the clearance equals the GFR. For substances with a net tubular secretion, the clearance exceeds the GFR. For substances with net tubular reabsorption, the clearance is less than the GFR.

17.10 B

Renal blood flow is increased by vasodilatation of the renal afferent arterioles. Noradrenaline or stimulation of the sympathetic noradrenergic nerves to the kidneys causes marked vasoconstriction and reduced renal blood flow. This is mediated via the adrenergic receptors, and partially explains the reduction in renal blood flow observed clinically in shock. Renin is released on stimulation of the renal nerves or by direct action of noradrenaline on the juxtaglomerular cells. It causes renal vasoconstriction with reduction in renal blood flow and GFR. Dopamine causes renal vasodilatation and an increase in renal blood flow. During exercise, blood is directed away from the kidneys. Changing from supine to standing position also slightly reduces renal blood flow.

17.11 E

The GFR is generally proportional to the body surface area. However, even after correction for surface area, the GFR is higher in men than in women, in adults than in neonates, and in younger adults than in the elderly. This is important clinically in prescribing, as smaller doses should be prescribed for neonates and the elderly. The normal GFR for an average man is 125 ml/min (i.e. 180 litres per day). This is about 60 times the plasma volume. Although inulin clearance is ideal for estimating GFR, creatinine clearance is often sufficiently accurate to be used in clinical practice.

17.12 –

In the proximal renal tubules, sodium ions are reabsorbed by primary active transport with energy derived from Na^+, K^+-ATPase. Some substances such as glucose, amino acids, lactate, citrate, phosphate, hydrogen and chloride ions are reabsorbed using secondary active transport via carrier proteins. For example, glucose and sodium ions bind to the common carrier SGLT 2, and glucose molecules are carried from the renal tubules into the cells as sodium ions move down its electrical and chemical gradient. Water is reabsorbed mainly by passive diffusion down the osmotic gradient created by the reabsorption of sodium ions. Mannitol acts as an osmotic diuretic, as it is not reabsorbed in the proximal convoluted tubule. Hence the osmotic pressure in the proximal renal tubules is increased, and less water is reabsorbed.

17.13 B E

Fluid at the glomerulus and proximal renal tubule is essentially plasma, and is isotonic. As it enters the water-permeable thin descending loop of Henle, water is drawn into the hypertonic interstitium. Hence the fluid becomes hypertonic. At the thick ascending loop of Henle, active transport of sodium into the interstitial fluid takes place but it is impermeable to water. Hence the fluid becomes hypotonic at the top of the thick ascending loop of Henle and the distal tubule. Water moves into the hypertonic interstitial fluid of the medulla at the medullary portion of the collecting duct. Hence it becomes hypertonic.

17.14 C

Vasopressin is produced by the posterior pituitary gland. It acts by increasing the permeability of the collecting ducts to water. Hence, in the absence of vasopressin (as in diabetes insipidus), the collecting ducts are impermeable to water. Therefore less water is reabsorbed from the collecting ducts, the urine volume increases and the urine osmolality decreases. As a result of water loss, the plasma osmolality increases.

17.15 A B D

Loop diuretics such as frusemide and bumetanide inhibit the transport of sodium and chloride ions at the medullary (thick) ascending loop of Henle. As a result, the countercurrent multiplier mechanism cannot function, and the normal hyperosmolality in the medullary interstitium is lost. Hence less water is reabsorbed in the collecting ducts, which results in the production of a large volume of dilute urine. As more sodium ions reach the distal tubule, they exchange with potassium ions, which leads to increased urinary potassium loss and hypokalaemia. Thiazide diuretics act by inhibiting sodium reabsorption at the cortical (thin) segment of the ascending limb of Henle.

17.16 A B

Spironolactone is a competitive inhibitor of aldosterone. Aldosterone increases the sodium reabsorption in exchange for potassium. Hence spironolactone increases urinary potassium loss and may cause hyperkalaemia. Spironolactone is a much less powerful diuretic than frusemide. However, it may act synergistically with a loop diuretic such as frusemide, as they act on different sites.

17.17 A C

If large quantities of solutes are present in the proximal renal tubules which cannot be reabsorbed, then the osmotic pressure increases and the amount of water reabsorbed increases.
This is known as osmotic diuresis. This may result from infusion of mannitol, sodium chloride or urea. Alternatively, the excessive solutes (e.g. glucose) may be produced in disease states (e.g. diabetes mellitus). In inappropriate ADH secretion, the urine volume is reduced. In diabetes insipidus, urine volume increases due to reduced reabsorption of water in the collecting ducts. The reabsorption of water in the proximal renal tubules is normal in compulsive water drinking.

17.18 A C D

Frusemide is an effective diuretic, and reduces the intravascular volume. Hence it is used in the treatment of congestive cardiac failure and pulmonary oedema. It increases the urinary loss of sodium, potassium and calcium by its action on the ascending loop of Henle, and is sometimes used in the emergency treatment of hypercalcaemia.

17.19 C

The extracellular fluid volume depends primarily on the amount of sodium in the body, which in turn depends on the sodium excretion from the kidneys. Hence sodium excretion is delicately controlled by several mechanisms. A reduction in extracellular volume (e.g. in hypotension, in shock and in massive gastrointestinal haemorrhage) results in a reduction of sodium excretion. A high-salt dietary intake results in increased sodium excretion. Aldosterone increases the tubular reabsorption of sodium.

17.20 A C

In dehydration, the kidneys attempt to compensate by increasing the urine concentration and decreasing the urine volume. This is achieved in two ways. Firstly, a reduction in renal blood flow leads to a decrease in the GFR. Hence less fluid is presented to the countercurrent mechanism, and the fluid flow rate in the loop of Henle decreases. The medullary interstitial fluid becomes more concentrated, and hence more water is reabsorbed from the collecting duct. Secondly, the secretion of ADH is increased due to an increase in plasma osmolality. This renders the collecting duct more permeable to water.

17.21 D E

Hydrogen ion is actively secreted into the renal tubular lumen mainly in the proximal and distal renal tubules. This occurs by secondary active transport. The Na^+, K^+-ATPase actively transports sodium from the renal tubule cell into the interstitial fluid. This lowers the concentration of sodium in the renal tubule cell, and sodium diffuses into the tubule cell passively from the tubular lumen in exchange for a hydrogen ion moving into the lumen. The source of hydrogen ions in the renal tubule cell is carbonic anhydrase, which catalyses the formation of H_2CO_3, which dissociates into hydrogen and bicarbonate ions. If the pH of the tubular fluid is less than 4.5, this transport mechanism fails. Hence the minimum possible urinary pH is 4.5.

17.22 A E

Acetazolamide is the most commonly used carbonic anhydrase inhibitor. Carbonic anhydrase is present in tissues secreting either acid or alkaline fluids, such as the gastric mucosa, renal tubule cells, the eye and the pancreas. It catalyses the formation of hydrogen and bicarbonate ions from water and carbon dioxide, which are essential in any acid or alkaline secretor processes. As acids are usually actively secreted in the renal tubular lumen, inhibition of carbonic anhydrase usually decreases urinary acid secretion and reduces the plasma pH. Acetazolamide is not commonly used as a diuretic. As the formation of aqueous humour depends on the availability of bicarbonate ions, acetazolamide reduces the formation of aqueous humour and is used clinically to lower the intraocular pressure in glaucoma. It is also occasionally used to facilitate acclimatisation at high altitude. Mountain sickness is caused by hypoxia, and the acidosis induced by acetazolamide may help to increase respiratory drive.

17.23 A C D

The secretion of acid into the tubular lumen cannot occur if the urinary pH is less than 4.5. However, excretion of acid may be increased if free hydrogen ions are removed from the urine in the tubular lumen by buffer systems. There are three main buffer systems: reaction with bicarbonate ions to form water and carbon dioxide; reaction with HPO_4^{2-} to form $H_2PO_4^-$, and reaction with ammonia to form ammonium ions.

17.24 B D E

Alkalisation of urine may be achieved either by sodium bicarbonate infusion or oral potassium citrate. Alkalisation of urine discourages bacterial growth in the urinary tract and reduces urinary tract inflammation, and is occassionally used to treat urinary tract infection in combination with antibiotics. Acidification of urine may be achieved by oral ammonium chloride. In poisoning by acidic drugs such as salicylate or phenobarbitone, alkalisation of urine increases the proportion of the ionised form of the drug in the tubular fluid which is lipid-insoluble and remains in the renal tubules. This increases its excretion in urine. Conversely, acidification of basic drugs such as amphetamine increases their urinary excretion.

17.25 B D E

Thiazide diuretics act by reducing sodium reabsorption at the cortical diluting segment between the ascending loop of Henle and the distal renal tubules. This leads to increased sodium excretion and a low plasma sodium level. The increased sodium at the distal renal tubule leads to increased Na^+–K^+ exchange at the distal tubule, and hence urinary potassium excretion is also increased. Potassium supplements may be required clinically. Both loop and thiazide diuretics may cause increased urinary excretion of magnesium, and may rarely cause cardiac arrhythmia. The urinary uric acid excretion is reduced for two reasons. Firstly, thiazide diuretics may compete for the transport of uric acid secretion into the renal tubules. Secondly, the volume depletion may lead to a reduction of GFR and an increased reabsorption of all solutes including uric acid. Both thiazides and loop diuretics may cause glucose intolerance due to prolonged hypokalaemia.

17.26 A C

In renal failure, the function of the kidneys is impaired, and the breakdown products of protein metabolism accumulate in the blood. Urea and creatinine are only two of many such substances. This clinical picture is known as uraemia, and symptoms may include anorexia, nausea, vomiting, lethargy, confusion and convulsions. As acid is normally actively excreted by the kidneys, abnormal accumulation of acid in the blood occurs in renal failure. Renal failure also results in failure to produce erythropoietin, which leads to anaemia. As the kidneys normally manufacture an active metabolite of vitamin D (1,25-dihydroxycholecalciferol), renal failure may be associated with renal rickets and a low plasma calcium level.

17.27 B C

Normally, large particles such as proteins and red blood cells are filtered by the glomeruli. Hence the presence of large quantities of blood and protein in urine is characteristic of glomerular disease. Smaller molecules (e.g. glucose and amino acids) are reabsorbed in the proximal and distal renal tubules. Thus the urinary excretion of these substances is increased in tubular diseases. As hydrogen ions are normally secreted in the renal tubules from the tubular lumen, renal tubular diseases are often associated with an abnormally high urinary pH and metabolic acidosis. The presence of urea in urine is normal.

17.28 A B C D E

There are numerous causes of glomerular diseases. They may be divided into immunological and non-immunological causes. Immunological causes may be primary (e.g. anti-glomerular basement membrane antibodies in Goodpasture's disease) or secondary to non-glomerular antigens (e.g. post-streptococcal glomerulonephritis). Non-immunological causes are usually secondary to diseases outside the kidneys (e.g. infections, metabolic diseases, vasculitis, drugs). Metabolic diseases which cause glomerular damage include diabetes mellitus and amyloidosis. Vasculitis may be caused by polyarteritis nodosa, systemic lupus erythematosus, and Henoch–Schönlein purpura. Drugs which may cause glomerular damage include gold and penicillamine.

17.29 A C D

Obstructive nephropathy may be due to any cause of urinary tract obstruction, and includes uretero-pelvic stenosis, ureteric stones, carcinoma of the bladder, carcinoma of the prostate and benign prostatic hyperplasia. The clinical and pathological features depend on the level of obstruction. If the obstruction is at the level of the ureter, the back-pressure causes dilatation of the renal pelvis and calyceal system. The kidney may become dilated, and the renal tissue may undergo atrophy due to compression. This is hydronephrosis. The bladder would not be affected as it is below the level of obstruction.

17.30 A B C D E

Pyelonephritis is defined as infection of the kidney. The infecting organisms may originate either in the bloodstream (i.e. in septicaemia) or from retrograde spread from the lower urinary tract. Ascending infection from the lower urinary tract may occur if the urine is infected and there is reflux of urine into the kidney. Urinary tract infection is commoner in women (due to short urethra), in pregnancy and following instrumentation of the urethra (e.g. urethral catherterisation). Reflux urine is more likely in patients with vesico-ureteric reflux, which may be due either to congenital abnormalities in children or to urinary tract obstruction in adults.

17.31 A C D

The commonest type of urinary calculi consists of calcium oxalate, followed by magensium ammonium phosphate and uric acid. The risk of calcium oxalate stones is increased in the presence of high urinary calcium, which may be due either to high serum calcium or idiopathic hypercalcuria (high urinary calcium with normal serum calcium). Magnesium ammonium phosphate calculi characteristically form large staghorn calculi. They are often associated with *Proteus* urinary tract infection, as *Proteus* breaks down urea to form ammonia. The formation of magnesium ammonium phosphate calculi is facilitated by alkaline urine. Gout is caused by an increased serum uric acid level, which also increases the risk of uric acid calculi formation.

17.32 C D

The commonest malignant tumours in men are bronchial carcinoma and colorectal carcinoma, and renal tumours are relatively uncommon. Amongst the primary malignant renal tumour, renal cell carcinoma is the commonest. Other less common histological types include Wilm's tumour (which occurs in children) and transitional cell tumour of the renal pelvis. Renal cell tumour has a small association with smoking, and occurs more frequently in a rare hereditary condition (Hippel–Lindau disease). Transitional cell tumours of the renal pelvis, like transitional cell tumours of the bladder, are associated with exposure to aniline dye and other chemical agents. Renal cell tumour may be associated with inappropriate erythropoietin secretion, which causes polycythaemia.

17.33 A

The empty bladder lies completely in the pelvis in adults, but rises to the hypogastric region of the abdominal cavity when it is filled with urine. Hence the empty bladder cannot be palpated through the anterior abdominal wall. However, in children under five years of age, the empty bladder lies partially in the abdominal cavity. The empty bladder is approximately pyramidal in shape, with its apex facing anteriorly and its base facing posteriorly. The ureters join the bladder obliquely at the superolateral angles of its posterior surface. This arrangement normally prevents the retrograde flow of urine from the bladder up the ureters.

17.34 C E

Micturition may be either a reflex action, a voluntary action, or a combination of both. Detrusor muscle forms the smooth muscular coat of the bladder, and is arranged in longitudinal, circular and spiral bundles. Its contraction helps to increase the pressure in the bladder during micturition. In voluntary micturition, the abdominal wall muscles also contract to increase the intra-abdominal pressure. The external urethral sphincter consists of skeletal (voluntary) muscles surrounding the membranous urethra. It is relaxed during micturition. It and the perineal muscles may be voluntarily contracted to postpone emptying of the bladder. The internal urethral sphincter consists of smooth muscles, and it plays no part in micturition.

17.35 A B C E

Micturition may occur as a spinal reflex action, as in a newborn baby. However, after about 18 months of age, it may be controlled and moderated by higher cortical centres. The bladder is supplied by both the sympathetic and parasympathetic nervous systems. Stimulation of the parasympathetic nerves causes contraction of the detrusor muscle and relaxation of the external urethral sphincter. This occurs during micturition. Conversely, stimulation of the sympathetic nerves causes relaxation of the detrusor muscle and contraction of the external urethral sphincter.

17.36 B C

Antimuscarinic agents (e.g. propantheline) relax the detrusor muscle, and may be useful in the treatment of incontinence due to detrusor instability. Tricyclic antidepressants (e.g. imipramine, amitriptyline) have antimuscarinic properties and may also be useful.

17.37 B C D

The bladder responds to increased pressure due to outflow obstruction by muscular hypertrophy. Causes of bladder outflow obstruction are abnormalities in the prostate gland and urethra. Abnormalities in the ureter and kidneys do not give rise to increased pressure in the bladder.

17.38 C D

Most bladder tumours are epithelial cell in origin, and the majority are transitional cell tumours. They frequently occur in multiples and are papillary in appearance. As they initially project into the bladder lumen before invading the bladder muscles, early diagnosis by cystoscopy is possible. A tumour near a ureteric orifice may cause urinary obstruction, and the back-pressure may result in hydronephrosis.

17.39 A D

Chemicals used in textile, printing, rubber and plastic industries are known to cause bladder tumours, and aniline compounds are thought to be responsible. Heavy smokers are also more prone to develop bladder tumours. Schistosomiasis infection is associated with squamous cell bladder tumour, but not transitional cell tumours. There is no evidence of association between either diabetes mellitus or excessive alcohol intake with transitional cell bladder tumours.

17.40 A B E

Bladder diverticuli are outpouchings from the bladder epithelium, and may be congenital or acquired. Congenital diverticuli are usually solitary, whilst acquired diverticuli are usually small and multiple. Acquired diverticuli are usually associated with bladder outflow obstruction, and occur between two ridges of hypertrophic muscles (trabeculae). As prostatic enlargement is a common cause of bladder outflow obstruction, bladder diverticuli occur more commonly in men than women.

17.41 C D

The prostate gland is shaped like an inverted cone, and lies below the neck of the bladder and above the urogenital diaphragm. Hence enlargement of the prostate gland may give rise to urinary obstruction. It lies just posterior to the symphysis pubis, and anterior to the rectum. Hence the gland can be palpated in a rectal examination. It surrounds the prostatic urethra, into which prostatic secretion is discharged. The prostatic secretion is alkaline and neutralises the acid in the vagina.

17.42 A D E

Benign enlargement of the prostate gland is due to hyperplasia of glandular tissue. It occurs in men over 50 years of age. The exact aetiology is unknown. However, it is thought that a reduction in androgen level and an increase in oestrogen level are important factors. There are often multiple circumscribed solid nodules and cysts. If the median lobe is involved, it often compresses the prostatic urethra and causes urinary obstruction. The bladder may respond by muscular hypertrophy and develop prominent bands of thickened smooth muscle (trabeculation).

17.43 B D

Although some drugs are effective in partially relieving symptoms of benign prostatic hypertrophy, surgery cannot be avoided once urinary retention has occurred. The prostatic stromal tissue is rich in α_1-adrenoceptors, whilst the glandular tissue is sensitive to androgens. α_1-adrenoceptor antagonists (e.g. prazosin) and 5 α-reductase inhibitors (e.g. finasteride) may reduce the prostatic volume, and are used to relieve the symptoms of benign prostatic hypertrophy. 5α-reductase inhibitors inhibit the conversion of testosterone into the more active dihydrotestosterone.

17.44 D

Prostatic carcinoma may be clinical or latent. Latent carcinoma may be found incidentally at histological examination after prostatectomy. The latent carcinoma appears to have a different natural history from the clinical types, and may remain latent for a long time. Unlike benign prostatic hyperplasia which occurs most commonly in the peri-urethral areas, clinical prostatic carcinomas mostly arise from the posterior lobe of the gland. Hence, if the median grove is obliterated on rectal examination, a diagnosis of prostatic carcinoma is likely. The prostate gland produces both acid phosophatase and prostatic specific antigen, and the levels of these substances increase in the presence of prostatic carcinoma. This is useful for diagnostic purposes, although screening for prostatic carcinoma using these biochemical markers is not currently recommended. Bone is the most frequent site for prostatic cancer metastasis, which typically causes a sclerotic lesion.

18. The nervous system
Questions

18.1 The following structures of the brain develop from the embryological forebrain (proscencephalon):

A Pons
B Cerebellum
C Cerebral cortex
D Thalamus
E Corpus striatum

18.2 The following structures contain fibres which link matching areas in the two hemispheres:

A Corpus callosum
B Anterior commissure
C Superior longitudinal fasciculus
D Posterior commissure
E The uncinate fasciculus

18.3 The following cranial nerves emerge from the pons:

A Oculomotor nerve
B Trochlear nerve
C Trigeminal nerve
D Abducens nerve
E Facial nerve

18.4 The following structures can be found in the midbrain:

A Substantia nigra
B Superior colliculus
C Cerebral peduncle
D Gracile and cuneate nuclei
E Fourth ventricle

18.5 The following statements about the cranial meninges are correct:

- **A** The venous sinuses lie between the dura mater and the arachnoid mater
- **B** The falx cerebri is a fold of dura mater
- **C** The tentorium cerebelli is a fold of arachnoid mater
- **D** Cerebrospinal fluid can be found between the pia mater and the surface of the brain
- **E** The middle meningeal artery can be found between the inner surface of the temporal bones and the dura mater

18.6 Meningiomas:

- **A** Are the commonest type of CNS tumours
- **B** Occur more frequently in children
- **C** Frequently invade the brain
- **D** Frequently invade the dura and skull bones
- **E** Usually have irregular edges

18.7 Adult bacterial meningitis is commonly caused by:

- **A** *Staphylococcus aureus*
- **B** *Salmonella*
- **C** Anaerobic organisms
- **D** *Streptococcus pneumoniae*
- **E** *Pseudomonas*

18.8 A cerebral abscess may result from spread of infection from:

- **A** The paranasal sinuses
- **B** The bloodstream
- **C** The lymphatics
- **D** The mastoid cavity
- **E** The middle ear

18.9 Cerebrospinal fluid (CSF):

- **A** Is secreted by the choroid plexuses of the lateral ventricles
- **B** Enters the third ventricle through the interventricular foramen
- **C** Enters the fourth ventricle via the aqueduct of Sylvius
- **D** Enters the subarachnoid space via the central canal in the spinal cord
- **E** Is returned to the blood via the lymphatic system

18.10 Causes of hydrocephalus include:

- **A** Obstruction at the fourth ventricle into the subarachnoid space
- **B** Obstruction at the aqueduct
- **C** Obstruction at the central canal of the spinal cord
- **D** Meningitis
- **E** Tumour of the choroid plexus

18.11 In most people, branches of the internal carotid arteries include:

- **A** Ophthalmic arteries
- **B** Posterior cerebral arteries
- **C** Basilar artery
- **D** Anterior cerebral arteries
- **E** Middle cerebral arteries

18.12 The following areas of the brain are supplied by the middle cerebral arteries:

- **A** The pons
- **B** The parietal lobes
- **C** The anterior limb of the internal capsule
- **D** The posterior limb of the internal capsule
- **E** The optic radiation

18.13 Factors which relax the arteriolar smooth muscle of the cerebral vessels include:

- **A** Increased pH
- **B** Increased carbon dioxide
- **C** Increased systemic blood pressure
- **D** Hyperventilation
- **E** Increased oxygen

18.14 Causes of a stroke include:

- **A** Intracerebral haemorrhage
- **B** Meningitis
- **C** Encephalitis
- **D** Cerebral infarction
- **E** Subarachnoid haemorrhage

18.15 Causes of cerebral infarction include:

- **A** Emboli from mural thrombus after a myocardial infarction
- **B** Atheroma of the intracranial arteries
- **C** Atheroma of the extracranial arteries
- **D** Thrombosis of the intracranial arteries
- **E** Cerebral hypotension following a cardiac arrest

18.16 Intracerebral haemorrhage:

- **A** Occurs more commonly in hypertensive subjects
- **B** May cause an increase in intracranial pressure
- **C** May cause cerebral herniation
- **D** Is commonly caused by rupture of arterial aneurysms at the circle of Willis
- **E** Is commonly caused by rupture at the bifurcation of intracerebral arterioles

18.17 The following statements about the blood–brain barrier are true:

- **A** The lining of the choroid plexus constitutes part of the blood–brain barrier
- **B** It is bound by tight junctions
- **C** Fenestrations occur frequently at the barrier
- **D** It modulates the entry of glucose
- **E** It prevents toxins from entering the CNS from the bloodstream

18.18 Significant quantities of the following drugs cross the blood–brain barrier:

- **A** Lipid-insoluble drugs
- **B** Lipid-soluble drugs
- **C** Inhaled anaesthetics
- **D** Alcohol
- **E** Chloramphenicol in the presence of meningitis

18.19 The following statements about neurones are true:

- **A** There are more neuroglial cells than neurones
- **B** Nissl bodies contain endoplasmic reticulum
- **C** Nerve impulses are conducted via the axon
- **D** There is usually one dendrite per neurone
- **E** Microtubules play an important role in neuronal transport

18.20 Retrograde neuronal transport:

- **A** Includes transport of substances from the cell body to the dendrites
- **B** Includes transport of substances from the axon to the cell body
- **C** Is the principal means of transporting synthesised neurotransmitters
- **D** Is the principal means of transporting neuronal waste products
- **E** Plays an important role in target cell recognition

18.21 In an action potential, the firing level:

- **A** Occurs when the membrane potential reaches 0 mV
- **B** Is associated with a sudden increase in the openings of sodium channels
- **C** Is associated with an increased K^+ influx into the cell
- **D** Is associated with an increased Na^+ efflux out of the cell
- **E** Is associated with a rapid increase in sodium conductance

18.22 Immediately after the spike potential of the action potential:

- **A** The sodium channels become inactivated
- **B** The potassium channels are gradually opened
- **C** The sodium conductance increases
- **D** The potassium conductance increases
- **E** There is a net movement of potassium out of the cells

18.23 The excitation threshold of the neurone to stimulation is increased:

A When the membrane potential is made more negative
B During the rising phase of the spike potential
C In the initial falling phase of the spike potential
D During the after-depolarisation period
E During the after-repolarisation period

18.24 The following statements about the chemical synapse are true:

A Neurotransmitters are released from the pre-synaptic membrane by exocytosis
B Neurotransmitters are transported from the Golgi apparatus to the synaptic boutons in vesicles
C The neurotransmitter receptor is located on the membrane of the target neurone
D Most synapses are dendrito-axonic
E Pre-synaptic inhibition may be achieved by axo-axonic synapses

18.25 Known inhibitory neurotransmitters include:

A Glycine
B Serotonin (5-HT)
C Noradrenaline
D γ-Aminobutyric acid (GABA)
E Glutaric acid

18.26 The following statements about the neuromuscular junction are true:

A Acetylcholinesterase can be found on the post-synaptic membrane
B Choline is transported from the synaptic cleft to the pre-synaptic neurone
C Each nicotinic receptor binds to two molecules of acetylcholine
D Binding of acetylcholine to its receptors results in the opening of sodium channels
E Cyclic GMP acts as the second messenger

18.27 Known second messengers for synaptic transmission include:

A Cyclic AMP
B Substance P
C Inositol triphosphate (IP_3)
D Diacylglycerol (DAG)
E Nitric oxide

18.28 Types of neuroglial cells in the brain include:

A Astrocytes
B Fibrocytes
C Ependymal cells
D Transitional epithelium
E Oligodendrocytes

18.29 Myelination:

A Is the function of microglial cells
B Increases the speed of nerve conduction
C Occurs in almost all nerve cells in the brain
D Is usually accompanied by deletion of potassium channels
E Never takes place in patients with multiple sclerosis

18.30 Multiple sclerosis:

A Occurs more commonly in tropical than temperate countries
B Is more common in males than females
C Affects both the peripheral and central nervous system
D Is characteristically associated with a loss of myelin in affected tissues
E Characteristically gives an oligodendrocyte-predominant histological picture

18.31 The following sensory phenomenon and the type of nerve endings in the skin are correctly matched:

A Sensation of heat – free nerve endings
B Sensation of vibration – Pacinian corpuscles
C Short-lasting touch sensation when clothes are put on – Ruffini endings
D Differentiating between smooth and rough table surface – Meissner's corpuscles
E Awareness of a fork held in the hand – Merkel cells

18.32 The following sites and their segmental innervation are correctly matched:

A Around the nipple – T8
B At the umbilicus – T10
C Inguinal region – L3
D Lateral side of the sole of the foot – S2
E The thumb – C8

18.33 Symptoms due to S1 nerve root compression by a disc prolapse include:

A Pain in the sole of the feet
B Tingling sensation in the sole of the feet
C Weakness of dorsifexion of the ankle
D Absent knee jerk
E Exaggerated ankle jerk

18.34 Consequences of damage to the radial nerve at the radial groove of the humerus include:

A Wrist drop
B Inability to extend the elbow
C Inability to extend the middle and distal phalangeal joints of the fingers

D Diminished sensation over the ulnar side of the dorsum of the hand
E Diminished sensation over the radial side of the palm

18.35 Consequences of damage to the ulnar nerve at the wrist include:

A Inability to abduct the thumb
B Inability to adduct the thumb
C Clawed hand appearance of the fourth and fifth fingers
D Loss of sensation on the ulnar side of the dorsum of the hand
E Reduced sensation in the ulnar side of the palm

18.36 The following statements about the knee jerk elicited in a clinical examination are true:

A Type Ia and type II muscle spindles in the quadriceps muscles discharge impulses to the spinal cord
B The nerve fibre from the muscle spindle synapses with the dendrites of α motoneurons supplying the quadriceps muscles
C Signals in the spinal cord are transmitted to the thalamus
D The nerve impulses must pass through two synapses before the knee jerk can occur
E Inhibitory impulses are sent to the α motor neurones supplying the hamstring muscles

18.37 The following statements about the posterior column–medial lemniscal pathway are true:

A The cell bodies of the first-order neurones lie in the anterior root ganglia in the spinal cord
B The first-order neurones cross the midline in the spinal cord a few spinal segments above
C The cell bodies of the second-order neurones lie in the nuclei gracilis and cuneatus in the posterior column
D The second-order neurone does not cross the midline
E The third-order neurone projects from the thalamus to the sensory cortex

18.38 The spinothalamic tract and the posterior column–medial lemniscal pathway show the following similarities:

A Both consist of three-order sets of neurones
B The second-order neurones cross over in both pathways
C Both pathways cross over in the spinal cord
D The third-order neurones project from the thalamus to the cerebral cortex
E The representations of different parts of the body in the cerebral cortex are similar

18.39 The following functions are lost in diseases affecting the posterior column – medial lemniscal pathway:

A Vibration sensation
B Temperature sensation
C Pain sensation
D Two-point discrimination
E Muscle power

18.40 The following lesions may cause loss in temperature whilst preserving joint position sensation:

A Peripheral neuropathy
B Diseases affecting spinal cord root ganglia
C Syringomyelia (cyst in and around the central canal of the spinal cord)
D Diseases affecting the thalamus
E A cerebral tumour affecting the sensory cortex

18.41 The following statements about neural transmission of pain are true:

A Sharp localised pain is transmitted by C fibres
B Dull diffuse chronic pain is transmitted by myelinated fibres
C Pain impulses for chronic pain travel slower than those for sharp pain
D Substance P is the neurotransmitter in the afferent pain fibres in the dorsal horn of the spinal cord
E Gating of pain impulses takes place at the dorsal horn cells of the spinal cord

18.42 Interventions for which the release of endogenous opioid neurotransmitters is a probable mechanism of pain relief include:

A Acupuncture
B Placebo
C Paracetamol
D Naloxone
E Transcutaneous nerve stimulation

18.43 The following drugs and their mechanisms of analgesic action are correctly matched:

A Diamorphine – μ-opioid receptor agonist
B Morpine – δ-opioid receptor agonist
C Non-steroidal anti-inflammatory drugs (NSAIDs) – cyclooxygenase inhibitor
D Corticosteroid – increased breakdown of prostaglandins
E Paracetamol – increased prostaglandin synthesis

18.44 Characteristic side effects of opiates include:

A Constipation
B Respiratory depression
C Dilated pupils
D Tachycardia
E Drowsiness

18.45 The following statements about the sympathetic nervous system are true:

A The pre-ganglionic fibres emerge from the cervical and thoracic segments of the spinal cord
B Most of the sympathetic ganglia lie in the sympathetic chain
C Some pre-ganglionic fibres synapse at the adrenal cortex
D Some post-ganglionic fibres synapse at the adrenal medulla
E The male genital tract receives sympathetic supply via the pelvic ganglion

18.46 Stimulation of the sympathetic nervous system causes an increase in:

A Heart rate
B Blood flow to the skin
C Blood flow to skeletal muscle
D Gut motility
E Sweating

18.47 Symptoms and signs of disruption of the sympathetic nerves immediately after their emergence from the superior cervical ganglion (i.e. Horner's syndrome) include:

A Ptosis (drooping of eyelid)
B Failure to abduct the eye
C Increased tear secretion
D A dilated pupil
E Reduced sweating on that side of the face

18.48 Pre-ganglionic parasympathetic fibres emerge in the following cranial nerves:

A Oculomotor nerve
B Trochlear nerve
C Trigeminal nerve
D Facial nerve
E Glossopharyngeal nerve

18.49 Actions of antimuscarinic drugs (e.g. atropine) include:

A Small pupils
B Dry mouth
C Increased heart rate
D Bronchoconstriction
E Diarrhoea

18.50 The following statements about the left corticospinal tract are true:

A It carries voluntary motor fibres
B It passes through the left internal capsule between the thalamus and the basal ganglia
C Most of its fibres cross over to the right side in the pons
D Most of its fibres descend in the right side of the spinal cord as the anterior corticospinal tract
E Less than 20% of its fibres descend in the right side of the spinal cord as the lateral corticospinal tract

18.51 Lesions at which of the following sites in the motor pathway usually result in a clinical 'upper motor neurone lesion'?

A Corticospinal tract
B Reticulospinal tract
C Corticonuclear tract
D Anterior horn cells of the spinal cord
E Peripheral nerve

18.52 Characteristic signs of lower motor neurone lesions include:

A Spasticity
B Absent tendon reflex
C Positive Babinski sign
D Fasciculation
E Pronounced muscle wasting

18.53 The basal ganglia include the following:

A Caudate nucleus
B Putamen
C Hypothalamus
D Substantia nigra
E Subthalamic nucleus

18.54 Parkinson's disease is associated with:

A A reduction in striatal activity
B A reduction in nigrostrial neurones
C Reduced activity of cholinergic neurones
D A loss of GABA-ergic pathway
E A reduction of MPTP (1-methly-4-phenyl-1,2,5,6-tetrahydropyridine)-like substance

18.55 Recognised drug treatments for Parkinson's disease include:

A Monoamine oxidase B inhibitors (e.g. selegiline)
B Phenothiazines (e.g. chlorpromazine)
C Levodopa with peripheral decarboxylase inhibitor
D Bromocriptine
E Anticholinergic agents

18.56 The neocerebellum:

- **A** Constitutes over 50% of the whole cerebellum
- **B** Includes the vermis
- **C** Receives afferent fibres from the pontocerebellar tract
- **D** Sends efferent fibres from the dentate nucleus to the contralateral motor cortex via the thalamus
- **E** Coordinates the movements of the limbs

18.57 Characteristic features associated with lesions in the vestibulocerebellum include:

- **A** Inability to stand upright without support
- **B** Finger – nose incoordination
- **C** Impaired articulation
- **D** Increased muscle tone in the limbs
- **E** Nystagmus

18.58 Characteristic features of neocerebellar lesions include:

- **A** Tremor at rest
- **B** Impaired 'heel-to-toe' walking
- **C** Impaired ipsilateral 'heel-to-shin' test
- **D** Uneven speech production
- **E** Staggering gait

18.59 The following functions and their corresponding cranial nerves are appropriately matched:

- **A** Sensation of the posterior third of the tongue – hypoglossal nerve
- **B** Phonation – spinal accessory nerve
- **C** Tongue protrusion – glossopharyngeal nerve
- **D** Mastication – facial nerve
- **E** Sensation to the forehead – ophthalmic branch of the trigeminal nerve

18.60 The mandibular division of the trigeminal nerve:

- **A** Originates from the Gasserian ganglion in the petrous temporal bone
- **B** Exits the skull base through the foramen rotundum
- **C** Innervates the tip of the nose
- **D** Mediates the jaw jerk
- **E** Supplies the teeth and gums of the upper jaw

18.61 The following functions and their corresponding cranial nerves are appropriately matched:

- **A** Taste in the posterior third of the tongue – glossopharyngeal nerve
- **B** Taste in the anterior two-thirds of the tongue – trigeminal nerve
- **C** Corneal reflex – maxillary branch of the trigeminal nerve
- **D** Attenuation of loud sounds – facial nerve
- **E** Parotid gland secretion – facial nerve

18.62 A unilateral upper motor neurone facial nerve palsy:
- **A** May be caused by a vascular stroke
- **B** May be caused by Bell's palsy
- **C** May be caused by compression of the nerve in its bony canal
- **D** Is associated with inability to close one eye
- **E** Is associated with inability to retract the lip

18.63 A unilateral lower motor neurone facial nerve palsy:
- **A** Is commoner than a corresponding lesion of any other cranial nerves
- **B** Is associated with inability to raise the eyebrow
- **C** Is associated with sensitivity to loud noise
- **D** Is associated with the inability to smile
- **E** Almost never recovers spontaneously

18.64 The oculomotor nerve supplies:
- **A** The lateral rectus
- **B** The superior rectus
- **C** The sphincter pupillae
- **D** The levator superioris
- **E** The superior oblique

18.65 Clinical features of a complete oculomotor nerve palsy include:
- **A** A constricted pupil
- **B** Inability to abduct the eye
- **C** Inability to close the eye
- **D** Reduced sweating on that side of the face
- **E** Inability to look upwards

18.66 The following statements about the medial longitudinal fasciculus (MLF) are true:
- **A** It connects the oculomotor, trochlear and abducens nuclei
- **B** It receives neural input from the vestibular nuclei
- **C** It is essential for maintaining visual fixation on a moving target
- **D** A lesion in the MLF may result in failure of abduction of the ipsilateral eye
- **E** A lesion in the MLF may result in nystagmus of the contralateral eye

18.67 The following are neural pathways involved in the direct pupillary light reflex:
- **A** The ganglion cells within the retina conduct impulses via the optic tracts to the lateral geniculate body
- **B** The lateral geniculate body conducts impulses towards the superior cervical ganglion in the sympathetic chain
- **C** The superior cervical ganglion conducts impulses towards the Edinger–Westphal nucleus

D The fibres from the Edinger–Westphal nucleus enter the oculomotor nerve and synapse in the ciliary ganglion
E Post-ganglionic fibres from the ciliary ganglion supply the sphincter pupillae in the iris

18.68 When a strong light is shone into the left eye, the right pupil constricts but the left pupil does not react. These clinical findings may be explained by a:

A Left optic nerve lesion
B Left oculomotor nerve lesion
C Right optic nerve lesion
D Right oculomotor nerve lesion
E Left sympathetic chain lesion

18.69 Cones and rods are the two types of photoreceptors in the retina. Compared to cones, rods:

A Are more numerous
B Are less sensitive to light
C Function less well in dim light
D Are mainly found in the fovea
E Are abnormal in patients with red – green colour-blindness

18.70 The following events occur in the photosensitive pigments of the retina in the presence of light:

A Conformal changes in the pigments occur
B Transducin (G_{t1}) is activated
C Phosphodiesterase is inhibited
D Intracellular cAMP is increased
E Sodium channels are opened

18.71 When an individual with normal vision moves from a very bright to a very dark room:

A The retina becomes less sensitive to light
B The changes in visual threshold occur more quickly than the reverse changes on moving from a very dark to a very bright room
C The initial changes in visual threshold are due to adaptation in the rods
D The later changes in visual threshold are due to adaptation of the cones
E The changes occur quicker if the individual had worn red-tinted glasses in the bright room

18.72 Myopia (short-sightedness):

A May be due to an abnormally short eyeball
B May be due to excessive curvature and convergence power of the cornea or lens
C Is associated with images formed in front of the retina
D May be corrected using concave lenses
E Is often genetic in aetiology

18.73 The following statements about the optic nerve are true:

A It develops from an outgrowth of the brain embryologically
B It is wrapped round by Schwann cells
C It can regenerate if damaged
D The cell bodies occupy the pretectal nucleus
E Almost all the fibres cross over to the lateral geniculate body on the opposite side

18.74 The following lesions in the visual pathway and their resulting visual field defects are correctly matched:

A Complete left optic nerve lesion – left homonymous hemianopia
B Optic chiasm – bitemporal hemianopia
C Left optic tract – right homonymous hemianopia
D Right optic radiation – right homonymous hemianopia
E Left occipital cortex – right homonymous hemianopia

18.75 Sound vibrations from outside the ear pass through the following to reach the acoustic nerve:

A Tympanic membrane
B Malleus
C Stapes
D The round window
E The inner hair cell of the cochlea

18.76 The auditory nerve impulses in the acoustic nerve pass through the following to reach the primary auditory cortex:

A Ipsilateral cochlear nuclei in the medulla
B Ipsilateral vestibular nuclei
C Ipsilateral lateral geniculate body
D Contralateral medial geniculate body
E Ipsilateral superior colliculus

18.77 The following features of sound waves and their associated qualities of sound are correctly matched

A Amplitude – loudness
B Frequency – pitch
C Wavelength – rhythm
D Harmonics – timbre
E Speed – duration

18.78 The differentiation between sound coming from:

A The left and the right side is partly due to the time difference between the arrival of stimulus in the two ears
B The left and the right side is partly due to the primary auditory cortex receiving signals produced by the stimuli only from the contralateral ear
C The left and the right side is partly due to the sound being louder on the side of the source

D The front and the back is partly due to the time difference between the arrival of stimulus in the two ears
E The front and the back is contributed to by the positioning of the pinna

18.79 The following statements about Wernicke's area are true:
A It is usually found in the right superior temporal gyrus
B Its main function is to understand speech
C Lesions in this area result in receptive aphasia
D It is connected to Broca's area by the arcuate fasciculus
E It is usually damaged by vascular occlusion of the left anterior cerebral artery

18.80 Alzheimer's disease:
A Is a metabolic disease
B Occurs more commonly in older people
C Is the second commonest cause of dementia
D May occur in families
E Is associated with the ApoE4 genotype on chromosome 19

18.81 Pathological features of Alzheimer's disease include:
A Cortical hypertrophy
B Small ventricles
C Neurofibrillary tangles
D Excessive cholinergic fibres
E Predominant cerebellar involvement

18.82 Benzodiazepines are:
A Antipsychotic
B Sedative
C Anxiolytic
D Anticonvulsants
E Muscle relaxants

18.83 Benzodiazepines:
A Act on three different subtypes of receptors
B Inhibit the effect of GABA
C Result in opening of chloride ion channels in target cells
D Act mainly on the reticular activating system
E Are antagonists at the neuromuscular junction

18.84 Phenothiazines are:
A Agonists of dopamine D_2 receptors
B Agonists of serotonin receptors
C Used to treat schizophrenia acutely
D Used as long-term maintenance therapy for schizophrenia
E Used as antidepressants

18.85 Characteristic side effects of phenothiazines include:

A Parkinsonian symptoms
B Akathisia
C Involuntary movement of the face and tongue
D Hypoprolactinaemia
E Insomnia

18.86 Drugs effective in the treatment of depression include:

A Lithium
B Benzodiazepines
C Barbiturates
D Butyrophenones
E Selective serotonin reuptake inhibitors (SSRIs)

18.87 Tricyclic antidepressants:

A Are muscarinic receptor agonists
B Act by increasing the synthesis of noradrenaline in the presynaptic neurone
C Are cardiotoxic
D Protect against convulsions
E Inhibit bladder contraction

18.88 Lithium:

A Increases the synthesis of phosphatidylinositol
B Is poorly absorbed in the gastrointestinal tract
C Is extensively metabolised by the liver
D Has a shorter half-life in patients with renal impairment
E Level increases when a diuretic is administered at the same time

18. The nervous system
Answers

18.1 C D E

In its embryological development, the closed neural tube expands to form three brain vesicles:- the forebrain (prosencephalon), the midbrain (mesencephalon) and the hindbrain (rhombencephalon). The proscencephalon form the adult cerebral cortex and corpus striatum, and the diencephalon forms the adult thalamus and hypothalamus. The mesencephalon forms the adult midbrain. The rhomencephalon forms the adult pons, cerebellum and the medulla oblongata.

18.2 A B D

Fibres which link matching areas in the two hemispheres are called commissural fibres. The main commissure is the corpus callosum. It spans from the genu linking parts of the frontal lobe to the splenium linking the occipital lobes. The anterior commissure connects the anterior parts of the temporal lobe, and the posterior commissure lies in front of the pineal gland. The commissure of the fornix links the two hippocampi. Fibres which pass from one part of a hemisphere to another are association fibres. Examples are the superior longitudinal fasciculus, which links the frontal and the occipital lobes, and the uncinate fasciculus, which links the frontal lobe with the occipitotemporal cortex.

18.3 C D E

The third (oculomotor) and the fourth (trochlear) cranial nerves emerge from the midbrain. The fifth (trigeminal), sixth (abducens), seventh (facial) and eighth (vestibulocochlear) nerves emerge from the pons. The ninth to twelfth nerves emerge from the medulla oblongata.

18.4 A B C

The two large cerebral peduncles lie in the ventral part of the midbrain, and consist of the substantia nigra and the crus cerebri. The superior colliculus lies in the dorsal part of the midbrain, and is responsible for the orientation of the head and body towards visual stimuli. The aqueduct of Sylvius, the periaqueductal grey matter surrounding the aqueduct, and the red nuclei can be found in the central part of the midbrain.

18.5 B E

Three layers of meninges lie between the periosteum of the skull bones and the brain: the fibrous dura mater, the arachnoid mater and the pia mater. Between the periosteum of the skull bones and the dura mater is the extradural space. The middle meningeal artery can be found between the inner surface of the temporal bones and the dura mater. Skull fracture in the temporal bone may tear this artery, resulting in extradural haematoma. This often leads to initial concussion with loss of consciousness, a lucid interval of several hours, followed by acute deterioration due to cerebral compression. An emergency burr-hole is a life-saving procedure. The dura mater is made of strong fibrous tissue. The falx cerebri and the tentorium cerebelli are two large and strong dural folds which stabilise the brain. Between the dura mater and the arachnoid mater is the potential subdural space. Rupture of superficial veins in transit from the brain to a venous sinus may lead to a subdural haematoma (an accumulation of blood in the subdural space). This may present acutely following a head injury in children. On the other hand, it may present with gradual deterioration in personality changes without a history of head injury in the elderly. Between the subarachnoid mater and the pia mater is the subarachnoid space, where cerebrospinal fluid can be found.

18.6 –

Meningiomas are extrinsic CNS tumours. As a group, they occur less frequently than intrinsic CNS tumours (e.g. glioblastomas). Unlike CNS tumours in adults, those in children are usually intrinsic and below the tentorium. Meningiomas are usually lobulated with smooth edges. They seldom invade the dura, skull bones or the brain. Hence they have a better prognosis, as surgical removal is usually curative.

18.7 D

Bacterial meningitis is caused by different organisms at different ages. In neonates, *Streptococcus* and Gram-negative bacilli are common. In children, meningococcus is a common cause. *Haemophilus influenzae* type B commonly caused bacterial meningitis in children in the past, but the incidence has declined sharply since the introduction of universal vaccination against *Haemophilus* type B. Pneumococcus and meningococcus are the commonest organisms causing meningitis in adults.

18.8 A B D E

A cerebral abscess may result from spread of infection locally (e.g. paranasal sinus, middle ear), via the sigmoid cranial sinus (e.g. middle ear or the mastoid antrum) or from the bloodstream. There are no lymphatics in the CNS.

18.9 A B C

Most of the CSF is secreted by the choroid plexuses into the lateral ventricles, the remaining being secreted by the choroid plexus of the third ventricle. The CSF passes through the interventricular foramen into the third ventricle. It then passes through the aqueduct of Sylvius and reaches the fourth ventricle. From the fourth ventricle, it enters the subarachnoid space via the median and the lateral apertures. Only a very small proportion of the CSF enters the central canal of the spinal cord. The CSF is returned to the bloodstream directly via arachnoid mater pouching through the dura of the superior sagittal sinus (arachnoid granulations).

18.10 A B D E

Hydrocephalus ('water in the head') is caused by the accumulation of CSF in the ventricles, which results in ventricular dilatation. The commonest cause is obstruction to the circulation of CSF. This may occur at the interventricular foramen, the third ventricle, the aqueduct, or the median and lateral apertures. Alternatively, obstruction may occur at the arachnoid granulations due to increased protein content of CSF (e.g. due to meningitis). A rare cause of hydrocephalus is excessive CSF production due to a tumour (papilloma) of the choroid plexus.

18.11 A D E

The internal carotid arteries enter the subarachnoid space in the roof of the cavernous sinus and give off ophthalmic, posterior communicating, and anterior choroidal arteries before dividing into their two terminal branches: the anterior and middle cerebral arteries. The basilar artery is formed from the two vertebral arteries, and divide into two posterior cerebral arteries at the upper part of the pons. The circle of Willis is completed by the posterior communicating arteries joining the posterior cerebral arteries, and the anterior communicating artery joining the two anterior cerebral arteries. In some people, the internal carotid arteries provide a significant proportion of blood to the posterior cerebral arteries via the posterior communicating arteries.

18.12 B D

The middle cerebral artery is the larger of the terminal branches of the internal carotid arteries. It gives off its central branches early on in its course. Deep to the lateral fissure, it divides into the upper and lower divisions. The upper division supplies the frontal and anterior parietal lobes. The lower division supplies the posterior parietal lobe, the temporal lobe and the middle of the optic radiation. It supplies about two-thirds of the lateral surface of the cerebral hemispheres. The central branches are important, and supply the corpus striatum, the thalamus and the posterior limb of the internal capsule. Hence blockage of this artery may cause paralysis of the opposite arm, leg and lower part of the face. The anterior limb of the internal capsule is supplied by the anterior cerebral artery. Blockage of the artery results in weakness of the opposite arm and face. The pons is supplied by branches of the basilar artery. The optic radiation is supplied by branches of the posterior cerebral arteries.

18.13 B

Cerebral blood flow is tightly regulated to maintain steady perfusion of the brain. Hence the perfusion of the brain remains relatively constant in spite of wide fluctuations in systolic blood pressure. An increase in acidity (a reduction in pH or an increase in carbon dioxide) leads to relaxation of the arteriolar smooth muscle of the cerebral vessels, and hence increases the cerebral blood flow. Increased systemic pressure leads to contraction of the arteriolar smooth muscle, so that blood flow to the brain can remain constant. Hyperventilation reduces carbon dioxide and hence reduces cerebral blood flow. Mechanical hyperventilation is sometimes used in treating patients with cerebral oedema. Oxygen concentration has relatively little effect on cerebral blood flow.

18.14 A D E

A stroke is a sudden disturbance of the functions of the CNS due to a vascular disease. Over 80% of strokes are due to cerebral infarction. Other causes include intracerebral haemorrhage and subarachnoid haemorrhage.

18.15 A B C D E

Cerebral infarction is due to a reduction of cerebral blood flow or cerebral oxygenation. Reduction in cerebral oxygenation may follow a respiratory arrest. Reduction in cerebral blood flow may be due to cerebral hypotension following cardiac arrest, occlusion of extracranial or intracranial arteries due to atheroma, thrombi or emboli. Other less common causes include head injury and venous thrombosis.

18.16 A B C E

Intracerebral haemorrhage occurs much more commonly in hypertensive subjects. It is caused by rupture at the bifurcation of intracerebral arterioles, and most commonly occurs in the basal ganglia, the brainstem, the cerebellum and the cerebral cortex. The resulting cerebral haematoma acts as an intracranial space-occupying lesion, and may therefore cause an increase in intracranial pressure or cerebral herniation. Rupture of arterial aneurysms at the circle of Willis causes subarachnoid haemorrhage.

18.17 A B D E

The blood–brain barrier exists to provide a chemically appropriate environment for the neurones to function optimally. It has two components: the ependymal lining of the choroid plexuses and the CNS capillary bed. In order to control substances entering and leaving the CNS, the cells lining the barrier are bounded by tight junctions, and fenestrations are absent. Functions of the blood–brain barrier include control of important metabolic substrate such as glucose, to prevent toxins and peripheral neurotransmitters from entering into the CNS, and to control ion movements.

18.18 B C D E

In general, lipid-insoluble drugs do not cross the blood–brain barrier easily, and their effect on the CNS is attenuated and delayed. Lipid-soluble drugs cross the blood–brain barrier easily, and their effect on the CNS is rapid. Inhaled anaesthetics and alcohol cross the blood–brain barrier, and produce CNS effects very rapidly. In the presence of meningitis, the blood–brain barrier is less effective. This can be made use of, as even drugs which usually do not cross the blood–brain barrier (e.g. gentamicin) can do so in the presence of meningitis. Chloramphenicol crosses the blood–brain barrier even in the absence of meningitis.

18.19 A B C E

Neurones are nerve cells whereas neuroglial cells are connective tissue supporting the nervous system. There are about 10 neuroglial cells to every neurone. Each neurone usually has many short dendrites which receive synaptic contacts from other neurones. However, each neurone only has one axon which conducts nerve impulses away from the neurone, although the axon may give rise to collaterals. Nissl bodies can be seen within the cytoplasm, and contain clumps of granular endoplasmic reticulum. Microtubules are intracellular organelles which can be seen in all parts of the neurone. They are involved in neuronal transport, and microtubule-associated proteins transport molecules along the outer surface of microtubules.

18.20 B D E

There are two types of neuronal transport: anterograde and retrograde. In anterograde transport, substances synthesised by the cell body move up the dendrites and axon. In retrograde transport, waste products from the axon and dendrites move to the lysosomes in the cell bodies to be destroyed. Retrograde transport is also important for target cell recognition. Axons constantly take up fragments of the plasma membrane of the target neurone and transport them back to the cell body. Retrograde transport may also be important for the transport of viruses to the CNS from the peripheral nervous system.

18.21 B E

At the resting membrane potential (–70 mV), there is continuous K^+ efflux and Cl^- influx to maintain the negative membrane potential. In an action potential, the firing level is reached when the membrane is depolarised by about 15 mV (i.e. membrane potential is depolarised from –70 mV to about – 55 mV). The voltage-gated sodium channels are suddenly opened at an increased rate as a result of positive feedback, and the sodium conductance increases. As the sodium concentration is usually higher outside than inside the cell due to Na^+,K^+-ATPase, sodium ions readily enter the cell. The membrane potential moves towards though does not reach the equilibrium potential for Na^+. This effect is much larger than the normal repolarising effect of the K^+ efflux and Cl^- influx.

18.22 A B D E

Immediately after the spike potential of the action potential, the sodium channels rapidly enter the inactivated state, and the sodium conductance rapidly decreases. The K^+ channels are gradually opened for a prolonged period of time, and the potassium conductance increases. There is a net movement of K^+ out of the cells, as the concentration of K^+ inside the cell is normally higher than that outside the cell. The prolonged opening of the K^+ channels also explains the after-hyperpolarisation phase.

18.23 A B C E

Before the firing level is reached, the excitation threshold of the neurone to stimulation is higher (i.e. less excitable) the more negative the membrane potential. The absolute refractory period lasts from the time when the firing level is reached until after the first third of the repolarisation. During this period, the neurone cannot be excited irrespective of the strength of the stimulus. The relative refractory period occupies the rest of the repolarisation. During this period, the neurone can be excited, although a stronger stimulus is required. The threshold for excitation is increased during both the absolute and relative refractory periods. During the brief after-depolarisation period which comes immediately after the repolarisation, the neurone is slightly more excitable. However, during the prolonged after-repolarisation period, the neurone becomes less excitable than in its normal resting state.

18.24 A B C E

A synapse is where one neurone meets another. In humans, most synapses are chemically mediated, although electronic synapses do exist. Neurotransmitters are manufactured and loaded into vesicles within the Golgi apparatus of the sending neurone. Neurotransmitters are released from the pre-synaptic membrane by exocytosis. The neurotransmitters diffuse across the synaptic cleft, and act on receptors located on the membrane of the target neurone. Most synapses are axo-dendritic. However, axo-axonic synapses may achieve pre-synaptic inhibition either by preventing the generation of impulses in the target axon or by preventing the release of neurotransmitters.

18.25 A D

GABA and glycine are the two main inhibitory amino acid neurotransmitters. GABA is found mainly in the cerebellum and the cerebral cortex, and glycine is found mainly in the spinal cord and brainstem. Most amines (e.g. dopamine, noradrenaline, adrenaline, 5-HT) are excitatory neurotransmitters. Glutaric acid is an excitatory amino acid neurotransmitter.

18.26 A B C D

At the neuromuscular junction, acetylcholine is synthesised in the cholinergic neurone from acetyl CoA and choline catalysed by the enzyme choline acetyltransferase. It is then taken into vesicles and is ready to be released into the synaptic cleft on the arrival of an action potential. After the acetylcholine vesicles are released, a proportion of the acetylcholine molecules bind to their receptors on the post-synaptic membrane. The nicotinic receptor is made up of five subunits: two identical α, one β, one γ and one γ subunits. Each α subunit binds to an acetylcholine molecule. When both α subunits are bound to an acetylcholine molecule, the sodium channel opens and depolarisation occurs. A second messenger is not required. To allow repolarisation to occur, the remaining acetylcholine molecules in the synaptic cleft are broken down into choline and acetic acid by acetylcholinesterase found on the post synaptic membrane. The choline is recycled and transported back to the pre synaptic neurone.

18.27 A C D

Most neurotransmitters exert their effects via a second messenger. Cyclic AMP is the commonest second messenger, followed by IP_3 and DAG. Nitric oxide is a neurotransmitter, and employs cGMP as the second messenger. Substance P is a neurotransmitter.

18.28 A C E

The types of neuroglial cells in the brain include astrocytes, oligodendrocytes, microglia and ependymal cells. Astrocytes maintain the structure of the capillary endothelium in the brain. Oligodendrocytes are responsible for myelination. Microglia are phagocytes in the brain. Ependymal cells line the ventricles and their cilia help the circulation of the CSF within the ventricular system.

18.29 B D

Myelination is the process of wrapping myelin sheaths around the axons of the neurones in the white matter of the brain, and is the main function of oligodendrocytes in the brain. Not all nerves are myelinated. For example, less than half of all peripheral nerves are myelinated. The axon is exposed at intervals between the myelin wrappings, and these are known as nodes. Myelination significantly increases the conduction of nerve impulses along the axon, as the impulses jump from node to node. During myelination, the potassium ion channels are deleted as they are no longer necessary. Multiple sclerosis is a disease characterised by patches of demyelination in the white matter, and usually occurs in young adults in the temperature latitudes. Since the potassium ion channels have already been deleted, nerve conduction is compromised. Multiple sclerosis causes a variety of neurological symptoms depending on the anatomical site involved.

18.30 D

Multiple sclerosis is the commonest demyelinating disorder of the CNS. It does not usually affect the peripheral nervous system. It occurs more commonly in temperate than tropical countries, and in women than in men. The aetiology of the disease is not entirely clear, although it has been hypothesised that it may be an autoimmune disorder triggered by viral infection in genetically susceptible individuals. Histologically, the chronic plaque characteristically shows a loss of myelin, scarcity of oligodendrocytes (which make myelin) and a predominance of fibrillary astrocytes.

18.31 A B D E

There are many types of receptors in the skin. As they have different speeds of adaptation and they are located in different areas, they detect different stimuli and perform different functions. Free nerve endings respond to variations in temperature and painful stimuli. Pacinian corpuscles are found especially on the fingers and the palms, and are particularly effective in detecting vibration. Follicular nerve endings detect touch, and are rapidly adapting. This explains the short-lived touch sensation when clothes are put on. Meissner's corpuscles are mainly found on the pulp of the fingers, and are rapidly adapting. They are responsible for the detection of the texture of objects. Merkel cells adapt slowly, and discharge continuously in response to constant pressure. This explains the continued awareness of an object (e.g. knife and fork) held in the hand.

18.32 B

Knowledge of the segmental nerve supply is sometimes important in making a diagnosis in neurological examinations. The correct answers are:

- Around the nipple – T5
- At the umbilicus – T10
- Inguinal region – L1
- Lateral side of the sole of the foot – S1
- The thumb – C6

18.33 A B

Nerve root compression in the vertebral canal commonly affects the cervical roots (e.g. due to cervical spondylosis) or the lumbosacral roots (e.g. due to intervertebral disc prolapse). It generally causes a feeling of numbness or tingling within that dermatome, referred pain in the muscles supplied by the relevant spinal nerves, weakness of muscles supplied by the spinal nerve and a loss of tendon reflex supplied by the spinal nerve. Hence compression of the S1 nerve root would cause pain in the sole of the feet, tingling or numbness in the area supplied by S1, weakness of the plantar flexion of the ankle and an absent ankle jerk. The knee jerk is unaffected, as its segmental level is L3/4.

18.34 A

Damage to the radial nerve at the radial groove of the humerus results in damage to the posterior interosseous nerve. Hence the long digital and carpal extensors are paralysed. The branch to the triceps is given off in the axilla. Hence extension of the elbow is unaffected. The middle and distal phalangeal joints of the fingers are extended by the interossei and lumbricals, and are therefore preserved. There may be diminished sensation over the radial side of the dorsum of the hand.

18.35 B C E

Damage to the ulnar nerve at the wrist results in paralysis of the adductor pollicis, the hypothenar muscles, and the third and fourth lumbricals. This results in inability of the thumb to adduct, and a clawed hand appearance. Sensation is diminished over the ulnar side of the palm, and over the palmar side of the little finger and the ulnar side of the fourth finger. However, sensation of the ulnar side of the dorsum of the hand is preserved, as the dorsal cutaneous branch is given off in the forearm.

18.36 A B E

When the hammer strikes the tendon of the quadriceps muscles, the muscle spindles in the muscle belly are passively stretched, and the type Ia and type II fibres discharge impulses to the posterior horn of the spinal cord. They then synapse with the dendrites of α motorneurones supplying the quadriceps muscles, and elicit contraction of the extrafusal muscle fibres. Most tendon reflexes involve only one synapse, and only occur at the spinal cord level. The muscle spindles also send inhibitory impulses simultaneously to the α motor neurones supplying the antagonist muscles (i.e. hamstrings). This is called reciprocal inhibition.

18.37 C E

The posterior column–medial lemniscal pathway is the larger of the two sensory pathways, and carries sensory fibres for joint position sense, vibration sense and discriminative touch. Like the spinothalamic pathway, it consists of three sets of neurones. The cell body of the first-order neurone lies in the posterior root ganglia. The fibres are projected from the sensory receptors to the nuclei gracilis and cuneatus, and the fibres are collected in the gracilis and cuneate fasciculi. Unlike the spinothalamic tract, the first-order neurone does not cross over. The cell bodies of the second-order neurones lie in the nuclei gracilis and cuneatus, and project to the ventral posterior nucleus of the thalamus. The fibres cross over at the level of the medulla oblongata, and the fibres form the medial lemniscus after crossing over. The cell bodies of the third-order neurones lie in the ventral posterior nucleus of the thalamus, and project to the sensory cortex.

18.38 A B D E

There are great similarities between the spinothalamic tract and the posterior column–medial lemniscal pathway. Both have three-order sets of neurones. The cell bodies of the first-order neurones lie in the posterior root ganglia. The second-order neurones cross over to the opposite side for both pathways. One major difference is that whilst the spinothalamic tract crosses over in the spinal cord, the posterior column–medial lemniscal pathway crosses over in the medulla oblongata. The cell bodies of the third-order neurones lie in the thalamus for both pathways, and the third-order neurones project from the thalamus to the sensory cortex. Moreover, the representation of different parts of the body on the cortex is similar for both pathways.

18.39 A D

The two sensory pathways are the posterior column–medial lemniscal pathway and the spinothalamic pathway. The posterior column–medial lemniscal pathway mediates joint position and vibration senses, as well as two-point discrimination. The spinothalamic pathway mediates pain and temperature sensation.

18.40 C

Dissociated sensory loss affecting temperature but not joint position sensation can only occur if the anatomical pathways for the two sensory functions are separate. As the nerves or their cell bodies relaying messages for these two functions run close to each other in the peripheral nerves, posterior root ganglia, thalamus and cerebral cortex, lesions at these sites are likely to produce abnormalities in both sensory modalities. However, as the posterior column and lateral spinothalamic tract run separately in the spinal cord, a cyst in the central canal (syringomyelia) may initially affect the spinothalamic tract whilst leaving the posterior column intact.

18.41 C D E

Sharp localised pain is transmitted by the larger and faster myelinated Aδ fibres, whilst dull diffuse chronic pain is transmitted by smaller and slower unmyelinated C fibres. This accounts for the delay between the feeling of a localised sharp pain and the diffuse dull pain which follows it.

Substance P is the neurotransmitter in the afferent pain fibres in the dorsal horn of the spinal cord. The dorsal horn cells act as 'gates' to the pain pathway: the synapse between the peripheral pain fibres and the dorsal horn cells can be modified by drugs, or by other fibres (e.g. collaterals from touch fibres) via pre-synaptic inhibition.

18.42 A B E

Endogenous opioid neurotransmitters (e.g. endorphins, enkephalins) in the spinal cord and the brain form the natural pain inhibitory system. The mechanism of action for acupuncture and transcutaneous nerve stimulation is thought to be the release of these endogenous opioid neurotransmitters, and placebo may also work in this way. The analgesic action of paracetamol is peripheral by inhibiting the synthesis of prostaglandin. Naloxone is an opioid antagonist.

18.43 A C

The correct mechanisms of analgesic actions for the drugs are:

- Opiates – μ-opioid receptor agonist
- NSAIDs – cyclooxygenase inhibitor, reduction of prostaglandin synthesis both centrally and peripherally
- Corticosteroids – prevention of prostaglandin synthesis by reduction of arachidonic acid release
- Paracetamol – same as NSAIDs, but, peripheral action predominant

18.44 A B E

Stimulation of μ_2-opioid receptors causes respiratory depression and reduced gastrointestinal motility. Opioids also stimulate vagal tone and reduce sympathetic drive, and bradycardia may result. This effect is useful in the treatment of acute left ventricular failure with excessive sympathetic drive. The increased predominance of parasympathetic over sympathetic drive may cause pupil constriction, and may help in the clinical diagnosis of opiate overdose.

18.45 B E

The pre-ganglionic fibres of the sympathetic nervous system emerge from the anterior nerve root of the thoracic and lumbar segments of the spinal cord, and enter the sympathetic chain. They may ascend or descend to supply various parts of the body. Most of the sympathetic ganglia are in the sympathetic chain (e.g. superior cervical ganglion, stellate ganglion, thoracic ganglion, lumbar and sacral ganglia), although some lie outside (e.g. adrenal medulla, coeliac ganglion, pelvic ganglion). The adrenal medulla develops from the neural crest embryologically, and acts as a sympathetic ganglion. The adrenal cortex does not receive innervation from pre-ganglionic sympathetic fibres, although it might receive post-ganglionic fibres from the renal ganglion. The male genitalia receive post-ganglionic fibres from the pelvic ganglion.

18.46 A C E

The sympathetic nervous system prepares the body for 'fright, flight and fight'. Effects include dilated pupils, increased heart rate, sweating, blood diverted from the skin and intestines to the skeletal muscles, reduced gut motility, and closure of sphincters for defecation and micturition. Hence, in patients with Raynaud's phenomenon with intermittent cold and painful fingers due to restriction of blood supply, interruption of the sympathetic nervous supply (sympathectomy) may be carried out. Similarly, the procedure might be considered in patients with serious excessive sweating of the hands.

18.47 A E

As the sympathetic nervous system normally dilates the pupils and increases sweating, interruption of the sympathetic nervous system after its emergence from the superior cervical ganglion would result in a small pupil and reduced sweating on that side of the face. Since the sympathetic nervous system also supplies the levator muscle of the upper eyelid, drooping of the eyelid (ptosis) may be seen in Horner's syndrome. Enophthalmos (sunken eye) may be seen in very severe cases. Eye movements are not affected, as the extraocular muscles are supplied by the third, fourth and sixth cranial nerves. Tear secretion is not affected. The lacrimal glands receive parasympathetic nervous supply from the pterygopalatine ganglion.

18.48 A D E

The pre-ganglionic parasympathetic fibres emerge from the cranial nerves and the sacral segments of the spinal cord. The cranial nerves carrying parasympathetic nerves include the oculomotor nerve (the post-ganglionic fibres from the ciliary ganglion supply the eye), the facial nerve (the post-ganglionic fibres from the pterygopalatine ganglion supply the lacrimal, submandibular and sublingual glands), the glossopharayngeal nerve (the post-ganglionic fibres from the otic ganglion supply the parotid gland) and the vagus nerve (the post-ganglionic fibres supply the heart and intestine).

18.49 B C

Acetylcholine is the neurotransmitter for the post-ganglionic parasympathetic fibres. Most of the post-ganglionic receptors are muscarinic, but different subtypes of muscarinic receptors have been found. Antimuscarinic drugs tend to block the parasympathetic effects, and cause dilated pupils, dry mouth, increased heart rate, bronchodilation, reduced gut motility and retention of urine.

18.50 A B

The corticospinal tract is the main voluntary motor pathway. Most of its fibres originate from the primary motor cortex in the pre-central gyrus, with contributions from the sensory cortex. It descends through the corona radiata and the internal capsule to reach the brainstem. It passes through the midbrain cerebral peduncles and the pons to form the pyramid in the medulla oblongata. About four-fifths of the fibres then cross over to the opposite side at the medullary decussation, and continue as the lateral corticospinal tract in the spinal cord. About one-fifth of the fibres remain uncrossed. Amongst these uncrossed fibres, half continue as anterior corticospinal fibres in the spinal cord, and half continue as uncrossed lateral corticospinal fibres. These uncrossed fibres may be important in the partial recovery of power in the affected limbs after hemiplegia caused by cerebrovascular accident.

18.51 A C

A clinical 'upper motor neurone lesion' is characteristically associated with weakness, increased muscle tone, spasticity, clasp-knife rigidity, exaggerated tendon reflexes and positive Babinski sign. It occurs when the upper motor neurone of the primary voluntary motor pathway is affected. These are the corticonuclear tract (for facial and lingual muscles) and the corticospinal tract. The anterior horn cells are the cell bodies of the 'lower motor neurones'. Periphery nerve lesions cause lower motor neurone lesions. The reticulospinal tract forms part of the extrapyramidal pathway responsible for posture and coordination of the limbs.

18.52 B D E

The distinction between upper and lower motor neurone lesions is important clinically, as it may give valuable clues about the aetiology of a neurological disease. The characteristic signs of a lower motor neurone lesion are weakness, wasting, reduced muscle tone, fasciculations and loss of tendon reflexes. Wasting occurs probably as a result of the loss of a factor produced by motorneurones. Fasciculations result from spontaneous discharge of motorneurones.

18.53 A B D E

The basal ganglia are concerned with the control of movement, and consist of a number of nuclei and nerve fibres at the level between the thalamus and the midbrain. They include the striatum (which include the caudate nucleus and the putamen of the lentiform nucleus), the globus pallidus, the substantia nigra and the subthalamic nucleus.

18.54 B

The main lesion in Parkinson's disease is a loss of dopaminergic neurones in the nigrostriatal pathway. The exact functions for each component of the basal ganglia are not yet entirely understood. However, it is generally accepted that there is a balance between the output of cholinergic and dopaminergic neurones in the striatum, and that the cholinergic output becomes unopposed in Parkinson's disease. The GABA-ergic neurones are reduced in Huntingdon's disease but not in Parkinson's disease. It was found that injection of the drug MPTP causes an acute clinical picture very similar to Parkinson's disease. MPTP is metabolised by monoamine oxidase B. Since monoamine oxidase B inhibitors (e.g. selegiline) appear to slow the progress of Parkinson's disease, it has been hypothesised that Parkinson's disease may be partly caused by the presence of a natural substance resembling MPTP.

18.55 A C D E

See question 18.54 above. Phenothiazines are dopamine antagonists, and tend to worsen Parkinsonian symptoms. Bromocriptine has dopaminergic agonist activity, and is sometimes useful in the treatment of Parkinson's disease.

18.56 A C D E

The cerebellum can be functionally divided into vestibulocerebellum, spinocerebellum and neocerebellum. The vestibulocerebellum consists of nuclei in the midline, and includes the vermis and fastigial nuclei. It communicates with the vestibular nucleus, and is important in maintaining balance. The spinocerebellum includes the anterior lobe. It receives fibres from the spinocerebellar tract, and is important in controlling gait and posture. The neocerebellum is the largest of all, and consists of the lateral parts of the cerebellum. It receives fibres from the pontocerebellar tract, and sends efferent fibres to the opposite cerebral cortex via the thalamus. Its main functions include coordination of the movements of the ipsilateral limbs and maintaining smooth contraction of the diaphragm and other speech muscles.

18.57 A E

The function of the vestibulocerebellum is most often impaired by midline cerebellar tumours. As the vestibulocerebellum communicates with the vestibular nuclei, vestibulocerebellar lesions usually result in the inability to stand upright without support (truncal ataxia) and nystagmus. Finger–nose incoordination and impaired articulation are characteristic features of neocerebellar lesions.

18.58 C D

See question 18.56 above. As the function of the neocerebellum is the coordination of ipsilateral limb movements and the maintenance of smooth contraction of speech muscles, characteristic features of neocerebellar lesions include impaired ipsilateral 'heel-to-shin' and 'finger-to-nose' tests and impaired articulation and phonation.

18.59 E

The correct cranial nerves responsible for the functions are:

- Sensation of the posterior third of the tongue – glossopharyngeal nerve
- Phonation – cranial accessory and vagus nerves
- Tongue protrusion – hypoglossal nerve
- Mastication – trigeminal nerve (motor root)
- Sensation to the forehead – ophthalmic branch of the trigeminal nerve

18.60 A D

The trigeminal nerve emerges from anterolateral surface of the pons, and enters the Gasserian ganglion in the petrous temporal bone. The three divisions emerge from the Gasserian ganglion and leave the skull through different foramina (the ophthalmic branch through the superior orbital fissure; the maxillary branch through the foramen rotundum; the mandibular branch through the foramen ovale). It has both sensory and motor functions. The motor branch innervates the muscle of mastication. The sensory branch supplies the dura mater of the middle and anterior cranial fossa, teeth and gums of the lower jaw, and the anterior two-thirds of the tongue. The mandibular division of the trigeminal nerve mediates the jaw jerk. The tip of the nose is innervated by the maxillary division.

18.61 A D

The correct cranial nerves responsible for the functions are:

- Taste in the posterior third of the tongue – glossopharyngeal nerve
- Taste in the anterior two-thirds of the tongue – facial nerve (via chorda tympani)
- Corneal reflex – (afferent limb) ophthalmic division of the trigeminal nerve; (efferent limb) facial nerve
- Attenuation of loud sound – facial nerve (branch to stapedius muscle)
- Parotid gland secretion – glossopharyngeal nerve (via otic ganglion)

18.62 A E

The nuclei of the facial nerve lie in the caudal part of the pons. Upper motor neurone lesion of the facial nerve is supranuclear, and is commonly caused by a vascular stroke which affects the corticonuclear fibres either in the cerebral cortex or the internal capsule. As the nuclei for the upper part of the face are bilaterally represented, a unilateral upper motor neurone facial nerve palsy affects only the lower part of the face, but spares the upper part of the face.

18.63 A B C D

The commonest cause of a unilateral lower motor neurone facial nerve palsy is Bell's palsy. It is caused by compression resulting from inflammation of the nerve inside the bony canal above the labyrinth between the geniculate ganglion and the stylomastoid foramen. This affects both the lower and upper parts of the face. As a result of loss of the stapedius function, the patient may complain of increased sensitivity to loud noise. Most cases resolve within a few weeks, although recovery in a few patients is incomplete.

18.64 B C D

All the extraocular muscles are supplied by the oculomotor nerve, apart from the lateral rectus (supplied by the abducens nerve) and the superior oblique (supplied by the trochlear nerve). In addition, the upper division of the oculomotor nerve also supplies the levator palpebrae. The oculomotor nerve also carries parasympathetic fibres to the eye to supply the sphincter pupillae (which constricts the pupil) and the ciliary muscle (for accommodation). The parasympathetic fibres originate from the Edinger–Westphal nucleus and synapse in the ciliary ganglion.

18.65 E

All extaocular muscles apart from the lateral rectus and superior oblique are paralysed in oculomotor nerve palsy. Hence the position of the eye is 'down and out'. Paralysis of the levator superioris results in complete ptosis due to the action of unopposed orbicularis oculi. Paralysis of the sphincter pupillae results in a fully dilated pupil due to unopposed action of dilator pupillae. Sweating is controlled by the sympathetic nervous system, which is unaffected in oculomotor nerve palsy.

18.66 A B C E

The MLF is a central brainstem nerve tract which connects the oculomotor, trochlear and abducens nuclei. It also receives neural input from the vestibular nuclei and the cerebellum. It is important for conjugate eye movement to ensure that the visual axes of both eyes are parallel, and to maintain visual fixation on a moving target. The MLF is often affected by multiple sclerosis. This results in internuclear ophthalmoplegia. The ipsilateral eye is unable to adduct, and nystagmus appears in the contralateral abducting eye.

18.67 D E

Direct pupillary light reflex describes the constriction of the pupil when light is shone onto the same eye, whilst consensual light reflex describes the constriction of the pupil when light is shone onto the opposite eye. Only the first-order neurone of the visual tract is involved. In direct pupillary light reflex, the ganglion cells within the retina conduct impulses along the optic nerve and the optic tracts to the pretectal nucleus near the superior colliculus in the midbrain. The pretectal nucleus is linked by internuncial neurones to the parasympathetic (Edinger–Westphal) nucleus. The pre-ganglionic fibres from the Edinger – Westphal nucleus enters the oculomotor nerve and synapses in the ciliary ganglion, and the post-ganglionic fibres supply the sphincter pupillae in the iris. Stimulation of the sphincter pupillae causes papillary constriction. For consensual light reflex, impulses are conducted from the pretectal nucleus to the opposite Edinger–Westphal nucleus via the posterior commissure.

18.68 B

The fact that the right pupil constricts in response to light shone onto the left eye indicates the pathway along the left optic nerve and the right oculomotor nerve are intact. A lesion in either the pathway along the left optic nerve or the left oculomotor nerve may explain why the left pupil fails to react in response to light shone on the left eye. Other explanations may include a lesion in the left Edinger–Westphal nucleus or paralysis of the sphincter pupillae (e.g. due to drugs). From these two deductions, the only given option which may explain the clinical findings is a left oculomotor nerve lesion.

18.69 A

The are two types of photoreceptor cells: the rods and the cones. The photosensitive compounds are contained in the outer segments, which contain regular stacks of membrane. In the rods, the outer segments are thin and rod-like, whilst those of the cones are more pointed. There are about 6 million cones in each eye, and they are mainly found in the fovea. On the other hand, there are about 120 million rods in each eye, and they are found outside the fovea. The rods are more sensitive to light than cones, and function in dim light. Hence they are important for night vision. However, they are not able to differentiate between different colours. The cones are important for vision in daylight. They are capable of distinguishing between different colours, and can achieve a higher level of visual acuity than rods.

18.70 A B

When the photosensitive pigments (opsin and retinene$_1$) are exposed to light, structural changes in the retinene$_1$ occur. This results in a conformation change of the photopigment, and activates an associated G protein-transducin (G_{t1}). This in turn activates a cGMP-associated phosphodiesterase, and hence causes a reduction in intracellular cGMP. This leads to a closure of the sodium channel, and hyperpolarisation of the photoreceptor occurs. This hyperpolarisation leads to an action potential in the ganglion cells in the retina.

18.71 E

When an individual with normal vision moves from a very bright to a very dark room, the visual threshold declines due to dark adaptation. The initial decline in visual threshold is mainly due to adaptation of the cones as the changes are tested at relatively high intensity of light when cones are active. The later changes in visual threshold are due to rod adaptation at a much lower intensity of light. The dark adaptation is due to the regeneration of the photopigments from their 'bleached' configuration. On the other hand, when a person moves from a very dark to a very bright room, the visual threshold increases due to the conversion of the photopigments into their 'bleached' configuration. This is a much faster process. If the individual had worn red-tinted glasses in the bright light, the rods would only be minimally stimulated as its peak sensitivity to light is at a lower wavelength of 505 mm. Hence the dark adaptation process would be quicker.

18.72 B C D E

Myopia is often genetic in origin, and is commoner amongst Chinese and Japanese than the Caucasians. It is due to an abnormally long eyeball, excessive convergence power of the cornea or lens, or a combination of the two factors. As a result, the images formed lie in front of the retina, and they appear blurred to the subject. It may be corrected by concave lenses, which tend to diverge the light rays and move the images further back onto the retina.

18.73 A

Both the retina and the optic nerve develop embryologically from an outgrowth of the brain (the optic vesicle). Hence the optic nerve is wrapped round by neuroglial cells (i.e. astrocytes and oligodendrocytes) and not Schwann cells as in peripheral nerves. The optic nerve is also surrounded by meninges. Whilst peripheral nerves can regenerate if damaged, the optic nerve cannot. The cell bodies of the optic nerve are in the ganglion layer of the retina. It synapses at the lateral geniculate bodies of the thalamus. The optic nerve is therefore homologous with the second-order neurone in the sensory pathway (e.g. spinothalamic tract). Whilst the fibres from the nasal side of the retina at the optic chiasma cross over to the opposite lateral geniculate body, those from the temporal side of the retina do not cross over, and join the ipsilateral lateral geniculate body.

18.74 B C E

Lesions before the optic chiasma will only affect vision in that eye. As the other eye is unaffected, the visual field with both eyes open is full. A lesion at the optic chiasma (e.g. due to a pituitary gland) may result in the fibres from the nasal side of the retina from both eyes being interrupted. This gives rise to bitemporal hemianopia. Lesions beyond the optic chiasma result in fibres of the temporal side of the retina from the ipsilateral eye and the nasal side of the retina from the opposite eye being interrupted. This gives rise to homonymous hemianopia in the visual field on the side opposite to the lesion.

The correct matches between the lesions and the resulting visual field defects are:

- Complete left optic nerve lesion – blindness in left eye
- Optic chiasm – bitemporal hemianopia
- Left optic tract – right homonymous hemianopia
- Right optic radiation – left homonymous hemianopia
- Left occipital cortex – right homonymous hemianopia

18.75 A B C E

Sound vibrations from outside the ear must enter the outer ear to set up vibrations in the tympanic membrane. The handle of the first ossicle (malleus) is attached to the back of the tympanic membrane, and the sound vibrations must pass through all three ossicles in the middle ear (malleus, incus, stapes) to reach the oval window. The foot plate of the stapes closes the scala vestibuli at the oval window, which separates the middle and the inner ear. The sound vibrations from the stapes stimulate the inner hair cells of the cochlea, which are the auditory sense organs.

18.76 A D

The axons of the neurones that innervate the inner hair cells form the auditory nerve, which synapse at the dorsal and ventral cochlear nuclei in the medulla. This is the first-order neurone. The second-order neurone runs from these nuclei to the contralateral medial geniculate body at the thalamus. It also sends fibres to the ipsilateral medial geniculate body through different pathways. The third-order neurone runs from the medial geniculate body to the primary auditory cortex in the superior temporal gyrus. Lateral geniculate bodies and superior colliculi are part of pathways for vision and visual reflexes.

18.77 A B D

The amplitude and frequency of sound waves determine the loudness and pitch of the sound respectively. The harmonics of the sound waves (i.e. the proportion of sound with harmonic vibrations) determine the timbre of the sound (e.g. the difference in sound quality of notes between different musical instruments of the same pitch). The speed of the sound is determined by the medium in which the sound is transmitted (e.g. faster in water than in air), but the sound appears the same. The wavelength can be calculated by the equation

Wavelength = Speed/Frequency

For a given speed of sound, the higher the wavelength, the lower the pitch.

18.78 A C E

Two factors contribute to the lateral localisation of sound. Firstly, there is a slight time difference in the arrival of stimulus in the two ears. This results in a phase difference in the sound waves on the two sides. Secondly, the sound is louder on the side of the source. These differences are interpreted by the auditory cortex. However, there is no time difference in the arrival of the sound from in front and behind in the two ears. Localisation is achieved by the shape and position of the pinna. The pinna also explains the localisation of sound coming from directly above or directly below the subject.

18.79 B C D

About 90% of the population are left hemisphere/right hand dominant. Amongst these people, Wernicke's area is found in the left superior temporal gyrus. Its main function is to understand speech. Hence lesions in the area result in receptive aphasia, and patients have difficulty in understanding the speech of others, retrieving the appropriate names of objects, and monitoring their own speech, although they might appear to speak fluently and they may not be aware of the gross errors in their speech.

Broca's area is usually found in the left inferior frontal gyrus. Its main function is to express what the subject wishes to say. Hence a patient with a lesion in Broca's area understands other people's speech. However, their own speech is slow, hesitant and telegraphic. Patients are well aware of their speech problem. The two speech areas are supplied by branches of the left middle cerebral artery. Broca's and Wernicke's areas are connected by the arcuate fasciculus.

18.80 B D E

Alzheimer's disease is the commonest cause of dementia. It is a degenerative condition, and therefore occurs more commonly amongst older people. Most cases of Alzheimer's disease are sporadic, and occur more commonly in individuals with the ApoE4 genotype on chromosome 19. However, a small proportion of cases run in families and appear to have an autosomal dominant inheritance. A gene on chromosome 21 appears to be involved in these cases.

18.81 C

Alzheimer's disease characteristically causes a severe loss of both white and grey matter. Marked cortical atrophy is characteristic, with consequent ventricular dilatation. The hippocampus, frontal and temporal lobes are most affected. This explains the clinical features of deterioration in personality, memory and cognition. Histologically, senile plaques and neurofibrillary tangles are characteristic, although the nature of these structures is not entirely known. Senile plaques are neuritic processes surrounding a central amyloid core. Neurofibrillary tangles are long corkscrew-like structures consisting of thickened fibrils within the neuronal cytoplasm. There is a reduction of cholinergic neurones in Alzheimer's disease. The effectiveness of drugs which enhance cholinergic activities in the CNS is currently being evaluated.

18.82 B C D E

Benzodiazepines have sedative, hypnotic, anxiolytic, anticonvulsant and muscle relaxant properties, and are used clinically for each of these properties. There are three different subtypes of benzodiazepine receptors. The traditional benzodiazepines act at all three subtypes. However, newer types of benzodiazepines might act selectively on one or two of these subtypes, and actions can be more specific.

18.83 A C D

Benzodiazepines act mainly on the reticular activating system (causing sedation and hypnosis), but also act on the limbic system. They act by attaching to a specific site on the GABA receptor/chloride channel complex. Their action is to potentiate the effect of GABA, which is an important inhibitory neurotransmitter. GABA acts by opening chloride ion channels in cells. The muscle relaxant properties of benzodiazepines are central and not peripheral.

18.84 C D

Neuroleptics are anti-schizophrenic agents. Schizophrenia is associated with excess dopaminergic D_2 receptors in the limbic system of the brain. Phenothiazines (e.g. chlorpromazine) belong to one of the traditional groups of neuroleptic drugs. Other neuroleptic drugs include butyrophenones (e.g. haloperidol) and thioxanthenes. They act mainly by competitively antagonising the dopaminergic D_2 receptors. However, phenothiazines also have other significant pharmacological actions, such as antagonists at serotonin, cholinergic, and α-adrenergic receptors. They are used to treat schizophrenia both in acute treatment and for maintenance therapy. Neuroleptics are not antidepressants.

18.85 A B C

As phenothiazines are antagonists of dopamine receptors, they may antagonise the dopamine receptors in the nigrostriatal tract and cause Parkinsonian symptoms. As dopamine inhibits the release of prolactin from the anterior pituitary gland, phenothiazines may cause hyperprolactinaemia. Tardive dyskinesia is a disorder characterised by involuntary movements of lips, tongue and face, and may occur after neuroleptics have been used for a few years. Akathisia (extreme restlessness of legs) may occur in about a fifth of the patients, but the exact mechanism of action is unclear. Phenothiazines are generally sedative. The newer types of neuroleptics (e.g. clozapine, risperidone) generally have fewer neurological side effects.

18.86 A E

The major types of antidepressants include tricyclic (e.g. amitriptyline), SSRIs (e.g. fluoxetine, paroxetine), monoamine oxidase inhibitors (e.g. phenelzine), and reversible selective MAO-A inhibitors (e.g. moclobemide). Lithium and carbamazepine are used in the treatment of manic-depressive illnesses, as well as mood stabilisers in unipolar depression. Benzodiazepines, barbiturates and neuroleptics have no place in the treatment of depression.

18.87 C E

Tricyclic antidepressants act by inhibiting the reuptake of noradrenaline into the neuronal stores. Hence, the sympathomimetic actions of adrenergic agonists (e.g. adrenaline and noradrenaline) are potentiated by tricyclic antidepressants. The cardiotoxic effects are also potentiated. Tricyclic antidepressants are antimuscarinics, and may cause blurred vision, urinary retention, dry mouth and raised intraocular pressure. The bladder inhibitory action is used clinically in the treatment of childhood enuresis. Tricyclics may also precipitate seizures as they lower the seizure threshold.

18.88 E

Lithium acts by reducing the recycling of free myoinositol for the synthesis of phosphatidylinositol, which is an important intracellular signalling molecule for regulating intracellular calcium concentration. As lithium has a narrow therapeutic window, a good understanding of the pharmacokinetics is important. Lithium is a small ion, and is therefore normally easily absorbed throughout the gastrointestinal tract. However, a sustained-release preparation may delay the absorption. It is not bound to plasma proteins, and it is not significantly metabolised by the liver. It is mainly eliminated by the kidneys, and the rate of elimination is proportional to the plasma sodium concentration. Hence the half-life decreases in patients with renal impairment, and lithium clearance is inversely proportion to sodium clearance. Thus lithium clearance decreases when a diuretic is administered at the same time.

19. The musculoskeletal system
Questions

19.1 The following statements about a typical long bone are true:

- **A** It is covered by a tough membrane made up of mainly fibrous tissue
- **B** Collagen makes up over 50% of its organic matrix
- **C** It is formed by ossification of membranes
- **D** When the rate of bone growth decreases, the epiphyseal plate widens
- **E** The linear growth rate increases sharply when the epiphyseal plate fuses with the shaft

19.2 Osteoblasts:

- **A** Make collagen
- **B** May differentiate into osteoclasts
- **C** Reabsorb bone
- **D** Are stimulated by parathyroid hormone
- **E** Are stimulated by corticosteroids

19.3 Predisposing factors for pathological fractures include:

- **A** Bone metastasis
- **B** Osteomalacia
- **C** Osteoporosis
- **D** Paget's disease
- **E** Myeloma

19.4 The clavicle:

- **A** Articulates with the first costal cartilage medially
- **B** Articulates with the coracoid process of the scapula laterally
- **C** Is essential for the abduction of the upper limb
- **D** Very rarely fractures
- **E** Fractures more commonly in its lateral than its middle third

19.5 The following statements about the shoulder joint are true:

- **A** The glenoid cavity is deep
- **B** It has a wider range of movement than the hip joint
- **C** Abduction is initiated by the supraspinatus
- **D** The axillary nerve runs anterior to the joint
- **E** Anterior dislocation is commoner than posterior dislocation

19.6 The rotator cuff muscles include:

A Supraspinatus
B Deltoid
C Latissimus dorsi
D Subscapularis
E Pectoralis major

19.7 The following muscles extend the elbow:

A Biceps
B Triceps
C Pronator teres
D Brachioradialis
E Extensor carpi radialis longus

19.8 The following statements about the scaphoid are true:

A It is a carpal bone in the distal row
B It is attached by the flexor retinaculum
C Most of the blood supply enters at the proximal end
D Fracture usually results from a fall on the outstretched hand
E Non-union is more likely after fracture of the tuberosity (distal part) rather than the waist of the scaphoid

19.9 The flexor retinaculum:

A Is a thickening of the palmar deep fascia
B Is attached to the hamate and the pisiform
C Gives origin to the muscles of the thenar eminence
D Forms the carpal tunnel
E Covers the median nerve

19.10 The following muscles of the hand and their actions are correctly matched:

A Abductor pollicis brevis – abduction of the thumb
B Opponens pollicis – extension of the thumb
C Dorsal interrosei – adduct the fingers
D Palmar interrosei – abduct the fingers
E Lumbricals – flex the proximal phalanx; extend the middle and distal phalanxes

19.11 The following statements about the hip joint are true:

A It has a deep acetabulum cup
B The associated ligaments are stronger than those of the shoulder joint
C Dislocation of the adult hip is common
D The sciatic nerve runs posterior to the joint
E It is commonly affected by osteoarthritis in older people

19.12 The following statements about the ligaments of the knee joint are correct:

A The anterior cruciate ligament passes from the front of the intercondylar area to the medial surface of the lateral femoral condyle
B The posterior cruciate ligament passes from the front of the intercondylar area to the lateral surface of the lateral femoral condyle
C The lateral collateral ligament passes from the lateral epicondyle of the femur to the head of the fibula
D The medial collateral ligament passes from the medial epicondyle of the femur to the head of the fibula
E The patellar ligament passes from the apex of the patella to the tibial tuberosity

19.13 The following statements about testing the stability of the knee joint are true:

A The knee should be fully flexed when the lateral collateral ligament is tested
B Excessive movement of the knee on varus testing indicates medial collateral ligament weakness
C The knee should be in half-flexed position when the medial collateral ligament is tested
D Anterior and posterior cruciate ligaments should be tested with the knee in full extension
E The patella should be tested by assessing the up-and-down movement when the knee is fully flexed

19.14 The following regions of the vertebral column and their corresponding number of vertebrae (before fusion occurs) are correctly matched:

A Cervical – 8
B Thoracic – 12
C Lumbar – 4
D Sacral – 4
E Coccygeal – 4

19.15 The following regions of the vertebral column are convex anteriorly (i.e. secondary curvature):

A Cervical
B Thoracic
C Lumbar
D Sacral
E Coccygeal

19.16 Osteoporosis is associated with:

A A reduction of total bone mass
B Gross histological abnormalities
C Gross biochemical abnormalities
D Increased susceptibility to fracture
E An excess of bone formation over resorption

19.17 Osteoporosis occurs more commonly in:

A Men than women
B Older than younger people
C Negroes than Caucasians
D After a period of bed rest
E Those on corticosteroid therapy

19.18 The following statements about the arrangements of filaments in the muscle fibre are correct:

A The overlapping patterns of the thick and thin filaments account for the characteristic striations seen on electron microscopy
B The thick filaments are made of actin
C The thin filaments are made of myosin
D Troponin binds to myosin
E Tropomyosin are located between filaments of actin

19.19 Which of the following events occur when an action potential in the skeletal muscle fibre leads to its contraction?

A The action potential is transmitted to different sarcomeres via the T tubules
B Calcium ions diffuse from the extracellular space to the thick and thin filaments
C Calcium ions increase the concentration of tropomyosin
D There is increased availability of troponin in the sarcomere
E There is increased formation of cross-linkages between actin and myosin

19.20 When the muscle fibre contacts:

A The length of the thick filaments decrease
B The length of the thin filaments decrease
C The length of the sarcomere decreases
D The overlap between the thick and the thin filaments increases
E Energy released from ATP is utilised

19.21 Compared to the red (type 1) muscle fibres, the white (type II) muscle fibres:

A Contract less rapidly
B Have a longer latent period
C Are smaller
D Contain more mitochondria
E Are richer in glycogen

19.22 The following substances which relax muscles and their mechanisms of action are correctly matched:

A *Clostridium botulinum* toxin – irreversible antagonist at the neuromuscular junction
B Tubocurarine – irreversible antagonist at the neuromuscular junction
C Suxamethonium – depolarisation of the motor end-plate
D Organophosphorus compounds – prevention of release of acetylcholine from pre-synaptic neurone
E Baclofen – glycine agonist in the spinal cord

19.23 Anticholinesterase drugs (e.g. neostigmine):

A Increase the synthesis of acetylcholine in the pre-synaptic neurone
B Increase the acetylcholine concentrationin the neuromuscular junction
C May be used to reverse the paralytic effects of tubocurarine
D May be used to reverse the paralytic effects of suxamethonium
E Are effective in the treatment of myasthenia gravis

19.24 Suxamethonium:

A Characteristically produces fasciculation before paralysis
B Normally has a half-life of less than 1 h
C Is usually metabolised by the enzyme acetylcholinesterase
D Is mainly excreted by the kidneys
E May have unusually prolonged effects in several members of the same family

19.25 The following statements about myasthenia gravis are true:

A It is an autoimmune disorder
B It is caused by a reduction of acetylcholine synthesis in the pre-synaptic neurone
C Edrophonium improves the symptoms for many months
D It is often associated with thymic abnormalities
E Corticosteroid is an effective treatment

19. The musculoskeletal system
Answers

19.1 A B

The bones are covered by periosteum, which is a tough membrane made up of fibrous tissue. Bone is mainly made up of a matrix of collagen, with microscopic crystals of hydroxyapatites (phosphates of calcium). Whilst the skull bones (other than the base of the skull) ossifies in membranes, the long bones are initially modelled in cartilage, and ossification starts in the shaft of the bone. In childhood, the ends of the long bones (the epiphyses) are separated from the shaft by a plate of actively proliferating cartilage (the epiphyseal growth plate). Linear bone growth is dependent on the formation of new bone laid down by this plate, and the rate of linear growth is proportional to the width of the epiphyseal plate. When the epiphyseal plate fuses with the shaft in adulthood, linear bone growth ceases.

19.2 A D

There are three types of bone cells: osteoblasts, osteocytes and osteoclasts. Osteoblasts are specialised fibroblasts which make collagen. They may differentiate into osteocytes. Osteoblasts are involved in the formation of new bones, and are stimulated by parathyroid hormones. On the other hand, osteoclasts are involved in breaking down bones. However, corticosteroids inhibit osteoblasts. Hence, if corticosteroids are given to children, growth may be stunted.

19.3 A B C D E

Any bone abnormalities which reduce the strength of the bones are predisposing factors for pathological fractures. They include primary or secondary malignancies, metabolic bone disease (e.g. osteoporosis, osteomalacia, Paget's disease), congenital bone disease (e.g. osteogenesis imperfecta) and infection of the bone (oeteomyelitis).

19.4 A C

The clavicle is a long bone which articulates with the manubrum of the sternum medially, and the acromion of the scapula laterally. It is convex anteriorily in its medial two-thirds, and concave anteriorly in its lateral third. It allows the upper limb to move away from the trunk, and it also transmits part of the weight of the upper limb to the trunk. It is very commonly fractured, especially in children and young adults. This usually occurs at the middle third of the bone.

19.5 B C E

The shoulder joint is a ball-and-socket joint. It has a wider range of movement than any other joint in the body. Hence the glenoid cavity is shallow, and the capsule is generally lax, especially inferiorly. The relative lack of muscles inferiorly also contributes to the frequency of downward dislocation of the shoulder after a fall on the hands with the arm abducted. As the head of the humerus which is forced out almost always moves up anteriorly due to the internal rotation – abduction force of the rotator cuff muscles, anterior dislocation is much commoner than posterior dislocation. The abduction of the shoulder is initiated by the supraspinatus and continued by the deltoid muscle. The supraspinatus is subject to the greatest mechanical strain compared to other rotator cuff muscles. Hence pain on active abduction of the shoulder is a common feature in the 'frozen shoulder' syndrome, especially between 90° and 135° abduction (the painful arc).

19.6 A D

The rotator cuff muscles are the short articular muscles of the shoulder joint which insert into the tuberosities of the humerus, and help to stabilise the shoulder joint. These muscles are affected in the 'frozen shoulder'. The rotator cuff muscles are the supraspinatus, infraspinatus, subscapularis and teres minor.

19.7 B

The triceps muscle is the only extensor of the elbow joint. The biceps and brachioradialis flex the elbow. The pronator teres pronates the forearm. The extensor carpi radialis longus extends and abducts the wrist.

19.8 B D

The scaphoid is a carpal bone at the lateral end of the proximal row. The flexor retinaculum (thickening of the deep fascia of the palmar aponeurosis) attaches to the tubercle of the scaphoid and the ridge of the trapezium laterally, and the pisiform and hook of the hamate medially. Fracture of the scaphoid often results in younger people from a fall on the outstretched hand. As most of the blood supply enters the scaphoid at the distal end, ischaemia may occur to the proximal end of the scaphoid after fracture of the waist of the scaphoid. This may lead to non-union or avascular necrosis. However, the blood supply to the scaphoid is preserved after fracture of the tuberosity.

19.9 A B C D E

See question 19.8 above. The flexor retinaculum is a thickening of the palmar deep fascia over the carpal bones. It is attached to the scaphoid and trapezium laterally, and the pisiform and the hamate medially. It gives rise to the origin of the muscles of the thenar and hypothenar eminence, and forms the carpal tunnel for the long flexor tendons. It also covers the median nerve. In the carpal tunnel syndrome, the median nerve is compressed by the flexor retinaculum, and pain and numbness in the distribution of the median nerve may occur. This may occur without any obvious cause, or may be associated with osteoarthritis of the wrist, hypothyroidism, pregnancy or rheumatoid arthritis. It may be treated initially by corticosteroid injection, but surgical decompression may be necessary.

19.10 A E

The correct responses are:
- Abductor pollicis brevis – abduction of the thumb (supplied by median nerve)
- Opponens pollicis – opposition of the thumbs to tips of fingers (supplied by median nerve)
- Dorsal interrossei – abduct the fingers (mnemonic: Dorsal aBduct, DAB) (supplied by the ulnar nerve)
- Palmar interrosei – abduct the fingers (mnemonic: Palmar ADduct, PAD) (supplied by the ulnar nerve)
- Lumbricals – flex the proximal phalanxes, extend the middle and distal phalanges (lateral two supplied by median nerve, medial two by the ulnar nerve). This explains the 'clawed hand' abnormality of the fourth and fifth fingers in ulnar nerve palsy

19.11 A B D E

The hip joint has a deep acetabulum cup, and the associated ligaments are strong. Hence grossly excess force (e.g. in a road traffic accident) is necessary to dislocate the hips, and hip dislocations are rare. As the sciatic nerve runs posterior to the hips, it may be damaged by posterior dislocation of the hip. Osteoarthritis of the hips commonly affects older people due to excessive cumulative wear and tear, and total hip replacement may be necessary.

19.12 A C E

The correct attachments of the important ligaments of the knee joint are:
- Anterior cruciate ligament – from front of intercondylar area to medial surface of the lateral femoral condyle
- Posterior cruciate ligament – from back of intercondylar area to lateral surface of the medial femoral condyle
- Lateral collateral ligament – from lateral epicondyle of femur to head of fibula

- Medial collateral ligament – from medial epicondyle of femur to upper medial surface of tibial shaft
- Patellar ligament – from apex of patella to tibial tuberosity

19.13 –

To test the collateral ligaments, the knee should be very slightly flexed whilst varus or valgus stress is applied. Excessive movement of the knee on varus testing may indicate lateral collateral ligament weakness. The cruciate ligaments should be tested with the knee flexed at 90°. The stability of the patella can be tested by assessing side-to-side movement when the knee is fully extended.

19.14 B E

The correct number of vertebrae in each region are as follows:
- Cervical – 7
- Thoracic – 12
- Lumbar – 5
- Sacral – 5
- Coccygeal – 4

The sacral and coccygeal vertebrae are fused in adults to form the sacrum and the coccyx.

19.15 A C

In the fetus, the vertebral column is flexed throughout its length (primary curvature). After birth, extension of the cervical region allows the head to be raised, and extension of the lumbar region allows the adoption of an upright posture.

19.16 A D

Osteoporosis is caused by an excess of bone resorption over bone formation, the result being a reduction of total bone mass. However, the bones are otherwise quite normal both histologically and biochemically. The main risk of osteoporosis is that it predisposes to fractures, especially of the femur and the wrist.

19.17 B D E

Men generally have greater bone mass than women. Hence women are more susceptible than men to osteoporosis. As the bone mass generally decreases with age, osteoporosis is commoner in the elderly. Negroes generally have greater bone mass than Caucasians. Hence osteoporosis is commoner in Caucasians than Negroes. Bone mass decreases with immobility. Other aetiology factors of osteoporosis include smoking, excess corticosteroids (either Cushing's syndrome or corticosteroid therapy), diabetes and excess alcohol.

19.18 A E

There are two types of filaments in the muscle fibre: the thick and the thin filaments. The overlapping patterns of the thick and thin filaments account for the characteristic striations seen on histology sections and electron microscopy. The thick filaments are made up of myosin. The thin filaments are made up of two long helical chains of actin. Tropomyosin molecules are located in the groove between the two chains of actin. Troponin molecules are located at intervals along the tropomyosin molecules.

19.19 A E

The correct version of events is:

- Depolarisation of the action potential spreads to other muscle fibrils through the T tubules, so that all sarcomeres in the muscle fibres contract at the same time
- Calcium ions are released from the terminal cisterns of the sarcoplasmic reticulum and diffuse to the thick and thin filaments in the sarcomere
- Calcium ions bind to troponin C, a subunit of troponin
- This causes movement of tropomyosin, and uncovers sites on actin which myosin can bind to
- Increased cross-linkages between actin and myosin occur, leading to shortening of the sarcomere

19.20 C D E

When the muscle fibre contracts, the thick and thin filaments slide over one another, and the overlap between the thick and thin filaments increases. However, the lengths of the individual filaments remain constant. Energy released from ATP is required for muscle contraction. The breakdown of ATP is catalysed by ATPase activity in the heads of the myosin molecules.

19.21 E

There are two types of muscle fibres: type I (red) and type II (white) muscle fibres. Type I fibres can contract for a prolonged period of time. Hence they are found mainly in the large muscles responsible for maintaining posture. They are mainly aerobic. Thus they contain more mitochondria and myoglobin and less glycogen store and glycolytic capacity. The high myoglobin content accounts for their red colour. They are smaller, contract slower, and have a longer latent period than type II fibres. On the other hand, type II fibres contract faster and are more suitable for fine, accurate movements. Hence they are found in the extraocular muscles and in the muscles of hands and arms.

19.22 C

The correct answers are:

- *Clostridium botulinum* toxin – prevention of release of acetylcholine from pre-synaptic neurone

- Tubocurarine – competitive antagonist at the neuromuscular junction
- Suxamethonium – depolarisation of the motor end-plate
- Organophosphorus compounds – irreversible antagonist at the neuromuscular junction
- Baclofen – agonist at GABA receptors in the spinal cord

19.23 B C E

Acetylcholinesterase (true cholinesterase) is an enzyme which normally destroys acetylcholine at the neuromuscular junction. Anticholinesterase increases the concentration of acetylcholine in the synapse by reducing its breakdown by inhibiting acetylcholinesterase. Hence it may be used to antagonise the paralytic effects of tubocurarine. It is also used in the treatment of myasthenia gravis caused by autoantibodies to acetylcholine receptors. However, as suxamethonim acts by depolarisation, anticholinesterase would, if anything, increase the effect of suxamethonium.

19.24 A B E

As suxamethonium acts by depolarisation, it causes stimulation to the motor end-plate before depolarisation block occurs. Hence fasciculation often precedes paralysis after suxamethonium is administered. Suxamethonium is destroyed by plasma pseudocholinesterases, and thus the half-life of the effect of suxamethonium is short (about 10 min). Therefore, suxamethonium is often used for short procedures (e.g. electroconvulsion therapy). However, pseudocholinesterase deficiency occurs as a hereditary disorder in about one in every 2500 individuals in the population. As they are unable to inactivate suxamethonium, the effect of suxamethonium may last for many hours. They often require artificial ventilation during this period.

19.25 A D E

Myasthenia gravis is caused by the presence of circulating antibodies to the nicotinic acetylcholine receptors. This prevents synaptic transmission at the neuromuscular junction. It is typical of autoimmune disease: it is commoner in women than men, it may be associated with thymic abnormalities, it is sometimes associated with other autoimmune disorders, and treatment with corticosteorid or other immunosuppressive drugs is often effective. Edrophonium is a very short-acting anticholinesterase, and is used as a diagnostic test for myasthenia gravis. The symptoms of myasthenia gravis improve dramatically following an intravenous injection of edrophonium, but the effect usually only lasts for minutes.